*Initial Management of the
Trauma Patient*

Initial Management of the Trauma Patient

Edited by

Charles F. Frey, M.D.

Professor and Vice Chairman
Department of Surgery
University of California, Davis;
Chief, Surgical Service
Veterans Administration Hospital
Martinez, California

LEA & FEBIGER   1976

Philadelphia

Library of Congress Cataloging in Publication Data

Main entry under title:

Initial management of the trauma patient.

    1. Wounds. 2. Medical emergencies. I. Frey, Charles F., 1929– [DNLM: 1. Hospital emergency services. 2. Wounds and injuries—Therapy. W0700 156] RD93.I54   1976   617′.1   76-20773 ISBN 0-8121-0519-2

Published in Great Britain by Henry Kimpton Publishers, London

Printed in the United States of America

Print number: 4   3   2   1

Preface

Since the publication of the National Academy of Science's White Paper on "Accidental Death and Disability: The Neglected Disease of Modern Society" in 1966, a definite change has occurred in the quantity and quality of emergency care available to the public in the United States. These changes have pervaded all aspects of emergency medical care, including access to the emergency medical care system, communications, equipment, and categorization of hospitals and their emergency departments and staffs. Concomitant with the rapid evolution of emergency medical care delivery, changes occurred in the education of the personnel required to operate an emergency care system. Training programs have been developed and implemented with remarkable speed and success for emergency department administrators, physicians, nurses and technicians. Physician-oriented programs have included programs for graduate, postgraduate, refresher and continuing education, as well as residency programs and course material for medical students. About the time of the publication of the White Paper, a required course in accident and emergency medical care was begun for freshman medical students at the University of Michigan Medical Center. This course, one of the first of its kind in the United States, has continued up to the present. The majority of authors of "The Initial Management of the Trauma Patient" contributed to this course over the years.

The emergency department is a triage station for the acutely injured. If the injury is serious, the patient will be admitted to the intensive care unit, or to a surgical or subspeciality service, or sent directly to the operating room. Probably no physician has a more complex or demanding task than the physician working in the emergency department. He must establish a diagnosis with a minimum of data, initiate resuscitation, and make judgments that can mean life or death or the difference between temporary or permanent disability and communicate them in a calm effective manner to the patient and the professional staff. This book reflects this reality and does not attempt to delineate the details of definitive operative techniques occurring to the patient after he has left the arena of the emergency department. The authors were asked to stress the early management of trauma to provide physicians and medical students working and learning in the emergency department with an understanding of the diagnostic techniques, the criteria for recognizing serious injury, the therapeutic techniques useful in the resuscitation of the injured, and indications for consultations and hospital admission. The authors of the chapters, most of whom are or have been members of the faculty of the University of Michigan Medical Center, have had wide experience with trauma patients in a hospital system that functions as a Regional Trauma and Referral Center.

The problem of injury and accidents is not likely to disappear from modern technological society. In presenting this volume, the authors hope to aid the emergency department "physician," be he medical student, house officer, or emergency department physician, to improve the care of the acutely injured.

The editor expresses his sincere appreciation to all the contributors, and to Odette Cassius, Dorothy DiRienzi, and Sue Petz, who aided him in making this book possible.

Martinez, California   CHARLES F. FREY, M.D.

Contributors

David Allan, M.D.
Professor of Anesthesia, University of Arkansas;
Medical Director, Anesthesia and Respiratory Therapy,
Ouachita Memorial Hospital, Hot Springs, Arkansas

H. Thomas Blum, M.D.
Director, Division of Emergency Medicine, Assistant
Professor of Medicine, Instructor in Environmental
Health, University of Cincinnati, College of Medicine;
Director, Emergency Department, Cincinnati General
Hospital, Cincinnati, Ohio

Richard W. Dow, M.D.
Chief of Department of Surgery
York Hospital
York, Maine

Calvin B. Ernst, M.D.
Professor of Surgery, Head of Vascular Surgery,
University of Kentucky Medical Center;
Senior Surgeon, University Hospital
Lexington, Kentucky

F. Robert Fekety, M.D.
Professor of Internal Medicine, University of
Michigan Medical School; Chief, Infectious
Disease Service, University Hospital,
Ann Arbor, Michigan

Irving Feller, M.D.
Clinical Professor of Surgery, University of Michigan;
Director of Burn Center, University of Michigan
Medical Center, Ann Arbor, Michigan

Earl R. Feringa, M.D.
Professor of Neurology, University of Michigan
Medical School; Chief, Neurology Service, United States
Veterans Administration Hospital, Ann Arbor, Michigan

Jay S. Finch, M.D.
Professor of Anesthesiology and Medical Director,
Respiratory Therapy Department,
University of Michigan Medical School;
Medical Director, Washtenaw Community College
Respiratory Therapy School, Ann Arbor, Michigan

Charles F. Frey, M.D.
Professor and Vice Chairman, Department of Surgery,
University of California, Davis; Chief, Surgical Service,
Veterans Administration Hospital, Martinez, California

Paul W. Gikas, M.D.
Professor of Pathology, University of Michigan Medical
School; Staff Pathologist, University of Michigan
Hospital, and Veterans Administration Hospital,
Ann Arbor, Michigan

Hank H. Gosch, M.D.
Clearwater, Florida

William C. Grabb, M.D.
Clinical Professor of Surgery (Plastic Surgery) and
Head of Section of Plastic Surgery, University of
Michigan School of Medicine; Staff Surgeon, University
of Michigan Hospital and St. Joseph Mercy Hospital,
Ann Arbor, Michigan

John W. Henderson, M.D., Ph.D.
Professor and Chairman, Department of
Ophthalmology, University of Michigan Medical School,
Ann Arbor, Michigan

Roland G. Hiss, M.D.
Associate Professor of Internal Medicine, and
Professor and Director, Office of Extramural Education,
Department of Postgraduate Medicine and Health
Professions Education, University of Michigan Medical
School, Ann Arbor, Michigan

Herbert Kaufer, M.D.
Associate Professor of Surgery, Section of Orthopaedic
Surgery, University of Michigan Medical School,
Ann Arbor, Michigan

Glenn W. Kindt, M.D.
Professor, Section of Neurosurgery,
University of Michigan Medical School; Neurosurgeon,
University Hospital and Mott Children's Hospital,
Ann Arbor, Michigan

Marvin M. Kirsh, M.D.
Professor of Surgery Section of Thoracic Surgery,
University of Michigan Medical School;
University Hospital, Ann Arbor, Michigan

George H. Lowrey, M.D.
Associate Dean of Student Affairs, Professor of
Pediatrics, School of Medicine, University of California,
Davis, California

Louis W. Meeks, M.D.
Clinical Instructor, Section of Orthopaedic Surgery,
University of Michigan Medical Center; Chief,
Department of Surgery, Beyer Memorial Hospital,
Ypsilanti; Attending Staff, St. Joseph Mercy Hospital,
Ann Arbor; Consultant, Wayne County General
Hospital, Michigan

Roger F. Meyer, M.D.
Assistant Professor, Director, Cornea and External
Disease Unit, Department of Ophthalmology,
University of Michigan, School of Medicine,
Ann Arbor, Michigan

Derek Miller, M.D.
Professor of Psychiatry, Northwestern University
Medical School; Chief of Adolescent Program,
Northwestern University Institute of Psychiatry,
Chicago, Illinois

Joe D. Morris, M.D.
Clinical Professor of Surgery, University of Michigan
Medical Center; Head, Thoracic Surgery Section,
St. Joseph Mercy Hospital, Ann Arbor, Michigan

William R. Olsen, M.D.
Professor of Surgery, University of Michigan Medical
School, Ann Arbor, Michigan

Robert M. Oneal, M.D.
Clinical Assistant Professor of Surgery (Plastic),
Department of Surgery, University of Michigan Medical
Center; Head, Department of Plastic Surgery,
St. Joseph Mercy Hospital, Ann Arbor, Michigan

Kathryn E. Richards, M.D.
Assistant Clinical Professor of Surgery,
University of Michigan; Assistant Director of Burn
Center, University of Michigan Hospital,
Ann Arbor, Michigan

Waldomar M. Roeser, M.D.
Clinical Instructor, Department of Surgery, Section
of Orthopedic Surgery, University of Michigan Medical
Center, Ann Arbor; Staff Physician, Orthopedic Surgery
Department, St. Joseph Mercy Hospital, Ann Arbor;
Staff Physician, Beyer Memorial Hospital,
Ypsilanti, Michigan

Eugene L. Saenger, M.D.
Professor of Radiology and Director, Radioisotope
Laboratory, University of Cincinnati College of
Medicine; Director, Nuclear Medicine, Cincinnati
Hospitals, Cincinnati, Ohio

Melvin L. Selzer, M.D.
Professor of Psychiatry, University of Michigan
Medical School; Director, University of Michigan
Alcoholism and Drug Abuse Clinic,
Ann Arbor, Michigan

Joseph Silva, M.D.
Associate Professor of Internal Medicine, University of
Michigan Medical School, Ann Arbor, Michigan

Herbert Sloan, M.D.
Professor and Head, Section of Thoracic Surgery,
Department of Surgery, University of Michigan
Medical Center, Ann Arbor, Michigan

Lawrence Stiffman, M.P.H.
Department of Health Planning and Administration,
University of Michigan School of Public Health,
Ann Arbor, Michigan

Jeremiah G. Turcotte, M.D.
Professor of Surgery and Chairman of the Department
of Surgery, University of Michigan Medical School;
University Hospital and United States Veterans
Administration Hospital, Ann Arbor; Wayne County
General Hospital, Eloise, Michigan

Condon R. Vander Ark, M.D.
Associate Professor of Medicine, Cardiovascular
Section, University of Wisconsin Medical School,
Madison, Wisconsin

Bruce A. Work, Jr., M.D.
Associate Professor of Obstetrics and Gynecology,
University of Michigan School of Medicine, Ann Arbor;
Consultant, Wayne County General Hospital
Eloise, Michigan

Contents

Accident Causation—
Motor Vehicular Accidents

1

The Impact of Injuries on the Medical System

Lawrence Stiffman

Accidents produce a variety of quantifiable costs, including the following:

1. *Medical costs of injuries,* principally involving the direct use of institutional and physician services (the direct economic costs).
2. *Additional costs* stemming from the loss or impairment of life, principally losses of future productivity and consumption (the indirect economic costs).
3. *Property damage,* mainly involving the costs of repairing and replacing property damaged in an accident.
4. *Administrative costs* incurred in insurance claims (the difference between premiums paid *to* insurance companies and claims paid *by* them).

By estimating these calculable economic costs of accidents, it is possible to compute the minimal amount of resources society can spend on safety without experiencing an economic loss. More importantly, approximate guidelines for allocating needed resources among medical service areas can be determined. As evaluation of accident countermeasure programs improves, these cost estimates are even more meaningful in the selection of program alternatives.

The scope of this chapter includes estimating the effect of accidents, primarily motor vehicular accidents, on in-patient hospital and physician services so that those directly involved in these services might gain insights into the relative magnitude of injuries affecting their workloads, the costs of this impact and therefore the benefits resulting from reducing accidents and injuries, and the planning of more efficient services in light of the trends in these factors with time.

Medical Service Requirements for Injuries

Table 1-1 summarizes the amount and cost of medical services, in and out of the hospital, required annually for injuries, including current injuries and the effects of old injuries.

Health Survey Findings. An evaluation of medical service requirements for injuries resulting from accidents is only as valid as the information available for the estimates of involvements and costs. The number of injuries was estimated from sample household surveys conducted by the National Center for Health Statistics (NCHS)–Health Interview Survey. The number of physician visits was estimated from the National Disease and Therapeutic Index (NDTI), a stratified random sampling of private physicians' services in 48-hour segments.

In the Health Interview Survey of NCHS, persons injured were classified according to the general class of accident causing the injury. Although most injuries are caused by accidents in the usual sense of the word, some result from other kinds of mishaps, such as adverse medical effects, overexposure, and nonaccidental violence—attempted homicide and suicide. The tabulated injuries (Table 1-1) include only those requiring medical attention or at least one day of restricted activity—the threshold of quantifiable injury effect.

Table 1-1. Annual Medical Services Required for Accident Injuries

Patient visits to private physicians (ref. 1)*	100,906,000
Persons receiving medical attention or experiencing one day or more of restricted activity (ref. 2)†	48,500,000
Persons hospitalized (ref. 3)‡	1,946,000
Hospital bed days required§	17,766,000
Hospital beds required for treatment‖	65,500
Total treatment costs	$2,003,000,000
Hospital care#	$1,297,000,000
Physician services**	$606,000,000
Nursing home care and other nursing care, 1963 (ref. 4)††	$100,000,000

* Refer to Table 1-9 to note stability of injury type over time.
† See Tables 1-2 and 1-3 for a breakdown of these injuries by class of accident.
‡ Only injuries in International Classification of Disease Adapted (ICDA) 800 to 898 are included. See Table 1-5 in which this table has been expanded to include bed days and the relative impact of discharges and bed days.
§ Based on Table 1-5. Number of discharges multiplied by length of stay for fractures, sprains and strains, head injuries, and lacerations.
‖ Hospital bed days/275 (at 75% occupancy).
Hospital bed days at $73/bed day.
** Patient visits at $6/visit.
†† For 1963, nursing home care totalled $73 million and nursing care totaled $31 million.

Table 1-2. Average Annual Number of Persons Injured and Number of Persons Injured per 1,000 Persons per Year, by Class of Accident: United States, July 1965–June 1967*

Class of Accident	Average Number of Persons Injured in Thousands	Number of Persons Injured per 1,000 Persons per Year
All classes	48,483	253.1
Moving motor vehicle	3,735	19.5
Traffic	3,481	18.2
Nontraffic	254	1.3
While at work	9,840	51.4
Home	20,406	106.5
Other	16,714	87.3

* Excluded from these statistics are all conditions involving neither restricted activity nor medical attention; the sum of the rates for the four classes of accidents may be greater than the total because the classes are not mutually exclusive.

Other measures of the impact of injuries on the medical system are disability requiring bed rest, need for hospitalization, and combinations of these. The need for medical attention characterizes the severity of injury to some extent, but it also reflects the economic status of the person involved, including the accessibility and availability of medical services, and the motivation to seek such services. Restricted activity

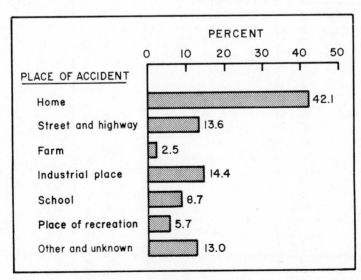

Fig. 1-1. Total number of persons injured according to place of accident.

Table 1-3. Percentage Distribution of Persons Injured, By Impact of Injury, According to Age: United States, July 1965–June 1967

Age	Total Injured	Medically Attended					Impact of Injury		
		Total	Without Restricted Activity	With Restricted Activity	Activity Restricting Only			Bed Disabling	Hospital-ized
All ages	100.0	86.3	46.6	39.7	13.7			21.8	3.9
Under 6 years	100.0	93.4	67.3	26.1	6.6			15.0	2.8
6–16 years	100.0	81.9	43.0	38.9	18.1			18.8	2.6
17–24 years	100.0	88.9	42.7	46.3	11.1			22.9	4.7
25–44 years	100.0	88.3	44.4	44.0	11.7			24.4	3.9
45–64 years	100.0	87.1	43.4	43.7	12.9			25.6	5.9
65 years and over	100.0	69.6	37.0	32.6	30.4			27.6	5.4

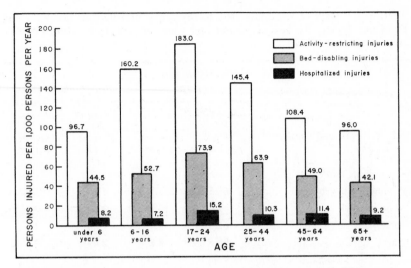

Fig. 1-2. Number of persons with activity-restricting, bed-disabling, and hospitalizing injuries per 1,000 persons per year, by age.

is also a highly variable factor and is also dependent on income, employment status, or usual activities involving varying risk exposure. About 46.6% of the annual average of 48.5 million persons injured receive medical attention without having any restricted activity. About 4%, or approximately 2 million persons, require hospitalization. Table 1-2 and Figure 1-1 show the number and percentage of people injured by place of accident. Table 1-3 and Figure 1-2 show the relative impact of injuries in terms of activity restriction, bed disability, and hospitalization by age of the victim.

Disability Days Due to Injury. Based on the Health Interview Survey during the 1965–1967 period, the average annual number of days lost because of injuries included 557,219,000 days of restricted activity, 143,855,000 days of bed disability, 102,012,000 days of work loss, and 11,925,000 days of school loss (ages 6 to 16). The days of bed disability, work loss, and school loss are considered to be days of restricted activity. Table 1-4 shows days of disability by sex of victim and class of accident.

For all classes of accidents, males experience more days of disability than females. Days of restricted activity and bed disability are more frequently caused by work accidents among males and home accidents among females, based on the entire population. When rates are computed per injury, however, moving motor vehicular accidents account for more days of disability for both males and females than does any other class of accident (see Table 1-4).

Table 1-4. **Days of Disability Due to Injury per 100 Persons per Year and Days per Injury, By Sex of Victim and Class of Accident: United States, July 1965–June 1967**

Sex of Victim and Class of Accident	Restricted-Activity Days		Bed-Disability Days	
	Days per 100 Persons per Year	Days per Injury	Days per 100 Persons per Year	Days per Injury
Male				
Moving motor vehicle	67.3	33.7	17.7	8.8
While at work	141.6	15.3	32.2	3.5
Home	62.3	5.9	14.6	1.4
Other	98.4	8.8	23.9	2.1
Female				
Moving motor vehicle	57.9	30.4	21.4	11.2
While at work	26.4	20.7	7.8	6.1
Home	110.4	10.2	29.3	2.7
Other	60.4	9.4	14.0	2.2

Estimates of Hospital Utilization. Based on the data presented in Table 1-5, hospital utilization by diagnostic class—20 International Classification of Diseases Adapted (ICDA) classifications—is highly clustered:

1. One of every six admissions is an obstetric case. The length of stay, however, is short—four days compared to a mean of 8.6 days for all admissions.
2. The leading nonobstetric discharges—diseases of the digestive and respiratory systems—account for 32% of nonobstetric discharges.
3. Five classes account for 65% of the nonobstetric discharges with injuries ranking third (see Table 1-6). The average length of stay for the five leading classes is 7.9 days compared with 9.9 days for all other nonobstetric conditions. Yet hospitalizations for the five groups account for a greater proportion of total conditions combined.
4. The five leading nonobstetric classes account for 75% of the inpatient discharges of children under 15 and for 60% of the discharges for each adult patient group.

Table 1-5. Number, Percent, and Rate of Discharges, Average Length of Stay, and Bed Days By Selected Conditions, All Ages. United States, 1965

Condition and ICDA Code (first listed)	Number of Discharges (000)	% of Total Discharges	Average Length of Stay	Bed Days (000)	% of Total Bed Days
Malignant neoplasms 140–205	1,002	3.5	14.8	14,829	13.0
Diabetes mellitus 260	342	1.2	12.4	4,241	3.7
Psychoneurotic disorder 324	292	1.0	10.9	3,183	2.8
Vascular lesions, central nervous system disorders 330–334	370	1.3	16.5	6,105	5.3
Arteriosclerotic heart disease 420	845	2.9	13.6	11,492	10.0
Respiratory diseases					
Acute upper respiratory disease	502	1.7	4.9	2,460	2.1
Pneumonia, all forms 490–493	875	3.0	9.0	7,875	6.9
Tonsils and adenoids 510	1,193	4.1	1.9	2,267	2.0
Digestive diseases					
Stomach and duodenal ulcers 540–542	478	1.7	9.6	4,589	4.0
Appendicitis 550–552	358	1.2	6.4	2,291	2.0
Inguinal hernia 560–561	496	1.7	7.2	3,571	3.1
Gastroenteritis 571	543	1.9	5.0	2,715	2.4
Cholelithiasis and cholecystitis 584–585	500	1.7	11.4	5,700	5.0
Disorders of menstruation 634	372	1.3	4.0	1,489	1.3
Obstetric conditions 640–659 06–07	4,793	16.6	4.0	19,172	16.8
Symptoms 780–789	794	2.8	5.9	4,685	4.1
Injuries					
Fractures, all sites 800–826	995	3.5	11.9	11,841	10.3
Sprains and strains of back and neck 846–847	327	1.1	7.9	2,583	2.3
Head injuries 850–856	300	1.0	6.2	1,560	1.4
Lacerations and open wounds 870–898	324	1.1	5.5	1,560	1.6
Total	15,701			114,430	

Table 1-6.   Rank Order of Discharge Rates for Five Leading Nonobstetric Classes, By Age: United States, 1965

Diagnostic Class (abbreviated title)	All Ages	Under 15 Years	15–44 Years	45–64 Years	65+ Years
Digestive	1	2	1	1	2
Respiratory	2	1	4	5	5
Injuries	3	3	2	4	4
Genitourinary	4		3	3	3
Circulatory	5			2	1

Excluding obstetric cases, patients with injuries spend more days in short-stay hospitals than do patients with any other conditions, and are second to deliveries in number of persons discharged. Figure 1-3 summarizes the impact of injuries relative to other selected diagnostic categories. The complete diagnostic category of injury and adverse effects is shown in Table 1-7.

Estimates of Private Physician Services. Estimates by the National Disease and Therapeutic Index reveal that injuries, or trauma, result in 100 million visits by patients to private physicians. Injury patients represent 7% of all physician visits, an increase of 5% since 1964. Tables 1-8 and 1-9 summarize these visits by type of injury (number and percentage distribution).

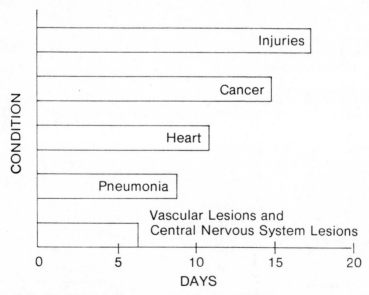

Fig. 1-3. Hospital bed days according to selected conditions and based on estimates from Table 1-5.

Table 1-7. Number and Percentage Distribution of All-Listed Diagnoses, By First-Listed and Additional Diagnoses for Inpatients Discharged From Short-Stay Hospitals, and Diagnostic Category: United States, 1965*

Diagnostic Category	Number of Diagnoses in Thousands				Percentage Distribution of All-Listed Diagnoses		
	All Listed	First Listed	Additional — In Same Class as First Listed	Additional — Not in Same Class as First Listed	First Listed	Additional — In Same Class as First Listed	Additional — Not in Same Class as First Listed
Injuries and adverse effects of chemical and other external causes ...800-999,Y10.0	5,127	2,923	1,520	683	57.0	29.7	13.3
Fracture of skull and face bones ...800-803	187	114	68	5	60.9	36.2	2.9
Fracture of radius and ulna (either or both) ...813	182	157	23	*	86.3	12.5	*
Fracture of neck of femur ...820	147	134	5	8	91.3	3.4	5.3
Fracture of other and multiple sites ...805-812, 814-817, 821-826	849	590	201	59	69.5	23.6	6.9
Dislocation without fracture ...830-839	133	108	14	11	81.0	10.5	8.4
Sprains and strains of back (including neck) ...846-847	453	327	86	40	72.1	19.0	8.9
Head injury (excluding skull fracture) ...850-856	508	300	186	22	59.1	36.6	4.3
Open wound of eye, ear, and face ...870-873	228	111	107	10	48.6	47.0	4.4
Laceration and open wound of other and multiple sites ...874-898	378	213	133	32	56.3	35.2	8.5
Burns ...940-949	121	91	19	11	75.3	15.4	9.2
All other injuries ...Residual 800-959, Y10.0	1,169	453	625	91	38.8	53.5	7.7
Complications of surgical procedures ...997-998	291	115	12	164	39.4	4.0	56.6
All other adverse effects of chemical and other external causes ...960-996, 999	480	211	42	227	43.9	8.8	47.3

*This excludes newborns. Diagnostic groupings and code number inclusions are based on the International Classification of Diseases Adapted, revised edition, December 1962. (From National Center for Health Statistics. *Inpatient Utilization of Short-Stay Hospitals by Diagnosis—1965*, Series 13, No. 6.

Table 1-8. Number of Patient Visits to Private Physicians By Type of Injury, as Estimated By the National Disease and Therapeutic Index: United States 1962–1966

Type of Injury	Number of Patients (in Thousands)				
	1962	1963	1964	1965	1966
Lacerations and open wounds	19,272	19,195	21,970	22,355	21,378
Sprains and strains of joints and adjacent muscles	18,315	20,853	18,534	20,622	23,806
Fractures of limbs	15,541	17,312	16,228	18,158	16,806
Superficial injuries, concussions and crushing with intact skin surface	11,592	13,190	13,133	13,423	13,322
Head injuries, excluding fractures	3,905	4,538	4,011	4,795	4,972
Burns	3,928	3,418	3,668	3,602	3,616
Fractures of spine and trunk	3,102	3,589	3,529	3,785	3,771
Effects of foreign bodies entering through orifices	2,385	2,269	2,407	2,196	2,110
Effects of poisons	1,355	1,225	1,688	1,726	1,378
Dislocations without fracture	1,394	1,280	1,276	1,084	1,480
Fractures of skull	1,248	1,187	998	1,404	1,426
Internal injuries of chest, abdomen, and pelvis	750	622	569	386	638
All other and unspecified effects of external causes	11,591	11,125	7,913	7,611	8,444
Total	94,378	99,803	95,924	101,147	103,147

In comparison to an average illness, most trauma cases are of short duration. The NDTI shows that, for all patient contacts in 1968, initial and follow-up visits were made in a ratio of one to three. Most types of trauma have a higher proportion of initial visits, thus indicating a shorter average duration of the disorder. For foreign body trauma, the proportion is nearly reversed. Burns and fractures are exceptions.

Slightly more than three-quarters of all trauma visits take place in a nonhospital treatment setting, a proportion comparable to that of the 1968 average for all patient visits. Table 1-10 shows different types of trauma and their deviation from this average. Table 1-11 shows the age distribution of visits by type of trauma. Table 1-12 shows trauma visits by specialty, indicating that general practitioners and surgeons treat 75% of all visits.

Table 1-9. Percentage Distribution of Patient Visits to Private Physicians By Type of Injury, as Estimated By the National Disease and Therapeutic Index: United States 1962–1966

Types of Injury	Percentage Distribution				
	1962	1963	1964	1965	1966
Lacerations and open wounds	20.4	19.2	22.9	21.1	20.7
Sprains and strains of joints and adjacent muscles	19.4	20.9	19.3	20.4	23.1
Fractures of limbs	16.5	17.3	16.9	18.0	16.3
Superficial injuries, concussions and crushing with intact skin surface	12.3	13.2	13.7	13.3	12.9
Head injuries, excluding fractures	4.1	4.5	4.2	4.7	4.8
Burns	4.2	3.4	3.8	3.6	3.5
Fractures of spine and trunk	3.4	3.6	3.7	3.7	3.7
Effects of foreign bodies entering through orifices	2.5	2.3	2.5	2.2	2.0
Effects of poisons	1.4	1.2	1.8	1.7	1.3
Dislocations without fractures	1.5	1.3	1.3	1.1	1.4
Fractures of skull	1.3	1.2	1.0	1.4	1.4
Internal injuries of chest, abdomen, and pelvis	0.8	0.6	0.6	0.4	0.6
All other and unspecified effects of external causes	12.3	11.2	8.2	7.5	8.2
Total	100.0	100.0	100.0	100.0	100.0

Table 1-10. Treatment Setting (1968)

Treatment Setting	Fractures	Lacerations/ Open Wounds	Abrasions	Contusions/ Crushing	Burns	Foreign Bodies	All Types of Trauma	All Diagnoses
Hospital	45%	12%	27%	14%	31%	6%	23%	22%
Nonhospital	55%	88%	73%	86%	69%	94%	77%	78%
Total	100%	100%	100%	100%	100%	100%	100%	100%
Bases (000)	22,248	19,368	9,319	8,308	3,520	1,963	94,148	1,343,464

Table 1-11.   Patient Age Distribution (1968)

Age	Fractures	Lacerations/ Open Wounds	Abrasions	Contusions/ Crushing	Burns	Foreign Bodies	All Types of Trauma	All Diagnoses
Under 2	1%	4%	4%	3%	12%	3%	3%	7%
3–9	8%	21%	16%	8%	11%	11%	10%	7%
10–19	19%	24%	17%	24%	15%	11%	19%	10%
20–39	17%	25%	26%	25%	28%	43%	26%	23%
40–59	21%	18%	22%	25%	22%	24%	25%	25%
60–64	6%	3%	4%	4%	2%	4%	5%	6%
65 and over	27%	5%	10%	11%	10%	4%	13%	22%
Total	100%	100%	100%	100%	100%	100%	100%	100%
Bases (000)	22,248	20,383	9,793	8,308	3,652	2,055	98,250	1,343,464

Table 1-12.   Trauma Visits By Physician Specialty (1968)

Physician Specialty	Trauma Visits	Visits/MD/Year
General practitioners	44%	775
Surgeons	30%	120
Osteopaths	11%	930
Internists	6%	250
Pediatricians	4%	390
Ophthalmologists	2%	305
All others	3%	—
Total	100%	
Base (000)	99,786	

Tables 1-8 through 1-12 are from *National Disease and Therapeutic Index Review,* 1(1):21, 1970, a publication of IMS America Ltd.

Estimates of Medical Costs of Motor Vehicular Accidents

The following projections are estimates of the medical cost of injuries in 1971 based, in part, on data from an unpublished report of the National Highway Traffic Safety Administration (NHTSA):

Motor vehicle injuries—3,800,000

Severity of injury[5]

    Permanent total disability—0.2%

    Permanent partial disability/disfigurement—6.5%

    No permanent injury—93.3%

Projections of the magnitude of medical costs are shown in Table 1-13, and total medical costs are given in Table 1-14.

Table 1-13. Average Medical Costs per Injury*

Severity of Injury	Average Hospital Cost/Injury	Average Other Medical Cost/Injury	Average Total Medical Cost/Injury
Permanent total disability	$5,015	$2,864	$7,879
Permanent partial disability/disfigurement	$1,599	$1,176	$2,775
No permanent injury	$ 113	$ 202	$ 315

* Based on figures in the National Highway Traffic Safety Administration Study and the Automobile Insurance Compensation Study.

Table 1-14. Total Medical Costs (in Thousands)*

Severity of Injury	Average Hospital Cost/Injury	Average Other Medical Cost/Injury	Average Total Medical Cost/Injury
Permanent total disability	$ 38,114	$ 21,766	$ 59,880
Permanent partial disability/disfigurement	$394,953	$290,472	$ 685,425
No permanent injury	$400,583	$716,090	$1,116,673
Total	$833,650	$1,028,328	$1,861,978

* Based on figures in the National Highway Traffic Safety Administration Study and the Automobile Insurance Compensation Study.

Estimates of Other Costs of Motor Vehicular Accidents

Given the out-of-pocket medical cost estimates presented in the preceding section, it must be realized that these figures represent only a small proportion of the true impact of accidents on society (see Table 1-15). This section attempts to provide at least a rough estimate of the less easily quantifiable costs of accidents, with gross motor vehicular accident statistics utilized to calculate the losses. Although economics are only one aspect of societal welfare, dollar estimates are used to assess whether trends in the cost impact of accidents are improving or worsening.

Societal welfare is worsened after a person is killed in an automobile crash. Earnings lost because of fatalities and permanent injuries represent the largest societal cost component. A victim's foregone output of goods and services is measured by his wages, with which he consumed goods and services and thereby contributed to both individual and public gain.

Table 1-16 lists the estimated wage losses by severity of accident. Since there is no market to test the monetary value of the services of a housewife, the average full-time earnings of women in the labor force are used as the relevant assessment on the estimates.

In addition to these costs, there are also severe opportunity costs stemming from vehicular repairs, insurance, and legal services. For example, the physician could be spending his time and talents offering preventive services; the lawyer could be developing programs in consumer protection; the auto body repairman could be involved in more useful work. At present, activities for the public good are hampered because of the time and resources necessary to treat the accident victims who are injured physically and hurt economically.

Obviously, pain and suffering, grief of family and friends, and children now lacking parental guidance and stimulation are real accident

Table 1-15.   Societal Costs of Motor Vehicular Accidents—1971

Cost Category	Annual Cost in Billions	Percent of Total Cost
Lost earnings	17.4	54.4
Property damage	7.2	22.5
Insurance overhead	4.4	13.8
Medical fees	2.0	6.2
Legal fees	1.0	3.1
Total	32.0	100.0

Table 1-16.   Estimated Total Wage Losses By Severity of Accident: United States, 1971*

Severity of Accident	Average Cost/Involvement
Fatalities	$132,000.00
Permanent and total disabilities	$139,000.00
Partial disabilities	$ 35,000.00
No permanent disability	$ 220.00
Property damage only	$ 10.00

* Based on unpublished data from the U.S. Department of Transportation.

costs, although quantification is extremely difficult. Even if an individual (or family) is more than adequately compensated by the insurance company so that he is in a better economic position than before the accident, there is still a societal loss—only the burden of costs has shifted to all those paying insurance premiums.

Based on various studies, the average property damage cost per highway accident has been estimated by the U.S. Department of Transportation at $710, yielding a yearly total cost of about $7.2 billion for all accidents. These figures are conservative in that it is estimated that there are more than 300,000 unreported accidents per year, with 90% of the costs being property damage.

The average person who is fatally injured would have lived 40 additional years. The average funeral cost in 1971 was $1,150. Assuming a 3% inflation increase per year and a discount rate of 7%, the present value of a funeral 40 years hence will be approximately $250. Thus $1150 − $250 = $900 worth of average funeral expense can be justifiably included in the societal cost estimate.

Legal costs have been estimated at about $1 billion per year, including court costs, legal fees, and police costs. The average legal and court cost of $2,700 per fatality (1971 dollars) and about $125 per injury has been estimated in a study by Wilbur Smith Associates.[7] The average legal cost per accident involving only property damage is low; only about 1% of such accidents incur legal and court costs and only 25% are reported to police. Insurance administrative costs of $4.4 billion per year have been estimated by the National Safety Council.[8]

Conclusion

Table 1-15 summarizes the estimated societal costs of motor vehicular accidents. While it is clear that medical costs represent a mere fraction of the total societal costs, motor vehicular accidents impose a substantial economic burden upon the medical care system.

References

1. N.D.T.I. Review 1970. Leading diagnoses and reasons for patient visits. *Nat. Dis. Therap. Ind.,* 1(1):21.
2. National Center for Health Statistics. 1970. *Persons Injured and Disability Days Due to Injury,* Series 10, No. 58, p. 1.
3. National Center for Health Statistics. *Inpatient Utilization of Short-Stay Hospitals by Diagnosis—1965,* Series 13, No. 6, p. 6.
4. Rice, D. 1966. Estimating the cost of illness. Health Economics, Series 6, USDHEW, PHS #947-6; Part I, May.
5. Automobile Insurance Compensation Study. 1970. *Automobile Personal Injury Claims,* Vol. I, U.S. Department of Transportation.
6. Automobile Insurance Compensation Study. 1970. *Economic Consequences of Automobile Accidents,* U.S. Department of Transportation.
7. Wilbur Smith Associates. 1966. *Motor Vehicle Accident Costs.*
8. National Safety Council. 1970. *Accident Facts.*

2

Vehicular and Highway Factors in the Pathogenesis of Fatal Injuries in Automobile Crashes

Paul W. Gikas

Accidents are exceeded only by heart disease, neoplasms, and cerebrovascular disease as a cause of death in all age groups in the United States. In 1974, there were 105,000 accidental deaths, of which 46,200 were attributed to motor vehicles. Between the ages of one and 24, motor vehicle accidents are the leading cause of death. More than 30,000 of deaths related to motor vehicles involve occupants of cars and trucks.[1] It is readily apparent that the highway is the major arena of violence in our society.

Since the greatest number of highway-related fatal injuries occur to occupants of cars and trucks, this facet of the problem is the subject of this chapter.

There are basically three approaches to the reduction of morbidity and mortality rates on the highways—crash prevention, injury prevention, and salvage of the injured victim. Salvage of the victim is the concern of emergency medical response systems and is discussed in subsequent chapters.

Previous attempts to prevent crashes alone have not reduced the morbidity and mortality rates. The causes of highway crashes are complex; there is no single common denominator. The three main factors are the driver, the vehicle, and the highway. Because of the lack of success and the complexity of the factors in crash prevention, a second endeavor is needed, and this is injury prevention. This approach assumes a crash will occur and involves provision for a crashworthy vehicle or safe package for the individual so he is not seriously injured

2

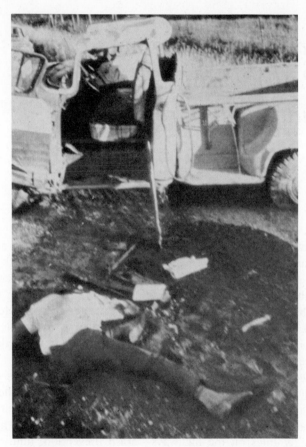

Fig. 2-1. Ejected driver on ground after truck had been righted. Note the lack of significant compromise of occupant space in the truck cab. (From Huelke, D. F., and Gikas, P. W. 1966. *Proceedings of the Tenth Stapp Car Crash Conference,* pp. 156–181. Copyright © Society of Automotive Engineers, Inc., 1966. All rights reserved.)

in the event. The concept of injury prevention is not a negativistic approach; it is merely realistic. The study of the mechanisms of injury to car occupants in fatal crashes has demonstrated that more than 50% of victims are dying under potentially survivable conditions. This means that these victims need not have died even though the crash occurred.

It is worthwhile to draw an analogy at this time and to compare these fatalities to deaths from other diseases. In our present state of medical knowledge, deaths from a Grade IV astrocytoma are tragic but essentially unpreventable. There is no known cure for this malignant cerebral neoplasm. In our society, a death due to smallpox, however, would be inexcusable. The tragedy in such a death is compounded by the fact that it need not have occurred in our present state of medical knowledge. The same pertains to 50% of deaths occurring to occupants of automobiles involved in crashes, because even though the crashes occurred, the deaths need not have resulted.

Causes of Death

Deaths in automobile crashes result essentially from two events. The victim dies either from injuries sustained when he is ejected from his vehicle or from injuries sustained in the second collision between him and the inside of the vehicle. The occupant is not killed when the vehicle strikes a tree; it is the second collision with the vehicle, manifested by the victim striking the inside of the car, that inflicts the fatal injury.

The following cases were selected to illustrate these two important mechanisms in the pathogenesis of automobile crash injuries.

Case 1. The driver of a pick-up truck lost control of the vehicle and it rolled over, ejecting him through the left door, which opened. He was trapped beneath the cab of the truck and suffocated (Fig. 2-1). This was a survivable crash. A seat belt or a better door latching mechanism could have prevented the fatal ejection.[2]

Case 2. A 1974 Chevrolet collided with a roadside abutment. The major impact was to the right front area (Fig. 2-2). There was adequate space remaining in the right front passenger area (Fig. 2-3). The occupant of this area sustained a fatal cranial injury when his head experienced a second collision with the right A pillar (Fig. 2-4). An upper torso–lap belt restraint would probably have prevented this fatal second collision.

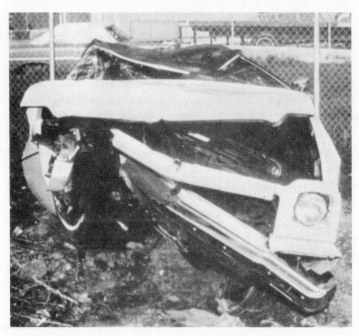

Fig. 2-2. Damage to right front area of car resulting from impact with abutment.

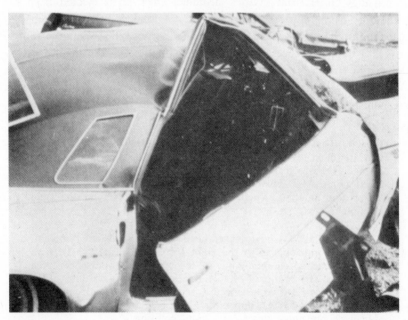

Fig. 2-3. Side view showing sufficient space in the right front seat to permit survival.

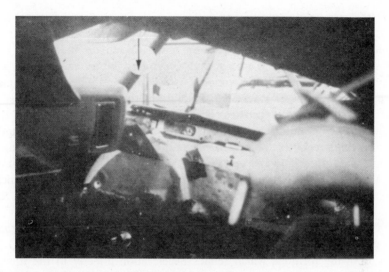

Fig. 2-4. Arrow points to impact area on A pillar inside passenger compartment where victim struck his head, receiving a fatal injury.

Case 3. A 1975 Monza was involved in a left front collision with another vehicle on a divided expressway. The Monza was traveling eastward in the westbound traffic lane. This vehicle sustained extensive damage with compromise of occupant space, trapping the driver in the car where he received fatal injuries (Fig. 2-5). A belt restraint system was not in use, and it is questionable whether it would have afforded adequate protection in such a severely damaged vehicle. Occupants of the larger car that was struck by the Monza survived.

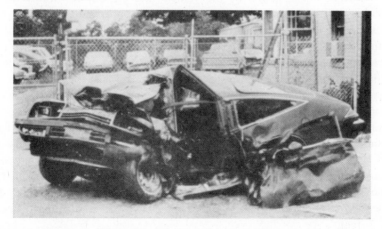

Fig. 2-5. Extensive deformation of the left front of the car with compromise of driver space.

The cases involving a second collision with the car emphasize vividly a law learned in high school physics. It is one of the laws of inertia, which states that a body in motion tends to remain in motion. Expressed another way, it states that occupants in an automobile are traveling at the speed the automobile is moving, and when the automobile suddenly stops as a result of a collision, the occupants do not stop but keep traveling at approximately the speed prior to the impact of the vehicle. They continue at this speed until they are decelerated abruptly against the interior of the vehicle. The only way this law can be violated is to fasten oneself to the vehicle by means of a restraint system, such as a lap seat belt and shoulder strap, so that one stops when the vehicle stops. The use of such restraining devices can prevent or attenuate the second collision, particularly if the impact is from the front.

The mechanical forces responsible for injury are generated by the sudden deceleration of the vehicle.[3] Deceleration is designated as G in the following formula, which relates deceleration directly to the square of the change in velocity and inversely to the stopping distance.[4]

$$G = \frac{V^2}{S.D. \times 30}$$

The number 30 is a constant that relates the velocity, measured in miles per hour, to the stopping distance, measured in feet.

It is readily apparent from this relationship that the forces of deceleration decrease as the stopping distance increases. In a crash such as that in Case 2, the stopping distance is equal to the amount of crush, or deformation, sustained by the vehicle and the object with which it collides. The deceleration of the occupant approximates that of the vehicle only if the occupant is fastened to the interior of the vehicle with a restraint system. If the occupant is not restrained, he does not take advantage of the stopping distance provided by the crush sustained by the anterior structure of the car, because he continues to travel forward after the car stops, only to experience the second collision within the car. As an example, if the occupant's head sustains a depressed fracture 1 inch in depth as a result of striking the A pillar, without significant deformation of the pillar, the stopping distance of the occupant's head would be only 1 inch. This would tremendously increase the G forces sustained by the passenger in comparison to the amount he would have experienced if he had been restrained and decelerated with the automobile, which may have had a stopping distance of 3 feet.

Safety Measures

In addition to the need for crashworthy attributes, an automobile should have operational safety features that are primarily directed to preventing crashes. Such operational safety attributes include visibility for the driver, braking ability, exterior lights, nonglare surfaces, steering ability, and adequate tires and suspension. Defects in these areas can contribute to a crash.

Motor vehicle inspection laws and particularly their proper enforcement can reduce the number of vehicles with operational defects on the highways. Although there is a federal safety standard that requires vehicle inspection programs in the individual states, there are several states, including Michigan, the home of the automobile industry, that do not have mandatory inspection. This deficiency emphasizes again the need for a crashworthy car to protect occupants when a crash results from an operational defect, such as poor brakes or defective tires.

The next group of cases emphasizes hazards in the highway environment that can contribute to a crash and complicate its outcome.

Case 4. A sedan was driven by an adult male who collided with a tree on the roadway (Fig. 2-6). This is an extreme example of poor highway planning manifested by failure to remove a tree from the path of traffic. The tree was finally sacrificed because of Dutch elm disease. The collision resulted in the death of the occupant of the vehicle.[5]

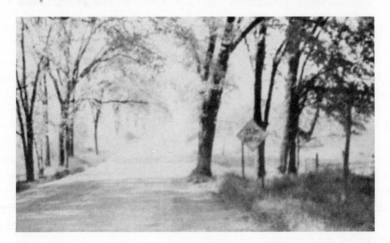

Fig. 2-6. Large tree on roadway with which a car collided, resulting in death of the driver. (From Huelke, D. F., and Gikas, P. W. 1967. *Highway Res. Rec.,* No. 152, pp. 103–119.)

Case 5. A car traveling at high speed went out of control while passing another vehicle on a two-lane roadway. The left side of the vehicle collided with a wooden bridge rail. A timber from the bridge (Fig. 2-7) penetrated the left vent wing, producing a severe laceration of the driver's shoulder, neck, and face. The injuries were fatal. This case demonstrates how an object at roadside can inflict injury when it penetrates the occupant area. This type of injury could have been prevented if a more crash-attenuating barrier had been in place.

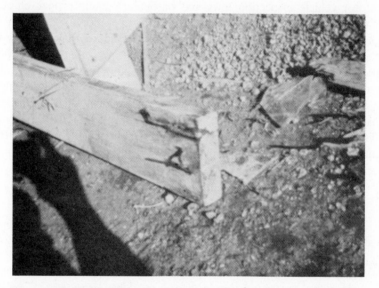

Fig. 2-7. End of bridge timber that penetrated the window on the driver's side of the car inflicting fatal injuries.

When one considers the mix of more than 90 million drivers on our highways and the spectrum of emotional and physical ailments that can afflict them at any one time, it becomes readily apparent that control of the driver is a most difficult endeavor. Revoking the driver's license is no assurance that a person will not drive. It has been estimated that at least 150,000 drivers in Michigan are without licenses and continue to drive. In another chapter, the problems associated with the alcoholic driver and the difficulty in attempting to impose restraints on this sick individual are discussed. Because of the futility of attempting to control 90 million drivers, the need for a crashworthy vehicle to compensate for driver error becomes obvious.

The highway environment is obviously in need of improvement. When new highways are constructed, obvious hazards should not be incorporated into the roadside. We witnessed the planting of trees, apparently part of a beautification program, in the immediate roadside area of an interstate expressway. Such acts violate the most rudimentary principles of safe highway design. Unprotected bridge abutments and sign supports can be shielded so that they decelerate a vehicle at a more tolerable rate or deflect it to attenuate the crash.

Restraint Systems. The greatest single step that can be taken by a car occupant today for the prevention of a crash injury is to use a restraint system, such as the shoulder strap and lap belt, which is provided in new cars. In a series of 177 car crash deaths studied at the University of Michigan, it was the opinion of the investigators that 40% of the victims could have survived if a simple lap seat belt had been worn, and 53% could have survived if a shoulder strap–lap belt combination had been worn.[6] Not all of those who would have survived by use of a lap belt alone, however, would have survived without injury. The belt itself may produce injury, but these injuries usually occur under severe crash conditions and are considered to be acceptable trade-offs for death. The lap belt should be worn snugly and low over the lap, not over the abdomen. Injury to the abdominal viscera and lumbar spine may result from flexion over the belt in a severe collision. If the belt is worn firmly over the lap, it is less likely to cause abdominal injury. The shoulder strap should never be used without the lap belt.

The seat belt has its greatest potential for preventing injury in the low impact collision, which is more likely to occur in the city. The high speed impact on the expressway is more likely to result in severe compromise of occupant space, which could preclude benefit from a restraint system. In high speed turnpike crashes involving side-swiping and rolling-over, however, the restraint system can be life-saving.

The argument offered by many that the seat belt will trap them in a burning or submerged car is invalid because seat belts and shoulder straps can prevent serious injuries that would preclude escape from such a vehicle. A person who is not seriously injured can release his seat belt and exit from a burning or submerged vehicle.

Unfortunately, the driving public has not accepted seat belts, which are now required by law. Since only a small percentage utilize these life-saving devices, a passive restraint system is obviously needed. One such device is the air bag restraint system, which has been the subject of considerable controversy. It offers passive protection by inflating suddenly when a sensor is activated as the result of a collision. The occupant of the vehicle then decelerates against the relatively soft bag and is prevented from a more abrupt deceleration against the hard interior of the vehicle. Some experts believe that such an air bag restraint system may allow persons to survive 60-mile an-hour, head-on crashes.

An embryonic form of this air bag restraint system was described in 1967 by Clark.[7]

Automobile Modifications. When we consider the three factors—driver, vehicle, and highway—involved in causing crashes, it becomes obvious that the vehicle is the easiest of the three to modify. Before the Federal Safety Standards were created, the concept of a crashworthy vehicle was relatively foreign to the automobile industry and the motoring public. As a result of the Federal Safety Standards, crashworthy improvements have been made in automobiles.

Why did the automobile industry not respond sooner to the need for a crashworthy vehicle so that many of the injuries and deaths could have been prevented even though the crashes occurred? The answer is obvious from the automobile industry's previous emphasis on styling rather than crashworthiness. The automobile stylists apparently had more influence than the safety engineers. For detailed descriptions of the conduct of the auto industry and the associated safety establishment, one is referred to Nader's excellent text, *Unsafe at Any Speed,* and O'Connell and Meyers' book, *Safety Last.*[8,9]

Organized medicine could have protested more vehemently the injury-producing attributes of automobiles. A few physicians did object to the uncrashworthy cars, and these men deserve much credit. In the 1930s Claire Straith, a Detroit surgeon, called the attention of the automakers to the hazardous interior features of cars. Fletcher Woodward, a former professor and Chairman of Otorhinolaryngology at the University of Virginia, was a strong proponent of safer interiors in the 1940s. Seymour Charles, a Newark pediatrician, founded Physicians for Automotive Safety, which picketed the automobile show at the Coliseum in New York City in 1965, protesting the indifference of automobile manufactureres to the need for crashworthy cars. Horace Campbell, a Denver surgeon, protested the trauma-producing features of automobiles. The greatest credit for the crashworthy changes in new cars goes to Ralph Nader, who emerged as the most articulate spokesman for the critics of the automotive industry. His book, *Unsafe at Any Speed,* catalyzed a national reaction that led to the Congressional Hearings in 1966 and the passage of the monumental National Traffic and Motor Vehicle Safety Act, which authorized the federal government to promulgate safety standards for automobiles.

Summary

Although a faulty driver may cause a crash, which is subsequently complicated by the highway environment, the vehicle usually produces the injury. From the evidence available it is apparent that the greatest potential for reducing morbidity and mortality rates lies in modification of the vehicle to make it more crashworthy, since it is the easiest to change.

In addition to the obvious physical trauma inflicted by the automobile, there is a more subtle, but just as real, threat to our health, *i.e.,* the assault on our bodies by the exhausts of the internal combustion engines, which are a major contribution to air pollution.

In the long-range solution to highway death and injury, the development of mass transit systems, which would reduce the dependence on the automobile, should be considered. The construction of superhighways and massive parking structures does not offer permanent relief from the obstipated corridors in and between population centers; it is only palliative and serves as a stimulus for the production of more cars and a greater dependence on this hazardous and air-polluting system of transportation.

References

1. *Accident Facts,* 1975. Chicago, National Safety Council.
2. Huelke, D. F., and Gikas, P. W. 1966. Ejection—the leading cause of death in automobile accidents, in *Proceedings of the Tenth Stapp Car Crash Conference,* Holloman Air Force Base. New York, Society of Automotive Engineers, pp. 156–181.
3. Gikas, P. W. 1972. Mechanisms of injury in automobile crashes. *Proc. Cong. Neurol. Surg.,* 19:175–190.
4. Gögler, E. 1965. Safety devices and safety in vehicle design, in *Road Accidents, Series Chirurgica.* Basle, Switzerland, J. R. Geigy, pp. 109–137.
5. Huelke, D. F., and Gikas, P. W. 1967. Non-intersectional automobile fatalities—a problem in roadway design. *Highway Res. Rec.,* No. 152, pp. 103–119.
6. Huelke, D. F., and Gikas, P. W. 1968. Causes of deaths in automobile accidents. JAMA, 203:1100–1107.
7. Clark, C. C. 1967. Airbag restraints and airlitter systems for the alleviation of highway injury, in *The Prevention of Highway Injury,* M. L. Selzer, P. W. Gikas, and D. F. Huelke (eds.). Ann Arbor, Highway Safety Research Institute, pp. 221–237.
8. Nader, R. 1965. *Unsafe at Any Speed.* New York, Grossman.
9. O'Connell, J., and Meyers, A. 1966. *Safety Last.* New York, Random House.

3

Preaccident and Postaccident Psychiatric Factors

Melvin L. Selzer

It is becoming increasingly obvious that traffic accidents are not sudden and totally unexpected phenomena that occur at random. Accident risk increases or decreases with the attributes of the roadway, the vehicle, and the driver. Although relatively little is known about most of the minor accidents, there is a growing body of literature documenting the importance of the driver's psychiatric and behavioral attributes in injury-producing and fatal accidents.

Preaccident Factors

Although a number of clinical reports clearly indicate a connection between certain emotional states or social stresses and accidents, these are usually considered to be isolated incidents, and their role in large numbers of serious or fatal accidents is ignored. In 1961, we undertook a 38-month study of drivers who caused fatal accidents in Washtenaw County, Michigan.[1,2] Fatal accidents were chosen as a prototype of serious accidents because all fatal accidents are reported, thereby insuring a random study. Ultimately, the study group consisted of 96 deceased and surviving drivers (henceforth F drivers) who were judged by the police to be responsible for 96 fatal traffic accidents resulting in 117 deaths between October 29, 1961, and December 31, 1964.

Washtenaw County is largely rural, with a population of 183,000 at the time of the study. Ann Arbor, its largest city, had a population of 80,000, including 30,000 University of Michigan students. Two four-lane expressways intersect the county, and 19 of the 96 fatal accidents occurred on these expressways. Omitted from the study were 19 accidents in which only pedestrians or motorcyclists were killed, 10 accidents in which the responsible driver lived in another state, and six accidents in which the drivers or other informants refused to be interviewed.

Some months after each fatal accident, the driver's family, friends, employer, family physician, and others who knew him were interviewed. If the driver survived, he too was interviewed. The interviews, which were conducted by social workers and senior medical students under my supervision, were informal but had a specific format. The number of interviews for each fatal accident ranged from one to eight, with an average of three. They were continued in each case until a clear picture of the driver's emotional state and characteristic use of alcohol emerged.

A control sample of 96 drivers matched to the F drivers with respect to age, sex, and county of residence was drawn from the state driver registration files. A matched alternate was drawn for each control and used if the original control refused to be interviewed or had left the state. Five controls refused to be interviewed and four had left the state; in each case the alternate control was cooperative. Three interviews were usually conducted with each control driver, although more were necessary in several instances because of contradictory findings. Control cases customarily involved separate interviews with the control driver, his spouse or other relative, and a close friend. The fact that all the controls were living introduced a bias, because 71 of the 96 F drivers had died as a result of the fatal accidents and respondents answering questions about a living relative or friend were understandably more circumspect. In addition, a living control driver was to some extent able to dictate who beside himself should be interviewed, an option not available to the deceased F drivers.

The arrest and driving records of all subjects were obtained from the Michigan State Police and the Michigan Department of State, respectively. If drivers had lived in other states for significant periods of their adult lives, records were obtained from traffic agencies in those states.

Statistical significance was determined by the chi-square test.

Of the 96 drivers responsible for a fatal accident, only 12 were women. Twenty-five of the 96 F drivers survived the fatal accident and 71 sustained fatal injuries.

Alcoholism. The definition of alcoholism used in this study was a variation of that proposed by Keller.[3] Alcoholism is a symptom of chronic, emotional illness characterized by repeated and excessive drinking in amounts sufficient to cause injury to the drinker's health or to his social or economic functioning. To establish the diagnosis the criteria outlined by Guze and others were used.[4] Thirty-six of the 96 F drivers, including two women, were alcoholics. Five of the 96 controls were alcoholics, but two of the five were arrested alcoholics (*i.e.,* no longer drinking). Alcoholics were therefore significantly overrepresented in the F group (p <0.005).

As in most attempts to determine the prevalence of alcoholism, the figures for the F and control groups are probably low.[5] It is likely that additional candor on the part of various respondents or additional respondents would have increased the number of subjects diagnosed as alcoholic.

Another group of drivers, although not meeting the definition of alcoholism, were distinguished by their use of alcohol more frequently and excessively than their fellows. These frequent, high quantity users were defined as persons who drank the equivalent of 8 oz. or more of 80 proof whiskey within a four-hour period at least once monthly. Eleven F drivers and 6 controls were in this category.

Of the 36 alcoholic F drivers, 11 had received treatment prior to the fatal accident. In a few instances this resulted in a temporary cessation or moderation of alcohol intake, in no case lasting more than six months. Three F drivers attended Alcoholics Anonymous meetings for periods ranging from two successive meetings to two years. Two men had been in a private hospital specializing in the treatment of alcoholism, and another had been committed to a state mental hospital because of his alcoholism. Two men had each visited a psychiatrist twice (with one using tranquilizers after that time), one man was treated by his family doctor, one had sought help from a clergyman, and one man was required to attend probation group counseling.

Age. Table 3-1 indicates that the 16- to 20-year-old F drivers were responsible for 20% of the accidents (although representing only 8% of Michigan drivers). The involvement of excessive numbers of young drivers in motor vehicle accidents is reflected in higher insurance rates for this group. Numerous factors have been suggested as contributing to their increased accident vulnerability.[6] Although inexperience appeared to be a factor in some of the fatal accidents of the younger drivers, the causes appear to be complex, often involving relatively small amounts of alcohol and a search for "kicks."

Table 3-1. Ages of 96 Drivers Responsible for Fatal Traffic Accidents

Group	Number of Drivers	Age					
		16–20	21–30	31–40	41–50	51–60	61+
Alcoholics	36	2	12	12	5	2	3
Nonalcoholics	60	17	17	8	8	4	6
Total	96	19	29	20	13	6	9

Table 3-2. Drinking Status of 96 Drivers Prior To Causing a Fatal Accident

Group	Number of Drivers	Drinking Number	%	Not Drinking Number	%	Unknown Number	%
Alcoholics	36	33	92	1	3	2	5
Nonalcoholics	60	23	28	35	58	2	3
Total	96	56	58	36	37	4	4

Drinking and Driving. As shown in Table 3-2, interviews and blood alcohol levels disclosed that 56 (58%) of the 96 F drivers had been drinking prior to the accident, 36 (37%) were abstinent, and the drinking status could not be determined in four cases. Only one of the 36 alcoholic F drivers was definitely abstinent prior to the accident (zero blood alcohol), whereas 35 (58%) of the 60 nonalcoholic drivers had not been drinking.

Postaccident blood alcohol levels were available for only 40 of the F drivers. In each case blood was drawn within four hours of the fatal accident and the alcohol level determined by the modified Nicloux method.[7] Since the blood specimens were obtained under diverse circumstances, the alcohol levels cannot be presumed to be typical of the entire F group. (Blood for alcohol determination was often drawn when the police suspected drinking to be a factor.) Table 3-3 shows that all but three of the 22 most heavily intoxicated drivers among the 40 were alcoholics. Not surprisingly, 19 (79%) of the 24 alcoholic drivers whose blood alcohol levels were known had levels of at least 0.15%.

One-Car Accidents. Of the 96 fatal accidents, 62 (64%) were single-vehicle accidents. The 36 alcoholic F drivers had 29 (81%) one-car accidents contrasted to 33 (55%) one-car accidents for the 60 nonalcoholics (p <0.02). Four accidents in which the driver's drinking status could not be determined involved only one-car.

Table 3-3. Blood Alcohol Levels of 40 Drivers After Fatal Accident

Group	Number of Drivers	Blood Alcohol Level 0.0–0.09%	0.10–0.14%	0.15–0.46%
Alcoholics	24	1	4	19
Nonalcoholics	16	10	3	3
Total	40	11	7	22

Time. Fifty (51%) of the 96 accidents occurred at night and 51 (52%) occurred on weekends (6:00 P.M. Friday to 6:00 A.M. Monday). The 36 alcoholic F drivers incurred 26 (72%) fatal accidents at night and 17 (47%) on weekends with corresponding figures of 24 (40%) and 34 (57%) for the nonalcoholic F drivers. There was a significant relationship of alcoholism to accidents occurring at night (p <0.01), but no similar relationship to accidents occurring on weekends.

Ten fatal accidents occurred between 6:00 A.M. and noon, but only one was caused by an alcoholic driver—who was sober (zero blood alcohol) but had a bad hangover at the time. Although alcoholics are apt to imbibe in the morning, they seldom do so to the point of intoxication.

Drunk-Driving and Nontraffic Drunk Arrests. This group of arrests is of particular importance because serious and chronic drinking problems are usually implied.[8] Twelve F drivers (10 alcoholics and two nonalcoholics) had a total of 24 drunk-driving convictions prior to the fatal accident. The two nonalcoholics each had one conviction, three alcoholics each had one, four had two, one had three, and two had four such convictions. Two alcoholic control drivers each had one drunk driving conviction.

Thirteen of the 96 F drivers, all alcoholics, had one or more convictions for drunk and disorderly behavior. Similar arrests were recorded for two alcoholic control drivers.

The combined traffic and arrest records of the 36 chronic alcoholics in the F driver group showed that 18 (50%) had at least one conviction for drunk-driving or drunk and disorderly conduct, a finding of considerable diagnostic and perhaps preventive importance because convictions are a matter of public record. Conversely, 50% had no such prior convictions, indicating that this form of case-finding assistance would not have been available for half the alcoholic F drivers.

Previous Accidents and Moving Violations. The 96 F drivers averaged 1.2 accidents and 3.1 moving violations each prior to the fatal accident as contrasted to 0.8 accident and 1.7 violations for the control drivers. The 36 alcoholic F drivers averaged 1.6 accidents and 3.5 moving violations, whereas the 60 nonalcoholic F drivers averaged 0.9 accident and 2.8 violations. Of special interest were the prior accidents that could be categorized as serious, *i.e.,* the vehicle overturned, the vehicle was totally demolished, or an occupant required medical attention or was killed. Details of accidents occurring many years earlier were not always available from informants, particularly for the deceased F drivers. Since official records revealed only that an accident occurred and did not indicate injury, the number of serious accidents attributed to the F group would probably have been higher if more drivers had been alive to provide details. The 96 F drivers averaged 0.34 serious accident per driver, with the 36 alcoholic drivers averaging 0.61 and the nonalcoholics 0.18 serious accidents. The 96 controls averaged 0.15 serious accident per driver. The difference between the F and control drivers, despite the incompleteness of the survey of previous serious accidents of the F drivers, was significant (p <0.001), but it is obvious the difference is attributed to the alcoholics in the F group.

Two alcoholic F drivers had been responsible for previous traffic deaths while driving in an intoxicated state!

Licensure. In addition to jail sentences and fines, suspension and revocation of the driver's license are favored methods of dealing with driver offenses. It has been pointed out that an addicted person is not likely to cease using the substance to which he is addicted when faced with conventional restraints.[9] The chronic alcoholic is seldom a solitary drinker and has a great need to drink with others, which in many areas necessitates use of a car to travel to a bar or tavern.[8] Lack of licensure alone is unlikely to prevent such travel. It is not surprising, therefore, that five of the F drivers were driving without valid licenses at the time they caused a fatal accident. Three of these drivers were alcoholics and two were nonalcoholics; all were diagnosed as having sociopathic or emotionally unstable personalities. In addition to the five F drivers who had no valid license at the time of the fatal accident, four more F drivers (all alcoholics) had previously been cited at least once for driving with a suspended or revoked license; three control drivers (two alcoholics) had been apprehended for the same offense.

Social Class. An earlier study of 67 persons arrested in Ann Arbor, Michigan, while driving in an intoxicated state revealed that 80% were in socioeconomic classes IV and V* as defined by Hollingshead and Redlich.[8,10] At that time we were unable to decide whether persons in the upper three social classes were less prone to alcoholism, drove less often when intoxicated, or drove more carefully even though under the influence of alcohol. We wondered whether police agencies are biased in favor of drivers whose socioeconomic positions reflect status and achievement. The present study suggests that police bias is not a major factor in drunk-driving arrests and confirms the impression that alcoholics in the upper social classes usually avoid causing serious accidents or are not revealed as alcoholics by the methods used in this study.

---

* The Hollingshead-Redlich socioeconomic index is a five point scale ranging from a high of I (i.e., dentist, plant manager) to a low of V (i.e., laborer). It is based entirely on education and occupation.

Seventy-five (77%) of the 96 F drivers were in classes IV and V (as were 84% of the 36 alcoholic F drivers and 75% of the 60 non-alcoholic F drivers). Only 52 (54%) of the 96 control drivers, however, were in classes IV and V, a difference significant beyond the 0.005 level. At the upper end of the social scale, 5% of the F drivers were in classes I and II, compared with 29% of the control drivers. None of the alcoholic F drivers was in class I or II.

Psychopathology. *Paranoia.* An earlier study of alcoholic drivers to determine if specific symptoms of emotional illness were related to traffic accidents unexpectedly revealed that paranoid thinking was the most highly correlated symptom.[11] We therefore sought evidence of paranoid ideation in the drivers in this study. Drivers were considered paranoid if they persistently and erroneously felt that others were intent upon doing them harm or that their wives were sexually interested in or involved with other men.

Table 3-4 shows that 22 F drivers and only four controls showed paranoid ideation, a greater than 5 to 1 disparity ($p < 0.01$). A salient finding here is that 50% of the 36 alcoholic drivers were paranoid compared to only 7% of the nonalcoholic F drivers and 4% of the controls. The suspiciousness of the alcoholic F drivers often centered on their wives' alleged sexual misbehavior and was apt to be present only when the drivers were intoxicated. When sober, they either did not entertain such thoughts or did not mention them.

Suicidal Proclivity and Depression. Drivers with a history of suicidal gestures or attempts, or of prolonged preoccupation with plans for self-destruction, were classified as suicidal. Drivers were classified as depressed if they experienced prolonged and frequent periods of deep despondency characterized by expressions of hopelessness, helplessness,

Table 3-4. Relevant Psychopathology in Drivers Responsible for Fatal Accidents and Control Drivers

Group	Number of Drivers	Paranoid Thinking		Suicidal Thoughts and Acts		Depression		Violence	
		Number	%	Number	%	Number	%	Number	%
Fatal accident group									
Alcoholics	36	18	50	5	14	11	31	14	39
Nonalcoholics	60	4	7	4	7	9	15	1	2
Total	96	22	23	9	9	20	21	15	16
Control group	96	4	4	1	1	7	7	9	9

and loneliness. As seen in Table 3-4, nine F drivers and only one control driver were suicidal (p $<$0.05).

Twenty F drivers and only seven controls suffered from depression (p $<$0.05). When considering the data on depression, it is important to note that 31% of the alcoholic F drivers but only 15% of the nonalcoholic F drivers and 7% of the controls were depressed.

Violence. Drivers involved in more than one unprovoked physical fight after age 18 were classified as violent. Table 3-4 disclosed that 15 F drivers, including 14 alcoholics, were violent, as were nine control drivers. The violence of the 14 alcoholic F drivers was more extreme in that they or their adversaries usually suffered more severe beatings.

Many alcoholic F drivers displayed more than one of the psychopathologic variables. Of the 36 alcoholic F drivers, 15 (42%) had two or more of the symptoms described as did only three (5%) of the 60 nonalcoholic F drivers and four (4%) of the control drivers.

In all, 40 (41%) of the F drivers and 16 (17%) of the control drivers had one or more of the symptoms listed in Table 3-4 (p $<$0.005). Within the F group, 25 (69%) of the 36 alcoholic F drivers and 15 (25%) of the nonalcoholic F drivers had one or more of these manifestations of emotional illness (p $<$0.005).

Social Stress. *Personal Crises.* Personal crises are defined herein as severely disturbing interpersonal events that occurred during the 12 months preceding the fatal accident (in the case of the F group) or during the 12 months preceding the personal interview (in the case of the control group) and that still affected the driver at the time of the fatal accident or the interview. The personal crises were either serious and disturbing conflicts with significant others (personal conflicts) or tragic events, usually a death or serious illness, involving persons close to the driver (personal tragedy).

Table 3-5. Stress Areas of Fatality and Control Drivers

Groups	Number of Drivers	Personal Conflict		Personal Tragedy		Vocational or Financial Stress		One or More Stresses	
		Number	%	Number	%	Number	%	Number	%
Fatal accident group									
Alcoholics	36	19	53	3	8	19	53	26	72
Nonalcoholics	60	12	20	6	10	16	27	25	42
Total	96	31	32	9	9	35	36	51	52
Controls	96	7	7	5	9	8	8	17	18

Table 3-5 reveals that 31 of the 96 F drivers experienced one or more personal conflicts during the 12 months prior to the fatal accident as did seven control drivers during the year prior to their being interviewed, a difference significant beyond the 0.005 level. Nineteen (53%) of the 36 alcoholic F drivers experienced personal conflict compared with 12 (20%) of the 60 nonalcoholic F drivers (p $<$0.01). The 9-to-5 difference in personal tragedy between the F and control groups was not statistically significant.

Vocational and Financial Stress. All disturbing vocational or financial difficulties that developed during the prior 12 months that were still a source of aggravation to the driver at the time of the accident or interview were included here. Among the vocational problems were actual or impending demotion, promotion, discharge, or job change as well as exasperating conflicts with foremen, employers, or fellow employees. Of the 96 F drivers, 35 experienced one or more vocational or financial crises as contrasted to eight of the control drivers (p $<$0.01). Nineteen (53%) of the 36 alcoholic F drivers experienced at least one vocational or financial crisis as did 16 (27%) of the 60 nonalcoholic F drivers (p $<$0.025).

Acute Preaccident Disturbance. In an appraisal of the F drivers' preaccident activity, 19 (11 alcoholics and 8 nonalcoholics) were found to have become acutely upset by events that occurred during the six hours immediately preceding the accident. This figure is minimal because in many instances a nonsurviving driver's preaccident activities could not be determined. Of the 11 alcoholic F drivers, eight men had quarreled with women, *i.e.,* their wives, girl friends, female drinking companions, and in one case a barmaid. Two men had fought with other men, and one man had become very upset because he could not have time off from work to go hunting.

In the group of eight nonalcoholics, one driver quarreled with his wife, one with his sister, one with a male friend, and one with his father; one woman driver quarreled with her husband. One driver alleged his money had been taken by a woman in a bar, one man became upset by his father's becoming intoxicated, and one man received news that his brother-in-law had been critically injured.

Although this study revealed that a number of factors were significant in the causation of fatal accidents, it was obvious that a driver's alcoholism played a more important role in overall etiology than did the other factors. If one uses the control drivers as a baseline, the relative risk of a driver who is alcoholic causing a fatal accident is 21 times that of the moderate user of alcohol.[12] On the other hand, the risk of a fatal accident increases only fourfold in the presence of psychopathology alone and independent of alcoholism, and it increases fivefold in the presence of social stress. These data clearly indicate that alcoholism is a more significant contributor, although it is often intertwined with the problems of social stress and psychopathology.

These statistical conclusions do contain a bias regarding the role of alcoholic drivers in fatal accidents because virtually all the alcoholics in the study had caused a fatal accident. Nevertheless, the need to find, restrain, and rehabilitate the traffic delinquent, alcoholic driver is readily apparent, particularly when one considers that most of them are unlikely to resolve their drinking-driving difficulties unaided.

Postaccident Factors

Psychiatric Disability. A number of accident victims subsequently suffer psychiatric disability. The precise number is unknown, but the symptoms frequently are severe enough to be uncomfortable and even disabling. Fortunately, most psychiatric sequelae of accidents are minor and the victims recover fairly rapidly. There does not appear to be any relationship between the severity of the injury and the degree of psychiatric impairment. Indeed, Modlin contends that psychiatric disability is much more likely to occur when the injury is minor.[13] He has theorized that the victim of a serious accident is immediately and continuously surrounded by rescue and medical workers who are helpful and sympathetic. Those suffering minor injuries, however, naturally get short shrift because their recovery is assured and they react to this lack of attention by developing psychological symptoms.

In general, psychiatric symptoms may develop after certain accidents as a function of the following: (1) the accident as a solution to a current life crisis; (2) the setting or context of the accident; (3) the unexpectedness of the accident; (4) the victim's previous mental adjustment; and (5) the person the victim views as being responsible for the accident.

If the victim is at a critical point in terms of certain life crises, the accident might unconsciously be seized upon as a solution to life problems. This does not imply any conscious intent on the victim's part, but symptoms may be desperately retained without awareness if the alternative is sufficiently degrading, humiliating, or futile.

Case 1. Mr. A., a 55-year-old married man, was driving his car home on a four-lane superhighway on October 7, 1963. He slowed to approximately 15 miles per hour to make a left turn and was impacted from the rear by another car driven at 50 miles per hour. He was rendered unconscious, but was conscious by the time he arrived at a nearby hospital. In addition to contusions and bruises of his face and head, he sustained several fractures of the right zygoma without displacement, which did not require special treatment. The diagnosis was cerebral concussion. He was discharged after four days but complained of almost continuous headaches and periods of dizziness. Attempts to return to work caused a marked exacerbation of the headaches and dizziness, and he soon abandoned the effort.

In January, 1965, his attorney sent him to a psychiatrist of the lawyer's choosing for psychiatric evaluation. The plaintiff's psychiatrist, Dr. Y., found Mr. A. "very much depressed." Other symptoms elicited from Mr. A. and his wife were irritability, restlessness, aloofness from others, insomnia, loss of appetite, and impotence—all dating from the accident. Dr. Y. concluded that the automobile accident "appears to have precipitated his current depressive reaction." He felt that Mr. A. had functioned at a reasonably adequate level prior to the 1963 accident.

Confronted with a $100,000 lawsuit, the attorney for the insurance carriers referred Mr. A. to a psychiatrist of *his* choosing, Dr. Z. In his letter to Dr. Z., the defendant's attorney referred to the "extensive rationalizations" of Dr. Y. and also offered *his* opinion: "My original reaction was that this is a pre-existing neurosis and an attempt to collect for a condition not a result of injuries suffered in this accident."

Dr. Z. interviewed Mr. A. and his wife on July 2 and 5, 1966. His report included the following information: "On July 2, Mr. A. appeared moderately tense and uncomfortable but was relaxed and affable on the later date. There was no evidence of depression. Both Mr. and Mrs. A. spoke of his headaches as being omnipresent and that as a consequence he had 'no interest in anything.' Since the accident he has suffered constant fatigue, dizziness when bending down, and inability to do any household chores, and has refused to leave the house or be around other people to whom he is rude and irritable if he cannot avoid them. Sexual activity ceased with the accident."

Dr. Z. also disclosed that Mr. A.'s background revealed he had worked at a number of poor-paying jobs until 1945 when he opened a small grocery store, which soon failed. He then started a catering business bringing sandwiches and coffee to factory workers. Although he enjoyed a meager prosperity for several years, business dwindled and he went bankrupt. He found employment in 1958 as a factotum in a store that arranged parties where he worked long hours for $1.50 per hour. Having owned his own business, it was ignominious to haul cases of soda and make deliveries. He was also a rather shy, misanthropic man who preferred solitude and television to the social and family amenities that were forced upon him.

The symptoms originating from the accident, particularly after his physical injuries had healed, were psychological and represented an honorable resolution of an intolerable, exhausting, and degrading job situation. Having been injured through no fault of his own and suffering headaches and dizziness, which prevented a return to gainful employment, he was able to sit in front of the television much like a wounded warrior nursing honorable wounds. He could at last avoid social activities that had previously been barely tolerable and yet have this "retirement" viewed sympathetically by his family.

Dr. Z. concluded his report to defense counsel with the statement that "there is no question but that he is psychologically disabled in terms of employability; he is not malingering despite the fact that his symptoms are resolving a conflict. His symptoms are psychic but real; he is not conscious of their neurotic nature. He would be unable to give them up even if his life depended on it."

Not surprisingly, many such cases reach the courts, and the possibility of a financial reward may complicate the situation. There is a curious notion held by some lawyers and doctors alike that the cash award in such cases is curative. The unconscious need for an illness is often too powerful, however, and at least one study has revealed that even when compensation by way of a lump settlement is provided, many of these psychologically disabled persons remain ill.

The setting or context of the accident can have a determinative effect upon the subsequent course of an accident victim's recovery. In the following case, the presence of the victim's children was believed to have been a critical factor.

Case 2. On May 29, 1959, Mrs. B., a 30-year-old housewife, was riding on a bus accompanied by her two children, ages 6 and 8. The bus impacted ladders extending from a parked truck and came to a sudden stop. Mrs. B. suffered injury to her neck as a result of the sudden jolt while her children's heads and faces were covered with shattered glass. She was immediately concerned that they might be blinded or disfigured because blood covered their faces, but they were found to be almost unharmed when the glass was brushed away. Immediately after the accident, Mrs. B. began complaining of a "burning sensation" in the back of her neck and was advised by the bus driver to consult her family physician. One hour later she was given medication by that physician. She continued to have moderately severe neck pain with restriction of neck motion until 1964, despite occasional efforts to seek relief. She also suffered headaches and periods of dizziness, which interfered with her previous activities.

Immediately following the accident she began to have a recurrent nightmare in which the accident was repeated. In the dream, her children were blinded and, as a consequence of their blindness, were taken from her. After each dream, which occurred frequently during the two years following the accident and less frequently thereafter, she would awaken crying and remain agitated for one or two days. She was phobic about leaving the house and discontinued her customary outside activities. She became chronically angry, irritable, and alternately indifferent and enraged at her children. Her husband's remonstrances met with angry denunciation.

She lost all interest in sexual activity for approximately nine months, and although permitting it thereafter, did not again find it gratifying until 1964. She was depressed and would sit for hours staring into space, irrationally convinced that no one cared about her. In her own words, "It was like I gave up life. I didn't want to be bothered living any more." During much of the period between 1959 and 1963, her husband had to assume the household chores because of her incapacitating anxiety and depression. In 1961, hampered by the neck pain and the feeling that she was helpless and would be a burden forever, she made an inconsequential suicide attempt.

Another disturbing factor was that one of the children also suffered nightmares for several months after the accident from which she frequently awakened insisting that "mommy was dead." The relevance of the children's involvement in the accident, became more apparent after another event in 1966, when Mrs. B. was driving her car with her sister as a passenger. She lost control of the vehicle and a very serious accident ensued in which Mrs. B. suffered multiple fractures, including a skull fracture. Although *barely surviving* these injuries, she suffered *no* psychiatric sequelae.

Although it can be postulated that the presence of the victim's children in the first accident contributed to her consequent serious psychiatric disability, other differences between the two accidents may also have contributed to the difference in sequelae. Indeed, sometimes minor factors may create psychological situations in which even trivial injury is converted into catastrophic psychiatric impairment. These phenomena are sometimes called symbolic injuries, because the actual injury is insufficient to explain subsequent reactions. Man is essentially a psychological creature and certain injurious events, because of the manner in which they are inflicted, or even the date upon which they occur, may revive long repressed psychological conflicts, which in turn disturb psychological equilibrium and result in an emotional illness.

There is evidence that if an accident is unexpected and the accident victim is totally unprepared for it, he is more likely to suffer a subsequent psychiatric disability.

A potentially instructive event involving a number of men occurred on March 7, 1957, when a gasoline tanker and a freighter collided in the Delaware River.[14] As a result of a series of explosions, the tanker's midship area sank immediately with loss of all command officers. Though deprived of leadership and surrounded by flames, both on the ship and on the water, 35 men of a complement of 45 lowered lifeboats and abandoned ship, incurring only minor physical injury. Since the circumstances were relatively homogeneous for all survivors, individual responses were an observable variable. When examined four years later, virtually every survivor still showed evidence that an impressive amount of psychological deterioration had taken place. Many of the survivors still suffered from headaches, gastrointestinal disorders, restlessness, depression, and phobic reactions. Indeed, 75% of them were in a worse state psychologically than they had been immediately after the accident. The examiners concluded that the nature of an accident is a more significant determinant of posttraumatic psychiatric disability than is preexisting personality.

Nevertheless, the preexisting personality of the accident victim may be of considerable importance, and it is obvious that some people are more vulnerable to psychiatric illness than others. Needless to say, the preexistence factor frequently becomes *the* critical issue if the accident victim's claim is brought into court or before a compensation board. Even when dealing with exclusively physical injuries, however, there can be clear parallels to preexisting personality problems. For example, let us hypothesize that two persons sustained identical trauma to their thighs in an industrial or traffic accident. One victim's femur was fractured and the other man sustained only a severe contusion. The first man was thin and frail, as were his bones. The second man had thicker, sturdier bones and more heavily muscled thighs and was therefore able to withstand the impact without femoral fracture. Yet no one would seriously suggest that the first man's case be dismissed because his preexisting bone and thigh structure were more vulnerable than the national norm. In cases of this kind, it need only be demonstrated that definitely inimical personality changes were initiated by the traumatic event.

There are times when an accident is converted, consciously or unconsciously, by the victim into a means of avenging himself for some long-held real or imagined grievance. In some instances, there are genuine resentments stemming from corporate indifference to working conditions. In other instances, the company or society at large has merely become a parent surrogate and is the object of long-held feelings of deprivation and frustration.

Reference is occasionally made in the literature to traumatic neurosis. An event may be traumatic as a result of diverse phenomena. Trauma can be a blow resulting in a fracture, but in some instances it consists of prolonged sensory deprivation, a loss of hope, or even a frightening statement or scene. The classic traumatic neurosis is apt to develop precisely at the time of the injury or threat in which the victim feels overwhelmed. The victim thereafter is extremely irritable and may even demonstrate a startle reaction to any noise or nuisance. Characteristically, the spouse complains that the accident victim can no longer tolerate the noise made by his children at play. The accident victim may have repetitive dreams of again being in the situation that precipitated his psychological illness. He is unable to return to the accident scene or similar settings. If he attempts to return, he develops symptoms such as dizziness, headache, and increased anxiety, and in effect exhibits a phobic reaction to the accident site. The victim exhibits marked anxiety, generally withdraws from his usual social activities, and loses interest in sexual activity. In actual practice, this classic syndrome is rarely seen, although elements of it are often present. In practice, we see that any psychiatric illness may appear following involvement in an accident. Hence, following certain accidents or other traumatic events of a physical or psychological nature, the victim may develop moderate to severe depression, psychoneurosis, or even serious schizophrenia.

Physicians can help to reduce the incidence of psychiatric sequelae following accidents. It is vital that one be sympathetic to accident victims, even though their injury may be minor, particularly when the victim obviously believes that his accident is a major event. This does not imply that an individual with little or no injury should be encouraged to believe that he has been grievously injured. One should be attentive and sympathetic and encourage family members to do the same, but no one should encourage the victim to believe that there is any underlying physical injury if none exists. In addition, it is important to encourage the victim to return to work as quickly as possible consistent with recognition of his feelings of injury and deprivation as a result of the accident. Above all, the physician should remain interested and attentive throughout the course of the victim's recovery.

The question of malingering occasionally arises but with remarkable infrequency considering the opportunity for such chicanery. The malingerer has no evidence of physical injury and usually insists on discussing the accident and his symptoms regardless of questions asked. Whereas persons suffering from genuine psychiatric illness following injury are more than willing to discuss their family life, problems at work, and other relevant factors, the malingerer is often impatient with this type of discussion and persists in repeatedly reminding the interviewer of his back pain, headaches, or other discomfort. Not surprisingly, a number of psychiatrists have pointed out that virtually all malingerers they have examined were people suffering from emotional illness. Despite their emotional illness, however, they were not suffering from physical postaccident symptoms.

Mourning. Physicians are often faced with the problem of an aggrieved family who has just lost a beloved person. The mourning process can be one of intense suffering, and one may be inclined or be importuned by a concerned family to intervene and relieve the mourner. Mourning is a natural process and is probably best dealt with by leaving the bereaved alone. His loss is real and it is natural that he should grieve. Mourning is essentially a healing process, a slow and painful adjustment to a loss. The lost person is given up memory by memory over a period of time; the leave-taking of the mourner from the person lost is piecemeal. Only if the sadness that accompanies mourning does not abate after a period of months must one consider the possibility of a critical depression, which requires treatment.

One additional and infrequent reaction to death may be encountered. Occasionally an individual who has lost a close family member may react with sufficient disbelief in the death to constitute an actual denial of the death. This person continues to reject the fact of death and refers to the deceased as still being alive. This denial reaction is usually short lived and passes within a day or two.

Conclusion

We have seen that 40% of the fatal accidents in our study were caused by alcoholic drivers, almost all of whom were under considerable stress at the time of the accident. Indeed, to *be* an alcoholic must of itself be a monumental stress.

The key to reducing fatal and serious accidents is to develop programs to determine who in the driving population has serious drinking problems, particularly among problem drivers. A number of demonstration programs are now in progress that stress rehabilitating the driver apprehended for driving while intoxicated rather than using punishment alone. We have little doubt that such programs will offer better long-term protection to the driving public than the previous exclusively punitive approach.

It is obvious that emotional stress is an important antecedent factor in accident causation and in development of postaccident psychiatric illness. Stress can be internal, familial, societal, or environmental. One can argue that stress is ubiquitous in the life of man. Nevertheless, there are times when stress increases, and accidents are more likely to occur at those times. Physicians are often aware of or are present when stressful events occur in the lives of patients. At the very least, persons under obvious stress should be warned of the increased risk of accident.

References

1. Selzer, M. L. 1969. Alcoholism, mental illness, and stress in 96 drivers causing fatal accidents. *Behav. Sci.,* 14:1–10.
2. Selzer, M. L., Rogers, J. E., and Kern, J. 1968. Fatal accidents: The role of psychopathology, social stress, and acute disturbance. *Amer. J. Psychiat.,* 124:1028–1036.
3. Keller, M. 1960. Definition of alcoholism. *Quart. J. Stud. Alcohol,* 21:125–134.
4. Guze, S. B., et al. 1962. Psychiatric illness and crime with particular reference to alcoholism: A study of 223 criminals. *J. Nerv. Ment. Dis.,* 134:512–521.

5. Mulford, H. A., and Wilson, R. W. 1966. Identifying problem drinkers in a household survey. Public Health Service Publication No. 1000, Series 2, No. 16.
6. Schuman, S. H., et al. 1967. Young male drivers. Impulse expression, accidents, and violations. *JAMA,* 200:1026–1030.
7. Muehlberger, C. W. 1954. Medicolegal aspects of alcohol intoxication, in *Legal Medicine,* R. B. H. Gradwohl (ed.). St. Louis, C. V. Mosby Co.
8. Selzer, M. L., et al. 1963. Alcoholism, mental illness, and the "drunk driver." *Amer. J. Psychiat.,* 120:326–331.
9. Schmidt, W., and Smart, R. 1959. Alcoholics, drinking and accidents. *Quart. J. Stud. Alcohol,* 20:631–644.
10. Hollingshead, A. B., and Redlich, L. C. 1958. *Social Class and Mental Illness.* New York, John Wiley & Sons, Inc.
11. Selzer, M. L., et al. 1967. Automobile accidents as an expression of psychopathology in an alcoholic population. *Quart. J. Stud. Alcohol,* 28:505–516.
12. Brenner, B., and Selzer, M. L. 1969. Risk of causing a fatal accident associated with alcoholism, psychopathology and stress: further analysis of previous data. *Behav. Sci.,* 14:490–495.
13. Modlin, H. C. 1967. Psychiatric reactions to accidents. *Washburn Law J.,* 6:317–323.
14. Leopold, R. L., and Dillon, H. 1963. Psycho-anatomy of a disaster: A long term study of post-traumatic neuroses in survivors of a marine explosion. *Amer. J. Psychiat.,* 119:913–921.

Management of the
Acutely Ill and Injured

4

Control of the Airway

Jay Finch

Although it is obvious that breathing is a very important body function, this fact is sometimes forgotten in the chaos surrounding an accident. Actually, control of the airway and reestablishment of a patient's natural spontaneous respiration or provision for artificial ventilation should be the first step in any rescue effort at the scene of the accident or in the emergency department. It makes very little sense to spend a great deal of time and energy attending to a patient's more obvious injuries only to discover that he has died anyway because someone forgot to breathe for him.

Situations involving rescue and resuscitation are usually panicky, with most observers not really accomplishing much. It is important, therefore, that at least one person involved in a rescue attempt be familiar with the basic principles of airway control and artificial ventilation. Only in this way is prompt restoration of breathing possible. Furthermore, it is useful that the rescuer have firmly in mind a reasonable sequence of procedures. This allows him to proceed in an organized manner and to reestablish ventilation as rapidly as possible with minimal wasted effort.

This chapter deals principally with management of the airway and ventilation in the acute situation. Basic upper airway physiology is reviewed and then an approach to management of airway difficulties is presented.

Physiology of the Upper Airway

The upper airway includes all extrapulmonary air passages and consists of both nasal and oral cavities, the pharynx, larynx, trachea, and origins of the right and left mainstream bronchi. The first and major

49

function of these structures is to transport respiratory gas to and from the lungs. The major portions of the upper airway, such as the nasal cavity and the larynx, are rigid or semi-rigid tubular structures that maintain their own intrinsic support. The oropharynx, however, is a muscular tube that is supported only by intrinsic and extrinsic muscle tension. In the conscious state, sufficient tone is maintained in the muscles of the neck and pharynx to maintain airway patency, even when expansile masses involving the neck and floor of the mouth deform the oropharynx.

Loss of this reflexly adjusted muscle tone is one of the major problems associated with loss of consciousness. Decrease in tone of the muscles attached to the hyoid (especially in the supine position) allows the unsupported tongue to fall into the oropharynx, blocking the middle portion of the supralaryngeal airway. The result may then be a patient who, while still capable of attempting inspiratory effort, cannot move air into the lungs because of oropharyngeal obstruction.

The second function of the upper airway is to protect the lower airway. Since the oropharynx is the common pathway for both respiratory and gastrointestinal systems, some mechanism must exist to separate the two functionally so that contamination of the lower respiratory tract with secretions or ingested material is prevented. The mechanism accounting for this protection is the laryngeal and pharyngeal reflexes. These range from the relatively complex reflexes involved in swallowing (in which the muscles of the tongue and soft palate and the constrictors of the pharynx and upper esophagus function in a coordinated manner) to simple closure of the glottic aperture when stimulated by foreign material.

These reflexes are depressed by a variety of insults, all of which have as a final common denominator a loss of consciousness. Absence of these reflexes creates the potential for contamination of the respiratory tract by upper airway secretions or regurgitated gastric contents. Their absence also allows inadvertent inflation of the stomach as a result of improperly applied positive pressure ventilation.[1]

Other protective mechanisms of the upper airway include mechanical removal of foreign bacteria and particulate matter and humidification. Although both of these airway functions are important in the total care of the patient, they are not significant in the acute resuscitative situation and will not be discussed here.

Types of Patients Who Need Airway Support

Patients who require external airway support may be classified into four categories.[3] The most common includes patients who are unconscious, including those with intracranial trauma, drug intoxication, or severe systemic toxicity. The underlying common factor in airway obstruction in this group of patients is relaxation of the parapharyngeal muscles.

It should be remembered that the unconscious patient has an unprotected airway. Intubation of these patients should be undertaken in the emergency room as soon as the problem is recognized and prior to their transport to other locations such as x-ray. This minimizes the risk of gastric contents being aspirated.

The second category of patients requiring airway support includes those with respiratory failure or insufficiency who require mechanical ventilation. The decision to support ventilation mechanically is an absolute indication for an artificial airway.

Included in this group of patients are those with the adult respiratory distress syndrome, which may have a variety of causes, including oxygen toxicity, drowning, fat embolization, shock with massive fluid and blood replacement, sepsis, and direct pulmonary trauma. These patients need airway control to allow institution of positive pressure ventilation with airway wave-form modifications, such as positive-end-expiratory pressure.

The third category includes patients who are unable to handle their secretions effectively. Here, blood gases may be within acceptable limits, and respiratory insufficiency may not yet have occurred. Included in this group are patients who have undergone upper abdominal and intrathoracic surgery, some patients with neurologic disease, and those with thoracic trauma, and related disorders.

The last category of patients present a very difficult management problem. This group includes patients with upper airway obstruction secondary to a space-occupying lesion in or about the upper airway and patients with laryngeal obstruction secondary to edema or inflammatory reactions. In these people, endotracheal intubation may be extremely difficult or impossible, and direct recourse to a tracheostomy is frequently necessary.

Palatal Valving. This is a cause of airway obstruction that is associated with manual bag and mask ventilation; inexperienced operators do not commonly recognize this condition. When a face mask is used for artificial ventilation, the patient's lips are usually approximated and the nasal air passages become the functional airway. In approximately one-third of patients receiving this type of ventilation, manual inflation is easy but passive exhalation is difficult. The mechanism at work here is a valvelike action of the soft palate. Recognition of this condition depends upon observance of a rhythmic rise and fall of the patient's chest with each excursion of the bag, as well as evidence of air entry and

3

egress. Correction requires the use of either a nasopharyngeal or an oropharyngeal airway, both of which are described later.

Once the airway has been satisfactorily established with endotracheal intubation (or tracheostomy in the rare situations in which it is indicated), disposition of the patient must be considered. In most cases, these patients are admitted to the intensive care unit for aftercare. Care of these patients in a ward setting is very difficult and usually does not lead to satisfactory results.

It is also important to realize that a set of baseline arterial blood gas values should be obtained in the emergency room as soon as the acute situation has been resolved. This allows intelligent interpretation of the patient's diagnostic data and serves as a baseline for additional therapeutic measures.

Initial Diagnosis of Respiratory Obstruction

A patient's respiratory adequacy in the emergency situation may be evaluated without instrumentation. Observation of the exposed chest and upper part of the abdomen reveals the presence or absence of coordinated respiratory movements. If respiratory movements are present, signs of air entry, such as audible passage of gas in and out of the nose and mouth synchronous with inspiratory movement of the chest, should be sought. Absence of suprasternal and intercostal retractions indicates that excess intrapleural negative pressures are not being generated and offers reassurance that ventilatory exchange is taking place.[2]

Initial Management of the Victim

Two steps must be taken prior to resuscitation. First the patient must be properly positioned for resuscitation, and then his pharynx must be mechanically cleared. Victims requiring resuscitation are found in an infinite variety of positions. In order to manage the airway adequately, the rescuer must place the victim in the supine position on a reasonably firm surface so that external cardiac massage can be given if necessary. This position allows the rescuer full access to the head and neck. While this is ideal and should be sought whenever possible, resuscitation efforts may be started with patients in awkward positions if time does not permit repositioning.

If foreign material within the upper airway is noted visually or aud-

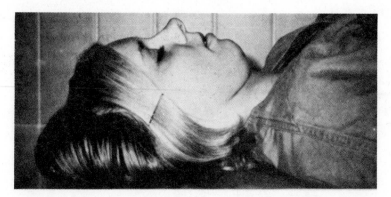

Fig. 4-1. Position of the head and neck in the unconscious patient.

ibly, it should be cleared rapidly by turning the victim's face to the side, forcing the mouth open, and wiping out the oropharynx with either the fingers or a cloth. If suctioning equipment is available, it should be used. Solid foreign material that cannot be removed by suction should be cleared manually.

Position of the Head and Neck. Figure 4-1 demonstrates the position of the head and neck in the unconscious patient. Here the head, neck, and trunk are all in a straight line with the head flexed on the neck because of relaxation of the parapharyngeal muscles. With the head and neck in this position, artificial respiration is impossible.

The classic head and neck position for airway resuscitation is shown in Figure 4-2. Here the neck is still in line with the thorax, but the tip of the mandible has been elevated markedly, extending the head on the

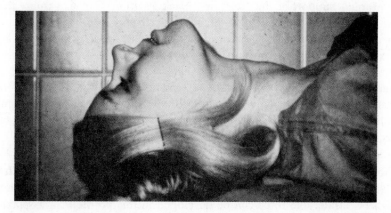

Fig. 4-2. Classic position of the head and neck **for** airway resuscitation.

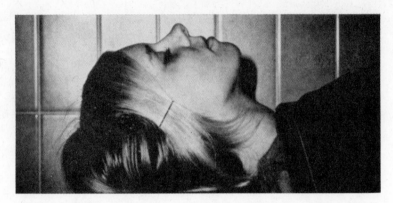

Fig. 4-3. The "sniffing" position for airway resuscitation.

neck. This increases the distance separating the jaw, tongue, and pharynx. The passageway between the nose and mouth above and the larynx below is then open. Another position for control of the airway that has been recommended more recently is shown in Figure 4-3. This is called the "sniffing" position. The head is elevated on a small roll or pillow so that the head is extended on the neck. The neck is then flexed on the thorax. Either of these positions permits adequate control of airway. Endotracheal intubation may be easier, however, in the "sniffing" position.

At this point, the patient's respiratory function should be reevaluated. The patient in whom inspiratory effort was not associated with signs of air entry prior to correct airway positioning may now be moving air satisfactorily. If this is the case, maintenance of this position is all that is required.

Manual Support of the Head and Neck Position. Let us assume that we have carried out the steps already described—positioned the victim in a supine position and extended the head. Although the patient appears to be making respiratory efforts, still no movement of air can be detected. Frequently, all that is necessary is to apply a slight amount of traction so that the head is further extended. One way of accomplishing this is by gently applying pressure to the rim of the mandible and pulling backward and then slightly upward (Fig. 4-4). At times, especially in patients with thick, heavy, short necks, more force is required than can be exerted with one hand on the mandible. Figure 4-5 shows one way of dealing with this problem. Here, the rescuer has placed both hands behind the angles of the jaw and is lifting up and back. Considerable force can be developed in this position. In a relaxed patient, it is possible to dislocate the jaw anteriorly.

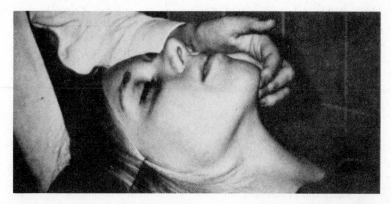

Fig. 4-4. The application of a slight amount of traction to further extend the head.

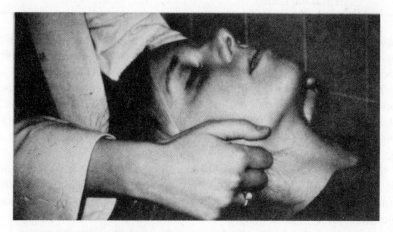

Fig. 4-5. The application of considerable force to extend the head.

Again the patient's ventilatory status should be reevaluated for signs of air entry.

Mechanical Airways

In a patient who is making spontaneous respiratory efforts, the application of traction to the mandible may be sufficient to open the airway and restore adequate ventilation. If this is not sufficient or if prolonged maintenance of the airway in the unconscious patient is desired, some mechanical device is required. These devices are divided into two categories: oropharyngeal or nasopharyngeal airways, which merely

Table 4-1. Suggested Equipment for Airway Control

Laryngoscope blades (curved and straight in various sizes)

Laryngoscope handle

Bite block

Oral airways (in various sizes)

Nasopharyngeal airway

15 mm. connectors (in various sizes)

Suction catheters (sterile)

Tonsil suction

Soft cuff endotracheal tubes (in various sizes)

Lubricant (water-soluble)

McGill forceps

Adhesive tape

Tincture of benzoin

---

hold the tongue out of the pharynx, and endotracheal tubes, which actually provide a secure airway. A complete list of suggested equipment for airway control is given in Table 4-1.

Oropharyngeal and Nasopharyngeal Airways. Figure 4-6 illustrates several mechanical airway devices. Typical of these are the white plastic Berman oropharyngeal airways. The nasopharyngeal airways are used in patients whose teeth are clenched tightly together so that insertion of an oropharyngeal airway is difficult or impossible.

The oropharyngeal airway is the more popular and perhaps the easier to introduce. An airway of the appropriate size is chosen and positioned using a tongue blade (Fig. 4-7). If it is simply slid into place without elevating the tongue, it may actually press the tongue more firmly into the posterior part of the pharynx, complicating the obstruction.

The oropharyngeal airway provides no guarantee of airway patency; it only facilitates its maintenance. Manual support of the chin may still be required, and continuous supervision is necessary because obstruction may occur at any time.

The oropharyngeal airway is also poorly tolerated by the patient who is partially reactive because it may stimulate the gag reflex or, if too large, it may actually provoke laryngeal irritation or laryngospasm.

Not infrequently one is faced with a patient requiring airway support in whom oral access is impossible. Patients in this group include those in the light planes of drug intoxication, some patients recovering from convulsive states who still have masseter muscle tone, and perhaps those with facial trauma preventing access through the mouth. In these patients, the nasopharyngeal airway may be a suitable alternative.

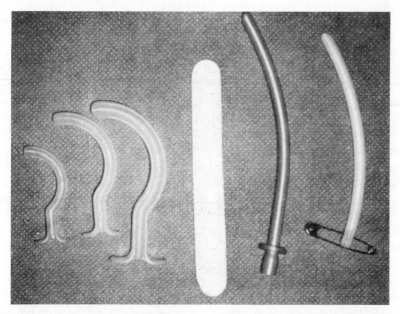

Fig. 4-6. Oropharyngeal (left) and nasopharyngeal (right) mechanical airway devices, and the tongue depressor (center) used for insertion of the oropharyngeal devices.

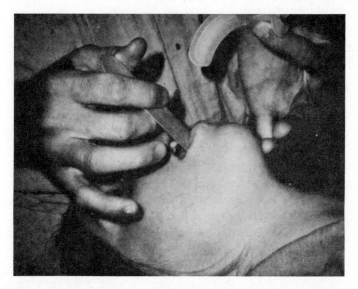

Fig. 4-7. Positioning of an oropharyngeal airway using a tongue blade.

The nasopharyngeal airway is a relatively soft, plastic or rubber tube with a device on the proximal end to prevent its disappearing into the nasal cavity. The nasopharyngeal airway should be well lubricated and inserted along the floor of the nasal cavity. Difficulty may be encountered at the angle between the nasal passage and the oropharynx. Gentle pressure and rotation may be necessary at this point, but care must be taken to prevent trauma to these structures or to the nasal conchae. When the nasopharyngeal airway is in proper position, its distal end is just above the tip of the epiglottis, and it satisfactorily holds the tongue off the posterior pharyngeal wall. Because the device does not stimulate the dorsal surface of the tongue, it can be tolerated by patients with an active gag reflex.

It should be emphasized again that although these devices maintain airway patency, they do not guarantee a truly patent system, and they do not isolate the lower airway so that aspiration is prevented.

Endotracheal Intubation. Up to this point, the steps described are relatively simple and may be performed without difficulty by the trained but inexperienced operator. These steps provide for maintenance of the airway and satisfactory access for artificial ventilation in most patients. If the steps however, do not promptly restore ventilation or if long-term ventilatory support is needed, endotracheal intubation is mandatory. This procedure is preferable to tracheostomy except in the most unusual circumstances.[5]

Since the manual airway support maneuvers already described serve to "buy time," orotracheal intubation should not be carried out as a "crash" procedure in most situations. Artificial ventilation and airway support should be carried out manually while a second operator is setting up the endotracheal equipment. This equipment should be laid out in an orderly fashion and checked for function before intubation is undertaken.

Minimal equipment to be used includes the appropriate size endotracheal tube and laryngoscope, a wire guide or stylet to stiffen the endotracheal tube, anesthetic lubricating jelly, a syringe to inflate the cuff, and a clamp to occlude the pilot tube to the cuff once it is inflated.

Selection of Endotracheal Tubes. Selection of the proper size of endotracheal tube is important to prevent the trauma associated with use of too large a tube and to eliminate difficulty with leaks from use of too small a tube. An approximate rule for the selection of pediatric tube sizes is that for children one year and older, add 18 to the child's age in years to determine the approximate French tube size. Selection and preparation of a tube that is the size indicated, plus one that is one size larger and one that is one size smaller, with final selection made after direct visualization of the glottic aperture, will secure a satisfactory fit.

Most mature adult females require a 34 French (8 mm. I.D.) endotracheal tube, whereas the adult male requires approximately a 36 French (9 mm. I.D.) tube. As with the pediatric tubes, preparation of tubes one size larger and one size smaller with final selection after visualization of the glottis will assure proper fit.

Problems of Wire Guide Use. For the inexperienced operator, use of a wire stylet or guide to stiffen the tube is mandatory. Two problems are associated with use of such a guide, however. The first is the possibility of direct laryngotracheal trauma from the guide. This may be obviated by securing the proximal end of the guide so that there is no danger of it slipping out the tracheal end of the tube. Perforations have been reported from improper use of such a device.

The second problem associated with use of a wire guide is due to "scuffing" of the anterior laryngotracheal area because of use of a tube that is too stiff. In many people, the longitudinal axis of the larynx and trachea is at an obtuse angle to the long axis of the endotracheal tube at the point at which it enters the larynx. Failure to withdraw the stylet partially after insertion of the tip of the tube into the glottic aperture may result in trauma to the anterior tracheal wall. If any resistance is felt after insertion of the tube into the glottis, the stylet should be partially or completely withdrawn prior to deeper insertion of the tube.

Selection of Laryngoscope. A variety of laryngoscopes are available for use in endotracheal intubation, but they can be divided into two categories. The first type is the one with a straight, or Miller, type of blade. With this type, the tip of the laryngoscope is used to elevate the free tip of the epiglottis directly, thereby exposing the glottic aperture. Because visualization of the aperture is usually better, this type of instrument is better suited for the inexperienced operator.

The second type of laryngoscope has a curved blade of which the MacIntosh blade is an example. The curved upward tip of the laryngoscope blade is inserted into the vallecula above the epiglottis and behind the posterior dorsum of the tongue, and by exerting upward traction on the base of the tongue, the epiglottis is indirectly elevated, exposing the glottic aperture. This blade is better tolerated in the partially reactive patient, because contact is not made with the exquisitely sensitive undersurface of the epiglottis, but full exposure of the glottic aperture is not possible in a large number of patients, and this blade is more difficult for the inexperienced operator to use.

Endotracheal Cuffs and Materials. Much attention has been turned recently to the materials used for the formation of endotracheal tubes and to the type of cuff used in adult tubes. Because of the possibilities of toxic substances—associated with either manufacture or sterilization —leaching out and producing a chemical laryngotracheitis, the only tubes selected for intubation are those that bear the imprint "IT," meaning that the material has been implant-tested in animals and found to be nonreactive. An equally acceptable indication is the imprint "Z-79," which refers to the committee of the U.S.A. Standards Institute, which has adopted similar testing procedures.

Considerable attention has also been directed to the problem of tracheal damage associated with high pressure cuffs. The standard slip-on endotracheal tube cuffs exert pressure on the tracheal wall in excess of 200 mm. Hg, which far exceeds capillary filling pressure. Various schemes, such as routine deflation schedules, or use of alternate cuff sites, have been suggested to attempt to obviate this problem, but none has worked satisfactorily. The present approach to the problem is to use one of a variety of low pressure cuffs. These are large, almost baggy cuffs, which use a large volume of gas rather than a high pressure to provide occlusion. Some have been found to have lateral tracheal wall pressures in the range of 4 to 20 mm. Hg.

Muscle Relaxants. The use of skeletal muscle relaxants for endotracheal intubation outside the operating room by the inexperienced operator is potentially hazardous. The use of an appropriate intravenous dose of succinylcholine will certainly produce total skeletal muscle relaxation and facilitate laryngeal exposure, but the use of such a pharmacologic adjunct is predicated upon the operator's skill at rapidly visualizing the larynx and inserting the tube. The obvious hazard with these agents is related to the total elimination of any residual respiratory activity on the part of the patient. If the experienced operator decides to use succinylcholine to facilitate endotracheal intubation, an intravenous dose of approximately 1 mg. per kilogram of body weight is appropriate.

Technique of Orotracheal Intubation. As with the steps described for manual airway support and artificial ventilation, the first step in orotracheal intubation is proper positioning of the head. Three positions are recommended. The traditional position is the one usually used by the bronchoscopist and consists of maximal hyperextension of the patient's unsupported head and neck over the edge of the bed or table. This is not a desirable position for simple orotracheal intubation because it considerably increases the distance between the mouth and the glottic aperture, and the operator is at a disadvantage because he has to look upward toward the glottis.

The classic position used in the operating room for anesthesia purposes for many years consisted of hyperextension of the patient's head and neck, which were still supported by the operating table. Although this position is not as extreme as the one previously described, it still has many of the same disadvantages. The currently recommended position for intubation is the "sniffing" position. This position, described in the section on manual airway support, facilitates intubation because the distance between the mouth and glottic aperture is shortest and the direction of visualization is downward, which is more comfortable.

After proper positioning of the head and neck and after manual ventilation of the patient to restore adequate oxygenation, orotracheal intubation may be performed.

If time is not a factor and if the patient is conscious, much can be gained from careful topical anesthesia of the mouth and pharynx. This may be accomplished by using a 4% lidocaine spray, carefully working one's way back from the dorsum of the tongue into the pharyngeal cavity, using the laryngoscope and spraying intermittently. Local anesthetics have a latent period, and time should be taken between exposure and spraying to allow the anesthetic agent to function. If time and facilities permit and the patient's condition can tolerate it, a great deal of benefit can be secured from direct translaryngeal topical anesthesia of the subglottic and tracheal area using either a Steiner needle or one of the commercially available kits (LTA Kit, Abbott). If the degree of airway obstruction is so great that periodic reoxygenation is not possible, or if the patient's level of consciousness does not require it, topical anesthesia should not be attempted.

With the laryngoscope in the operator's left hand, the mandible should be opened with the right (Fig. 4-8A). The blade is inserted along the right side of the tongue, with the shoulder of the blade being used to push the tongue to the patient's left. Every attempt should be made to visualize the various anatomic structures of the oropharyngeal cavity as the laryngoscope is advanced. Advancement of the laryngoscope across the dorsum of the tongue with gentle upward traction visualizes the tip of the epiglottis lying against the posterior pharyngeal wall. If a straight blade is used, the tip of the epiglottis should be picked up; if a curved blade is used, the tip is inserted in the vallecula. Direct upward traction should then be applied to the handle of the laryngoscope blade, bringing the glottic aperture into view. Placement of the endotracheal tube may then be accomplished under direct vision (Fig. 4-8B). It is frequently helpful to have an assistant to pull the right corner of the patient's mouth out slightly to facilitate bringing the tube in from the side rather than blocking the operator's vision by passing it down the laryngoscope.

Inexperienced operators frequently make the mistake of utilizing the laryngoscope as a prying rather than a lifting device to secure exposure of the larynx. This may result in trauma to the maxillary central incisors and does not facilitate laryngeal exposure.

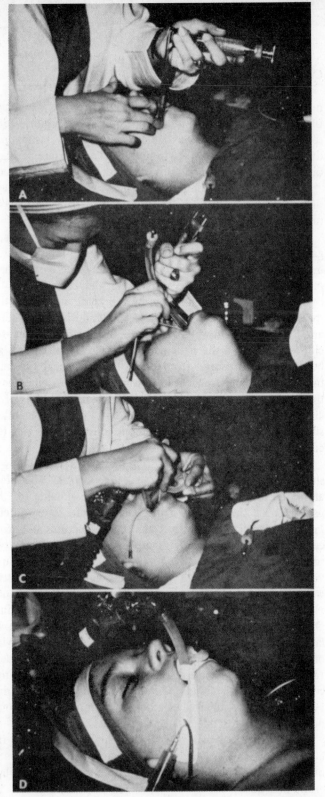

Fig. 4-8. Technique for orotracheal intubation: A, insertion of laryngoscope; B, passage of endotracheal tube; C, insertion of bite block; and D, endotracheal tube attached to positive pressure device.

Another mistake is failure to identify the anatomy as the laryngoscope blade is inserted, in which case the blade is usually inserted too far and all that is seen is the esophagus. Structures should be carefully identified as the laryngoscope is inserted.

In adults, the endotracheal tube is inserted until the proximal end of the cuff is just seen to disappear below the glottic aperture. The tube is fixed at this point, and the laryngoscope and stylet (if still in position) are removed. The endotracheal tube is attached to a mechanical ventilator or a self-inflating bag, and positive pressure is applied. Visual proof of chest wall excursion and evidence of satisfactory breath sounds confirm the proper placement of the tube. Attention should also be paid to equal ventilation of both sides of the chest in order to prevent endobronchial intubation.

Following this initial check, the cuff should be inflated, the oropharyngeal airway inserted as a bite block, and the tube taped in place (Fig. 4-8C and D). If the tube has been inserted in a patient requiring long-term ventilation, a chest x-ray to confirm tube position is usually considered to be mandatory.

Technique of Nasotracheal Intubation. In cases in which oral access to the larynx is not possible, orotracheal intubation may not be feasible. In these cases, nasotracheal intubation may be an acceptable alternative. In the spontaneously breathing patient, a suitable topical anesthesia is applied to the nasal cavity, preferably with an agent containing a vasoconstrictor, and then a well lubricated tube is inserted through the more patent nostril. Manipulating the patient's head and neck into varying positions and listening to air entry through the proximal end of the tube frequently permit blind tracheal intubation. If blind tracheal intubation not be feasible, a nasotracheal tube may be inserted into the larynx under direct vision with conventional laryngoscopy, using a McGill forceps to direct the tube.

Nasotracheal intubation is much more difficult than orotracheal intubation, particularly in the hands of the inexperienced operator. It usually takes longer, has a higher potential for trauma, and usually involves use of a tube one size smaller and somewhat longer than the one used orally. Moreover, nasopharyngeal bacteria may be passed into the lower airway when nasotracheal intubation is employed.

Surgical Approaches to the Airway

There are basically two surgical approaches to the airway—cricothyreotomy and tracheostomy. In the emergency situation in which surgical access to the airway is needed because of a failed endotracheal intubation, cricothyreotomy is the procedure of choice. If time is not a consideration, the surgical procedure of choice is the standard tracheostomy (preferably after an airway has been established with an endotracheal tube).

Cricothyreotomy. Cricothyreotomy may be carried out rapidly with almost any sharp instrument. The cricothyroid membrane is identified with the index finger of the operator's left hand and the larynx supported with the middle finger and thumb. A horizontal skin incision approximately 1 inch long is made over the cricothyroid membrane. The larynx is stabilized and the operator's knife is pressed into the membrane in the midline. The opening is extended laterally with blunt force, and the airway may be maintained by rotating the instrument 90 degrees or by inserting a small tube. If a tracheal cannula is needed after 24 hours, cricothyreotomy should be shifted to a standard tracheostomy site.

Tracheostomy. Except in very rare circumstances, tracheostomy is not the approach of choice for airway problems. It therefore will not be discussed in detail here.

It has become obsolete to consider tracheostomy a highly dramatic emergency procedure to be performed on a patient with an airway problem as soon as it comes to mind. Most surgeons recognize that this procedure is best done in the operating room with assistants and with adequate lighting and instruments. It should be done after the airway has been established by endotracheal intubation, if possible, so that there is no question of urgency. The problems associated with improper positioning of the tracheal stoma, tracheal stenosis and erosion associated with improperly selected cuffs, tube length, and similar factors are well known and will not be discussed in this chapter.

Artificial Ventilation

If respiratory gas exchange is still not occurring after the airway has been reestablished with an airway device or an endotracheal tube, artificial ventilation is mandatory.

The type of ventilatory assistance selected depends largely on the circumstances at the time of the rescue attempt. The decision may be made to use expired air resuscitation or, if more equipment is available, to use a self-inflating manual bag and mask combination. The point to be stressed here is that no equipment is necessary, and time should not be wasted waiting for it.

Exhaled Air Ventilation. Exhaled air ventilation has been well accepted as the technique to be used when equipment is not available since it has been proved that exhaled gas is adequate for resuscitative purposes and that exhaled air ventilation is superior to manual chest pressure–arm lift maneuvers, and since airway patency is a *sine qua non*.

Direct mouth-to-mouth or mouth-to-nose ventilation may be performed by several techniques. The first step is to secure an airway by placing the head and neck in the appropriate position as previously described. The rescuer should then seal his mouth around the patient's mouth in a wide circle and blow. Leakage of gas through the nose is prevented by using either the rescuer's cheek or a free hand to occlude the patient's nose. If attempts to blow into the mouth fail, it is sometimes helpful to close the patient's lips and blow into his nose.

Intermittent positive pressure ventilation with the rescuer's exhaled air can maintain normal arterial oxygen and carbon dioxide tensions provided that inflation volumes are approximately double the normal tidal exchange. The operator is thus capable of increasing his exhaled oxygen concentration from the usual approximate of 16% to 18%. If, in the average adult, tidal volumes of approximately 1 liter are used at a rate of at least 12 times per minute, blood gas levels are kept within normal ranges for prolonged periods.

The necessary hyperventilation results in a moderate respiratory alkalosis of the rescuer, whose end tidal carbon dioxide concentrations decreases to between 3 and 4%.

Direct mouth-to-mouth or mouth-to-nose ventilation can be made more aesthetically pleasing by using a handkerchief over the patient's mouth and nose, by using an artificial device, such as an S-tube airway, or by blowing directly into a face mask if one is available.

Artificial Ventilation with a Bag and Mask Unit. A variety of bag and mask units are available that can be used for artificial ventilation. The most common problem with such a unit, particularly for the inex-

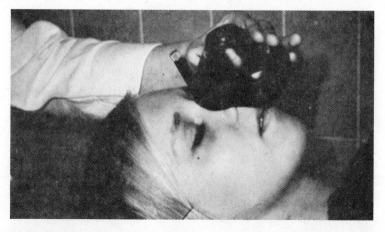

Fig. 4-9. The face mask is seated firmly at the bridge of the nose and rocked forward onto the face.

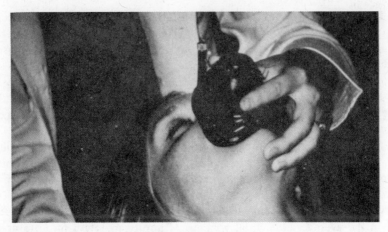

Fig. 4-10. Correct way of holding the face mask with the fingers applying traction to extend the head and neck.

perienced operator, is that of securing a satisfactory mask-to-face seal. This is facilitated by selecting an appropriate size mask, seating it firmly at the bridge of the nose, and rocking it forward onto the face (Fig. 4-9). The mask is held between the thumb and the index finger, and the remaining fingers of the hand are used to extend the head and neck by applying traction to the rim of the mandible (Fig. 4-10).

Figure 4-11 is an example of the wrong way to hold such a mask. Here the mask is supported only by the thumb, with the fingers applying pressure to the floor of the mouth. This results in a large air leak at the bridge of the nose. The pressure on the floor of the mouth may push the tongue back into the throat and further obstruct the patient's airway.

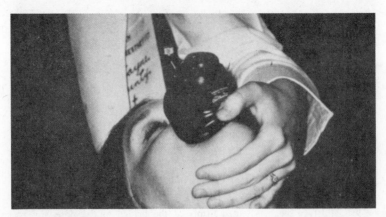

Fig. 4-11. Improper way of holding the face mask.

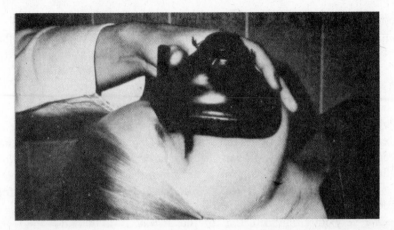

Fig. 4-12. Use of a face mask that is too large. Note that the edge of the mask rests on the eyes.

Figure 4-12 shows use of a mask that is too large; the edge of the mask actually rests on the eyes, and corneal abrasion or other ocular damage may result. A properly selected and fitted mask rests a considerable distance from the eyes.

The principal working part of a self-inflating resuscitation bag is a nonrebreathing valve. Ideally, this valve, when used to deliver positive pressure ventilation, should have no forward or backward leak, a low resistance, a small dead space, and a minimal opening pressure. It should be transparent, easy to clean and sterilize, durable, and reliable. It should aso permit spontaneous inhalation from the bag. Figure 4-13

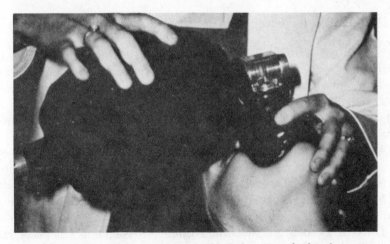

Fig. 4-13. Proper use of a self-inflating resuscitation bag.

shows the use of such a bag. Effective long-term respiratory support can be given by holding the mask and supporting the airway with the left hand and rhythmically squeezing the bag with the right hand.

After-Care of the Artificial Airway

After the artificial airway has been established and the emergency is over, attention should be directed to the after-care.[4] Appropriate management of the patient with an artificial airway involves provision for sufficient humidification, control of secretions, and prevention of infection. These areas are interrelated and must be managed together for effectiveness.

One very important function of the airway is to humidify and air condition the inspired gas mixture. Inspired room air usually has a low relative humidity, and medical compressed gases have no humidity. Failure to add humidification to an artificial airway results in rapid drying of the tracheal mucosa. Secretions become more viscous and tenacious, and atelectasis rapidly follows. Moisture may be delivered to the inspired gas mixture by a wide variety of devices ranging from heated humidifiers to the more efficient ultrasonic nebulizers.

Intimately related to humidification is the control of secretions and prevention of infection. Removal of the liquefied secretions using a sterile suction technique is important to prevent atelectasis and unnecessary contamination of the lower airway. Prevention and treatment of infection of the airway involves monitoring the bacterial flora of the upper airway at least every other day.

Complications Associated With Use of Artificial Airways

Possibly the most frequent complication of use of such a device is obstruction with secretions. This is usually associated with inadequate humidification and improper attention to suction. Secretions may inspissate and gradually circumferentially occlude the internal lumen of a tube. The diagnosis may be made by noting an inability to pass a suction catheter past the distal end of the tube.

An endotracheal tube is also frequently obstructed by herniation of the cuff over the bevel of the tube. This may produce an expiratory obstruction with wheezing and expiratory resistance, mimicking an episode of bronchospasm. Diagnosis of this condition may be made by deflating the cuff and noting the disappearance of the problem.

Tracheal stenosis and tracheal erosion are long-term complications and will not be discussed here.

Esophageal Obturator Airway

Recently, a new instrument for airway management in the emergent situation has been developed, especially adapted to use by the rescuer who is not experienced in endotracheal intubation.[6] This device (Fig. 4-14) is a large bore tube with a very large cuff and a plug or obturator in the distal end. A series of side-holes are at the proximal shaft of the tube, at about the level of the oropharynx.

The tube is inserted into the esophagus, with the distal cuffed end lying just below the level of the carina. When the cuff is inflated, a seal is formed, isolating the airway from the possibility of gastric reflux. The seal also allows positive pressure to be applied to the airway for ventilation without the risk of gastric distention.

The device seems capable of providing a fairly safe, secure airway for the inexperienced operator, although some potential problems are associated with its use. Accidental endotracheal intubation must be guarded against. Gastric reflux and aspiration are possible when the cuff is deflated prior to removal of the tube. It has been recommended that a more secure airway be obtained with conventional orotracheal intubation before removing the esophageal obturator. Finally, esophageal rupture has been reported.

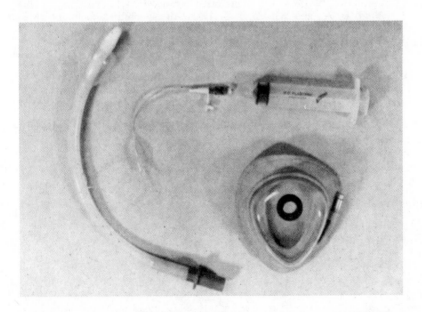

Fig. 4-14. Esophageal obturator airway, composed of a large bore cuffed tube with a plugged distal end, a face mask that fits the tube, and a syringe to inflate the cuff.

At this time, the esophageal airway is too new to be considered proven as safe and effective as its promoters claim; more experience is needed to confirm this.

Summary

In this chapter we have reviewed the problems associated with control of the airway in a variety of clinical situations. An important point to recall is that control of the airway does not require mechanical equipment and that the airway may be established and maintained and artificial ventilation instituted only by totally manual means. If equipment is available, reestablishment of the airway and effective bag and mask ventilation should be instituted before endotracheal intubation is attempted.

The final principle is that tracheostomy is not, except in the most unusual circumstances, an appropriate way of providing an airway, and endotracheal intubation is to be preferred.

References

1. Spoerel, W. E. 1973. The unprotected airway. *Int. Anesth. Clin.*, 10:1–35.
2. Peltori, D. A., and Whalen, J. S. 1973. Airway obstruction in infants and children. *Int. Anesth. Clin.*, 10:123–149.
3. Ashbaugh, D. G. 1972. Establishment and care of the airway, Chapter 2 in *Intensive and Rehabilitative Respiratory Care*, T. Petty (ed.). Philadelphia, Lea & Febiger.
4. Meyes, J. A. 1972. Care of the recent tracheostomy, Chapter 13 in *Ventilators and Inhalation Therapy*, A. Dobhirs (ed.). Boston, Little, Brown & Co.
5. Brigg, B. D. 1970. The clinical development of prolonged endotracheal intubation. *Int. Anesth. Clin.*, 8:781–784.
6. Farley, M. 1973. The esophageal obturator airway. *Respir. Ther.*, 3:95.

5

Shock and the Accident and Trauma Victim

William R. Olsen

Shock is a frequent result of severe injuries and is the most common preventable cause of death in accident victims. Physicians caring for the injured must understand the diagnosis and pathophysiology of shock and be proficient in its treatment if a reasonable survival rate is to be obtained.

Although shock may be caused by a variety of conditions, the resultant circulatory derangements are similar. The common denominator is inadequate nutritive capillary blood flow.[1-4] Capillary perfusion is not sufficient to maintain normal cellular function. If shock persists, cells die and, with sufficient cellular death, the shock becomes irreversible; *i.e.,* there are not enough viable cells to sustain the person's life. Hypotension, *per se,* is not shock. Shock can exist with normal or elevated blood pressure, especially if the patient is receiving vasopressors, and in some circumstances capillary perfusion may be adequate despite a low mean arterial pressure.

Causes of Shock After Accidents or Trauma. The most common cause of shock after accidents or trauma is hemorrhage, which may be obvious but usually is at least partially occult. Retroperitoneal hematomas and hemoperitoneum from lacerations of the spleen, liver, and mesentery are frequent causes. Bleeding into injured soft tissue may be severe in any patient who has suffered blunt trauma. A fractured femur in an adult causes a 500- to 1,000-ml. hemorrhage into the musculature of the thigh. Patients with multiple abrasions and contusions, with or without fractures, lose a significant but unmeasurable amount of blood into their soft tissues.

Contusions and fractures are associated with intrastitial edema, which occurs within hours of injury. The resultant depletion of plasma volume may be sufficient to cause shock and death. If burns accompany other trauma, the problem is compounded.

Cardiac tamponade or tension pneumothorax may interfere with ventricular diastolic filling, reducing cardiac output with dramatic rapidity, and the patient may die within minutes if not treated promptly. In rare instances a cardiac contusion may interfere sufficiently with ventricular contractile force to diminish cardiac output and cause cardiogenic shock.

Head injuries do not produce shock except terminally. Although many patients with severe head injuries are in shock, the shock is almost always due to loss of circulating blood volume and indicates a major injury elsewhere.[5] Frequently, the signs and symptoms of the injury causing the hemorrhage may be obscured by the unconsciousness caused by the head injury. Beware of the patient with a head injury and shock—he is bleeding somewhere!

Pathophysiology of Shock

Hemorrhage is followed by various compensatory mechanisms, some of which are more vestigial than useful. As blood volume decreases, venous return to the heart decreases with associated incomplete ventricular diastolic filling and a decreased cardiac output. Baroreceptors in the aortic arch, carotid sinus, and perhaps elsewhere respond and trigger the release of epinephrine from the adrenal gland and norepinephrine from the sympathetic postganglionic nerve endings. These catecholamines stimulate adrenergic receptors throughout the body, resulting in constriction of arterioles and veins (alpha adrenergic response) and tachycardia (beta adrenergic response). The alpha adrenergic receptors of the venous system are probably more sensitive to minimal cathecholamine stimulation than are those of the arterioles.[6] Therefore, early hypovolemia is followed by selective venoconstriction.

The venous (capacitance) system normally contains about 70% of the circulating blood volume but can expand or contract rapidly to accommodate larger or smaller volumes without altering the internal pressure appreciably. The arterial (resistance) system cannot change capacity to accommodate volume changes. Arterial volume changes are therefore reflected in changes in arterial blood pressure. The selective venoconstriction that accompanies early hypovolemia causes a shift of blood to the arterial portion of the circulation.[7] This compensatory mechanism allows the young patient to maintain a fairly normal cardiac output, arterial blood pressure, and nutritive capillary flow despite the loss of 10 to 20% of the blood volume.

If the hemorrhage is limited or occurs slowly, the plasma volume may be maintained by the inflow of fluid and protein from the interstitial space with resultant anemia.[8-10] In accident victims in shock, however, the blood loss has been too massive and this compensatory mechanism has occurred too slowly to be of benefit. The hematocrit is a poor guide to replacement therapy in acute hemorrhage.

As hemorrhage approaches 30 to 40% of blood volume, the venous compensatory mechanism is no longer adequate, venous return to the heart is reduced, cardiac output decreases, catecholamine release is accentuated, and arteriolar constriction predominates. The resultant increase in peripheral resistance diminishes capillary flow but is insufficient to maintain arterial volume. The arterial pressure decreases and the capillary flow is further diminished to dangerous levels. If the condition is untreated, capillary sludging, thrombosis, and cellular death follow, with eventual death of the patient.

Blood vessels in different vascular beds[11] and in different parts of the same organ[12] react differently to the same degree of hemorrhage. A blood volume loss sufficient to produce ischemia in one organ therefore may not produce ischemia in another. This may allow selective perfusion of some vital organs, perhaps the central nervous system, in early shock and allow temporary maintenance of life. Other structures, for example the distal renal tubule, become ischemic in early shock and, if sufficiently damaged, may not function well enough to sustain life in the late postshock period. It is necessary to understand the capillary flow changes produced by hemorrhage on *specific tissues* to understand the effects of hypovolemia and to use a logical approach to its treatment.

Attempts to study the flow changes in shock have been hindered by the lack of methods to measure capillary flow. Many investigators have attempted to estimate capillary flow by measuring the flow in large vessels, usually by operative methods in anesthetized dogs. Dogs are not good animals for the study of clinical shock because they develop splanchnic congestion following hemorrhage, a response not seen in humans.[13] Furthermore, methods of measuring flow in large vessels fail to differentiate nutritive capillary flow from flow through arteriovenous pathways. These methods frequently fail to consider the significant hemodynamic variables introduced by anesthesia,[14-20] operative manipulation,[17,18,20,21] and the frequently resultant mild hypothermia[14,22] and hypovolemia, making their validity questionable. Radioactive methods can be used to determine nutritive capillary flow without introducing the variables associated with anesthesia or operative manipulation.[12,19,23-26] Although much work remains to be done in this field,

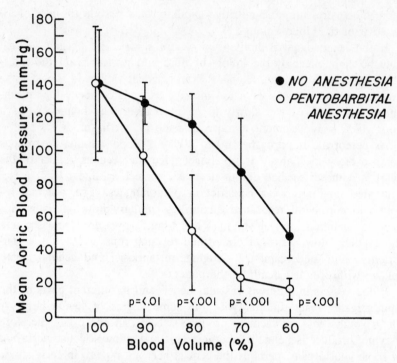

Fig. 5-1. Blood pressure response to graded hypovolemia in the pig. Note the difference between the anesthetized and unanesthetized states. (From Olsen, W. R., and Simon, M. A. 1969. *Arch. Surg.*, 99:634–636.)

correlation of the results of studies measuring capillary flow in animals with clinical studies[27,28] allows us to formulate opinions regarding human responses to hemorrhage.

Figure 5-1 illustrates the blood pressure responses to graded arterial hemorrhage in the pig,[19] an animal that does not develop splanchnic congestion after hemorrhage. These pressure curves are similar to those seen in humans after hemorrhage. When correlated with data regarding capillary perfusion following hemorrhage,[12,19] several generalizations can be made.

In the nonanesthetized state, a mild hemorrhage (10 to 20% of blood volume) produces little change in aortic blood pressure and no significant change in capillary flow to tissues other than the stomach. The venous, cardiac, and arteriolar compensatory mechanisms seem to be sufficient to maintain a fairly normal microcirculation.

The protective compensatory mechanisms are no longer adequate after a hemorrhage of 40% of blood volume. The arterial blood pressure decreases, peripheral vasoconstriction is accentuated, and significant decreases occur in capillary blood flow to the renal cortex, stomach, skin, and skeletal muscles. Interestingly, adrenal blood flow is increased after hemorrhage. The differences in the degree of ischemia of various tissues is thought to represent local differences in reactivity to the adrenergic stimulation of hemorrhage, with varying degrees of local arteriolar constriction.

It is of particular interest that, although studies on *anesthetized* animals have shown the detrimental effect of hypotension on coronary artery flow,[16,19,29–32] this does not seem to occur in the *nonanesthetized* state.[12]

Sodium pentobarbital has a pronounced effect on the local distribution of nutritive capillary blood flow after hemorrhage.[19] A hemorrhage of 20% of blood volume under pentobarbital anesthesia causes hypotension and ischemia of the stomach, skin, and skeletal muscles. A hemorrhage of 40% of blood volume causes a decrease in capillary flow to the myocardium, stomach, small intestines, and skin. As in the nonanesthetized state, an increase in adrenal blood flow occurs. Under pentobarbital anesthesia, the arterial blood pressure is as low after a hemorrhage of 20% of blood volume as it is after one of 40% in the nonanesthetized state and becomes a more sensitive indicator of the blood volume.

The differences in responses of the anesthetized and the nonanesthetized animal are emphasized for two reasons: first, to caution the clinician against undue reliance upon experimental data derived from *anesthetized animals,* usually dogs, when evaluating and treating shock in *nonanesthetized* humans, and second, to emphasize to the clinician the dangers of anesthetizing a patient in hypovolemic shock. Although a patient may appear to be fairly well compensated and to have a reasonable arterial blood pressure following a hemorrhage of 20% of blood volume, anesthesia will convert him to a poorly compensated state, interfering with local capillary blood flow and causing the arterial blood pressure to decrease precipitously. Since this mechanism may be responsible for some instances of cardiac arrests that occur in hypovolemic patients when general anethesia is instituted, it is important, when feasible, to make sure that the blood volume has been restored before anesthesia is induced.

The compensatory mechanisms and local capillary flow changes of cardiogenic shock are similar to those of hypovolemic shock. A deficiency of nutritive capillary flow is the basic pathophysiologic defect in both. A low arterial blood pressure results from a decrease in cardiac output due to deficient ventricular contractile force. A compensatory adrenergic response, clinically indistinguishable from that of hypovolemia, occurs with an increase in peripheral vascular tone and a further decrease in capillary flow. The patient with hypovolemic shock usually has a decreased central venous pressure, but the patient with cardiogenic shock has an adequate blood volume that is not being propelled through the heart, resulting in an overloading of the capacitance vessels and, usually, an increase in the central venous pressure. It is extremely important to differentiate cardiogenic shock from hypovolemic shock and to detect a cardiogenic element in hypovolemic shock. Whereas rapid fluid administration is essential to the correction of shock in the patient with hypovolemia, it may be the *coup de grace* to the patient with cardiogenic shock.

Recent evidence indicates that acidosis is usually the result rather than the cause of the failing circulation in shock in humans and indicates that clinical acidosis is rarely a potentiating factor in shock.[33-35] Sepsis is not a factor in shock in the early postinjury period and will not be discussed here.

Initial Management of the Injured Patient

The accident or trauma victim offers a unique clinical challenge. He is usually young (80% of our automobile accident victims are less than 40 years old) and, except for a disturbingly high rate of alcoholic intoxication, in good health. If he survives his life-threatening injuries, he can anticipate a reasonably long, productive life. There are few areas in medicine in which prompt and resourceful treatment is so liberally rewarded or in which delays and mistakes can lead to such tragedy. Proper care of these patients demands mature judgment, prompt action, and a conditioned awareness of priorities of treatment, which is acquired only through knowledge and experience. It is unfortunate that emergency department responsibility is often delegated to the least experienced members of the physician team.

Rapid and simultaneous evaluation and resuscitation is the first task in the care of these patients. The airway should be cleared and maintained, external hemorrhage controlled, and fractures immobilized.

While the most urgent and life-threatening problems are being cared for, associated problems should be assessed and treatment begun. Injuries must be evaluated according to their seriousness and an order of sequential therapy established. As soon as possible, blood should be drawn for typing, cross-matching, and making blood gas and other important and urgent laboratory determinations. If shock is present or the nature of the injuries indicates that hypovolemia may occur, a large intravenous route should be established.

As soon as possible, responsibility for the management of the severely injured patient should be assumed by the person who will care for him through the operative and convalescent phases of his hospitalization. When this physician assumes control early, he is better able to coordinate diagnostic and therapeutic efforts of the many members of the team required for sophisticated care of these patients. The practice of transferring physician responsibility after resuscitation and evaluation of the patient causes unnecessary delay and confusion, which interferes with successful therapy.

The evaluation and treatment of shock should begin as soon after the injury as possible and continue through the phases of resuscitation, evaluation, preoperative preparation, operation, and early convalescence. Unfortunately, adequate specific therapy is rarely available before the patient reaches the emergency room. This time lag may be detrimental, and physicians should become more active in improving the in-transit care of the injured patient.

One of the most important factors in survival of the severely injured patient is the degree of urgency with which the physician evaluates and treats hypovolemia. A sense of compulsive urgency, or an urgent sense of compulsion, is mandatory if one is to treat shock successfully. Patients do not live long in shock. The natural course of the disease is progressive deterioration and death unless the cause is reversed by adequate treatment. There is a direct relationship between the duration and severity of shock and survival. If treated promptly and adequately, a patient will recover from a hemorrhage of 40 to 60% of blood volume without sequelae. If therapy is delayed, the same patient will die from a less extensive hemorrhage, especially if he is aged or has associated problems. Treatment of these patients cannot wait. The cause of shock and any contributing factors must be rapidly assessed, and treatment must be initiated and sustained until the causal factors are controlled. A physician who is not willing to exercise the degree of dedication necessary to provide this type of care should not assume responsibility for the care of accident victims.

Since shock is a dynamic condition that is either improving or worsening, it is important that the patient's circulatory system be monitored during evaluation and treatment. The cardiac output, peripheral vascular tone, capillary flow (tissue perfusion), blood volume, and adequacy of the pulmonary and tissue oxygen exchange are of special interest. Sophisticated, computerized monitoring systems are being developed, but they lack the ease of application and portability needed for use in most acute injuries. Adequate approximations of these important values can be obtained and most patients can be successfully treated using only the equipment available on any nursing station provided the physician understands shock.

The best way to evaluate the severity of acute shock due to injury and to determine the adequacy of treatment is to examine the patient repeatedly. The clinical signs and symptoms of shock appear sequentially and disappear in the reverse order with treatment. The first sign of hypovolemia is oliguria. Signs and symptoms of more severe oligemia proceed from poor peripheral venous fill to pallor, tachycardia, diaphoresis, agitation, thirst, hypotension, dyspnea, confusion, cyanosis, coma, and death.

A good estimation of myocardial adequacy can be made from the strength of the pulse and the arterial pressure. Although a normal myocardium cannot maintain a strong pulse in the presence of severe hypovolemia, a strong pulse and normal blood pressure indicate that the myocardium is functioning adequately and excludes the diagnosis of cardiogenic shock.

The status of the peripheral vascular tone is best determined by examining the patient's skin and mucous membranes. Coldness and pallor of the skin indicate vasoconstriction from an alpha adrenergic sympathetic response. In accident and trauma victims, this is usually due to hypovolemia, although hypothermia from exposure may produce similar signs. Accompanying signs are piloerection and iris dilatation (alpha adrenergic responses) and sweating (a cholinergic sympathetic response). Cyanosis indicates more deficient perfusion and capillary stasis. The change in color of the ocular conjunctivae may be more noticeable than the skin color change, especially in pigmented patients.

The urinary output is a very sensitive indication of the adequacy of the blood volume and should be monitored closely in all patients in shock. An indwelling urinary catheter should be inserted on admission and the urinary output recorded every 15 minutes. In adults with normal renal function, a urinary output of about 50 ml. per hour is an indication of adequate renal perfusion and can be assumed to indicate adequate perfusion to other tissues as well. Small deficits in blood volume are followed promptly by oliguria before other clinical signs appear. A urinary output of less than 30 ml. per hour is a cause for concern because it may indicate renal ischemia and is usually an indication to alter treatment to improve renal perfusion. Vasopressors and diuretics increase urinary output in the presence of severe hypovolemia and, if they do not lull the physician into a false sense of security regarding adequacy of his treatment, they at least deprive him of this valuable guide to therapy. The urinary output should be maintained with adequate fluid replacement, not vasopressors or diuretics.

There are various means of measuring blood volume quantitatively, usually with radioisotopes. These methods are cumbersome, expensive, and time consuming, and the determinations are subject to the errors inherent in the use of complex equipment and the problems of availability of trained personnel. Until more practical bedside methods are developed, blood volume determinations remain of limited clinical value.

Central Venous Pressure Monitoring

This is a simple, reliable, and far less expensive means of estimating fluid needs than the methods already mentioned. The results are available immediately and the determination can be repeated as often as desired. More importantly, this monitoring device determines the aspects of blood volume that are most important to the physician, *i.e.,* the relationship of the effective circulating blood volume to myocardial adequacy, which helps distinguish cardiogenic shock from hypovolemia, and whether or not the patient can tolerate more fluid. We really do not need to know the precise blood volume. We need to know only if the patient can tolerate more fluid or if it is apt to cause congestive failure and pulmonary edema. In early injuries, central venous pressure monitoring can be used for this determination whereas radioisotopes cannot. In the complicated situation, especially when pulmonary and cardiogenic factors necessitate monitoring the patient for several days, more sophisticated monitoring, including pulmonary artery pressure, is important.[36] Central venous pressure monitoring has been extremely valuable in the management of volume replacement in a variety of clinical situations. In patients with manifest or imminent shock, regardless of cause, a catheter should be placed in the intrathoracic innominate vein and superior vena cava and the central venous pressure monitored. In accident and trauma victims, this is done in the emergency department by percutaneous subclavian venipuncture at the time of admission.[37-40] Although supraclavicular and internal jugular venipuncture are acceptable and safe in skilled hands, we believe that they are harder to learn and more dangerous for the inexperienced operator. We therefore advise use of the subclavian technique.

With the patient recumbent, the skin of the upper part of the chest and base of the neck is prepared and draped using careful sterile technique, including masks and gloves. The patient is then placed in the Trendelenburg position (one of the few uses for this position) to distend the veins. A finger is placed in the suprasternal notch, and a large needle, usually attached to a syringe, is inserted 1.5 cm. below the clavicle at its midpoint and passed horizontally below the clavicle, aiming toward the tip of the finger over the sternum (Fig. 5-2). The direction of the needle is perpendicular to the long axis of the patient, or slightly more cephalad, and parallel to the surface on which he is lying.

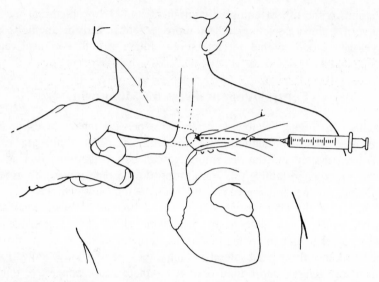

Fig. 5-2. Technique of percutaneous infraclavicular subclavian venipuncture. The needle is passed perpendicular to the long axis of the patient, or slightly more cephalad, and parallel to the surface on which he is lying. Caudad or posterior insertion increases the chance of pneumothorax and subclavian artery injury.

When the vein is entered, blood is withdrawn for necessary laboratory determinations. A catheter is threaded through the needle into an *intrathoracic* vein. Peripheral venous pressure is misleading and of no value in determining shock therapy.[38]

Care must be taken to prevent air embolism during removal of the syringe and passage of the catheter. A radiopaque catheter should be used so that the position of the catheter can be determined on subsequent x-rays. If radiopaque catheters are not available, fill the catheter with a small amount of radiopaque contrast material and obtain a chest x-ray. The catheter is connected to tubing containing an electrolyte solution and attached to a manometer via a three-way stopcock.

Passage of the catheter through peripheral cutdowns or venipunctures is more time consuming and, if the catheter is to remain in place for some time, is associated with a higher rate of suppurative thrombophlebitis. The cephalic and external jugular veins are not satisfactory because they enter the axillary subclavian veins at nearly right angles. Catheters inserted through these veins frequently impinge on the opposite wall of the larger vein and cannot be advanced into the chest. Veins of the leg should not be used because of the frequency with which deep thrombophlebitis occurs from inlying catheters and intravenous infusions in the legs. The subclavian vein is an ever present route for fluid therapy, even in profound shock. In the very rare instance in which the patient is in deep shock and fluids must be administered rapidly to maintain life, but the type of injury precludes use of an upper extremity vein, a saphenous vein cutdown may be used until the urgency is passed and the catheter can be moved to a more satisfactory site.

It is important to position the tip of the catheter in the superior vena cava 2 or 3 cm. above the heart. Catheters resting in the heart may cause arrhythmias, or repeated cardiac contractions against the catheter may cause myocardial erosion with pericardial tamponade and death.[41-43]

After passage of the catheter, a chest x-ray, portable if necessary, should be obtained to determine the position of catheter and to check for pneumothorax. If the catheter is near or in the heart, or in an extrathoracic vein, it should be repositioned.

Sepsis is one of the most common complications of indwelling intravenous catheters.[44-46] It is essential that these catheters be passed under aseptic conditions and that the skin around the catheter be kept sterile.

Serious complications of subclavian venipuncture, such as pneumothorax, hemothorax, hydrothorax, brachial plexus injury, and subclavian artery puncture, although infrequent, are usually the result of improper technique particularly introducing the needle with too great a posterior or inferior angulation.[38,47]

Special care should be taken to prevent shearing off the intravenous catheter with resultant catheter embolization.[48] This usually occurs while attempting to withdraw a catheter inserted through a needle that is still in the vein. The catheter is transected by the needle point and passes to the right ventricle or pulmonary artery. If it is necessary to withdraw the catheter, always remove the needle first! The incidence of breakage and embolization of catheters after final positioning can be reduced by suturing the catheter to the skin and by using a catheter in which the flange is permanently attached. If catheter embolization occurs, the catheter may be removed by passing a snare through a peripheral vein under fluoroscopic control.[49]

There are very few worthwhile means of diagnosis and treatment that do not carry risk if used improperly. The possible complications of subclavian venipuncture should not discourage its appropriate use. They are listed here to emphasize the need for caution and proper technique in performing this extremely useful procedure. With such forewarning, we believe any physician should be able to catheterize central veins repeatedly with few problems.

Consistency in positioning the manometer is important. A mark is made at the midaxillary line with a pen or marking pencil and this mark is used repeatedly as the zero reference point for determining the venous pressure. The head of the bed is lowered to the horizontal position and respirators, which cause falsely high readings, should be momentarily disconnected. The manometer is filled to the top with an electrolyte solution, all bubbles are run out of the system, the stopcock is turned, and the fluid is allowed to find its level. If the catheter has been inserted recently, the fluid will fluctuate with respirations, assuring that the tip is in an intrathoracic vein.

After a few days, a thrombus and fibrin sleeve forms around the catheter and may interfere with this fluctuation. In time the sleeve may form a flap valve, which usually does not interfere with the continued use of the catheter for fluid administration but may invalidate the venous pressure reading. Our experience in the laboratory and in patients indicates that heparin does not prevent thrombus or sleeve formation. Although a single fibrin sleeve is rarely harmful to the patient, multiple catheter insertions, and therefore multiple fibrin sleeves, may cause complete venous thrombosis. It is usually better to maintain one catheter than to use multiple injection sites.

Proper interpretation of the venous pressure is as important as careful technique in its measurement. One must remain aware that the central venous pressure is a measure of the right ventricular filling force, and therefore it is of value only in indicating the ability of the right side of the patient's heart to propel the blood being presented to the right atrium. It does not indicate blood volume nor does it necessarily measure the adequacy of the left side of the heart. It is of value only in judging the ability of the patient to tolerate fluid replacement and in helping to prevent cardiac overloading during therapy. Central venous pressure therefore must never be considered in isolation but should always be used in conjunction with other estimates of cardiac output and peripheral perfusion.

If the midaxillary line is used as the zero reference point, the normovolemic patient will have a central venous pressure of 3 to 8 cm. H_2O. If the central venous pressure is normal or low, fluid may be administered safely but only if other signs indicate the need. One should not use a seemingly low central venous pressure *per se* as an indication for fluid administration. If the central venous pressure is high, too much fluid has been administered, the myocardium is failing, or there is pulmonary interstitial edema. In any case, the patient will not tolerate more fluid. Always remember that the central venous pressure *may* not be elevated in left heart failure, especially in the early stage. When the left side of the heart is incapable of pumping blood normally, pulmonary venous pressure increases before the central venous pressure does. The chest x-ray and auscultation of the chest may indicate pulmonary congestion and a Swan-Ganz catheter indicates increasing pulmonary arterial pressure before the central venous pressure rises.

Fluid Replacement

Since most early postinjury shock is due to hemorrhage, normal capillary perfusion can be restored most effectively by rapid blood transfusion. Unfortunately, it takes 45 to 60 minutes to obtain crossmatched whole blood. Since patients frequently will not tolerate such delays without irreparable sequelae, emergency resuscitation must be started with other methods of blood volume expansion.

The shock position (Fig. 5-3), with the trunk and head elevated 5 degrees and the legs elevated 30 degrees, allows more rapid return of venous blood from the extremities which, in effect, constitutes an internal transfusion of several hundred milliliters. The Trendelenburg position (head down, legs up, and hips straight) accomplishes the same thing but impairs cerebral perfusion, interferes with respiration and should not be used.

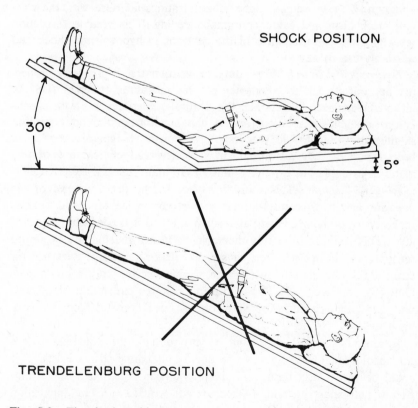

SHOCK POSITION

30°

5°

TRENDELENBURG POSITION

Fig. 5-3. The shock position speeds venous return from the legs, thereby improving cardiac output during the resuscitative period of shock therapy. The Trendelenburg position accomplishes the same thing but, because it impairs respiration and cerebral perfusion, should not be used.

Types of Fluids. Emergency resuscitation areas must be kept stocked with satisfactory blood substitutes for use until whole blood can be obtained. These substitutes must be safe and effective and should be relatively stable and easy to store (long shelf life).

The Dextrans. Use of the dextrans as emergency blood substitutes has been the subject of intensive laboratory and clinical investigation, which has been well summarized by Atik.[50] Six percent Dextran 70 (clinical dextran; average molecular weight 70,000) and low molecular weight dextran (Dextran 40, Rheomacrodex; average molecular weight 40,000) are osmotically active and have fluid-expanding properties. Dextran 40 has the added advantage of reducing the viscosity of whole blood when it is abnormally high, as in clinical shock, which improves tissue perfusion. The dextrans, however, must be used with caution. They may produce severe allergic reactions and, although they are relatively safe if administered in the recommended dose of 10 to 15 ml. per kilogram of body weight, higher concentrations interfere with the clotting mechanism and cause abnormal bleeding. This volume restriction severely limits the usefulness of the dextrans in hypovolemic shock and we rarely use them.

Hydroxyethyl Starch. This amylase resistant starch possesses properties appropriate for an emergency plasma substitute. It remains in the intravascular space longer than the dextrans, interferes less with coagulation, is stable in solution, and is eliminated from the body without significant tissue storage reactions.[51] Although allergic reactions have been reported, they are infrequent.[52] Widespread clinical use of this material as a plasma expander must await more clinical experience.

Ringer's Lactate. This solution is free of the disadvantages of the dextrans and hydroxyethyl starch and is our choice for rapid volume replacement in hypovolemic patients when blood is needed but not available. This solution is readily available, is stable indefinitely, needs no refrigeration, is pyrogen-free, causes no allergic reactions, does not interfere with the clotting mechanism, is inexpensive and, most importantly, is effective.[8,53-55] Rapid infusion restores circulating blood volume and capillary perfusion and decreases the eventual blood requirement.[56]

Because Ringer's lactate contains no protein, the potential risk of dilutional hypoalbuminemia and secondary interstitial edema exists. This could be particularly harmful if this mechanism potentiated the formation of pulmonary interstitial edema as one would expect by application of Starling's hypothesis. Recent work suggests, however, that the transcapillary exchange of fluid and protein is controlled by much more complex autoregulatory mechanisms and that the interrelationships of circulating protein, oncotic pressure, and blood volume vary greatly in sick patients, especially those in shock and those with contused tissues.

Marty has recently indicated that excessive albumin therapy may accentuate interstitial edema and interfere with pulmonary mechanics and gas exchange.[57] In young, healthy patients, the serum albumin is not significantly lowered following mild hemorrhage and rapidly returns to normal after massive hemorrhage treated with protein-free electrolyte solutions,[8,58,59] indicating that albumin enters the vascular space rapidly after hemorrhage. Clinical studies indicate that, if care is taken to prevent iatrogenic fluid overload, peripheral and pulmonary interstitial edema occur infrequently when hemorrhage is treated by protein electrolyte solutions.[8] More work is necessary before the need for protein in emergency resuscitation fluids is clarified and can be recommended.

Some surgeons have been concerned that the hepatic threshold for metabolizing lactate may be overcome by large volume infusions of lactate-containing solutions, causing lactic acidemia and rendering the blood lactate levels useless. Clinical studies now show that this does not occur.[53]

Blood. An acute hemorrhage of less than 15% of blood volume usually can be treated with prompt volume replacement of an erythrocyte-free solution without impairment of oxygen-carrying capacity. With more severe hemorrhage, particularly if the hematocrit is less than 30 or the hemoglobin less than 10, whole blood should be transfused. Although cross-matched blood of the same type is preferable, massive hemorrhage or the need for rare blood type may deplete the available supply. In such an instance, blood from the same ABO type should be transfused whenever possible. The same Rh type is preferable, but Rh negative blood is tolerated well by Rh positive patients and Rh positive blood may be given to Rh negative patients for a few days. However, Rh positive blood should not be given to sensitized Rh negative patients or to Rh negative women in the childbearing age.

Remember that the low pH and high potassium content of banked blood may cause cardiac arrhythmias and lead to arrest, especially when accentuated by hypocalcemia secondary to the calcium-binding capacity of citrate and hypothermia if the blood, and the patient, are not warmed. Banked blood also is deficient in platelets, some clotting factors, and 2,3-diphosphoglycerate, which leads to abnormal bleeding and impaired oxygen release at the tissue level after massive transfusions. Transfused blood causes at least 30,000 cases of overt hepatitis and 1,500 to 3,000 deaths in the United States per year with a significantly higher rate from blood from paid donors as opposed to blood from volunteers.[60,61] It seems evident that whole blood should be used only for specific indications and not in excess of the quantity needed.

Amount of Fluid Replacement. The amount of fluid necessary to restore the normal hemodynamic state is equal to the loss caused by the injury and can be determined only by the clinical response of the patient. In other words, replacement must be continued until the clinical signs of shock disappear, and they do so in the reverse order to which they appeared, the urinary output being the last to return to normal.

The first indication that the patient will need fluid therapy is the severity of the injuries. A badly injured patient requires fluid. The alert physician anticipates the requirement and begins fluid therapy promptly, often before the clinical signs of shock occur. His patients endure less hypovolemia for shorter periods of time and reap the benefit in decreased morbidity and mortality rates.

Remember that none of the signs taken out of context is sufficient to indicate normovolemia. Most patients maintain a normal blood pressure with a volume deficit of 1,000 ml. and, in acute hemorrhage, the hematocrit is misleading. Each patient must be considered a unique pathophysiologic model and monitored and treated until the circulatory derangements are corrected.

The relative amounts of Ringer's lactate and whole blood needed are dependent upon the type of injury. Whole blood loss requires whole blood replacement in nearly equal amounts. Because of the logistical delays and the need to begin to replace third space loss into injured tissues, most of our patients admitted in hemorrhagic shock receive 2,000 to 4,000 ml. of Ringer's lactate before type specific or cross-matched whole blood is available. This allows us to reduce the amount of fluid replaced, decreasing the risks of transfusion reactions and hepatitis. The resultant posttherapy anemia usually requires no treatment.

If there is significant soft tissue injury, and there usually is after automobile accidents, more Ringer's lactate is needed. It must be remembered that the fluid sequestered in injured tissues is released into the venous capillaries as the tissues heal. Several days after injury this reabsorption of fluid may equal or exceed the patient's daily fluid requirement. This reabsorption should be anticipated and fluid therapy altered accordingly or hypervolemia and secondary pulmonary problems may ensue. Watch the hourly urinary output. When it increases to greater than 70 ml. per hour, the rate of intravenous fluid administration should be reduced.

After estimating the relative proportions of crystalloid and colloid solutions needed, one administers the fluid rapidly while observing the patient, monitoring the urinary output and central venous pressure, and auscultating the chest repeatedly until the signs and symptoms of shock disappear and the urinary output returns to normal (indicating satisfactory reestablishment of a normal blood volume) or until there is evidence of imminent fluid overload or edema.

If the central venous pressure increases to greater than 10 cm. H_2O, fluid overload is imminent. If this occurs before the signs and symptoms of shock disappear, the shock may be at least partially cardiogenic. Fluid replacement must be stopped while efforts are made to improve cardiac output by increasing the strength of ventricular contraction. This may require isoproterenol (a potent beta stimulator that must be administered cautiously to prevent excessive tachycardia), digitalis (especially useful in patients with preexisting cardiac disease and in patients with a pulse exceeding 120 per minutes), or a combination of an adrenergic agent and an alpha blocker.

Occasionally, pulmonary interstitial edema occurs, as signified by the portable chest film or auscultation. Pulmonary contusions, aspiration, or embolization of particulate matter (a frequent problem with massive transfusion therapy) may be the cause, but excessive fluid administration is usually at least partially to blame. Repeated determinations of the central venous pressure and arterial blood gases and frequent chest films and chest auscultation should detect difficulties before edema becomes fulminant. Pulmonary edema from acute left heart failure frequently is not accompanied by an increase in the central venous pressure. Measurement of pulmonary arterial pressure by means of a Swan-Ganz catheter is very helpful in such isolated instances. Once pulmonary edema has occurred, fluid restriction and diuretics are indicated, and controlled respiration may become necessary.

Central venous pressure monitoring is most useful in preventing excessive transfusion during the rapid administration of fluid to healthy, young patients. As long as the central venous pressure is not elevated and the chest is clear, fluid can be administered as rapidly as desired with little fear of fluid overload. When the central venous pressure increases, the blood volume is approaching the maximum that can be tolerated by the heart, and the rate of administration must be decreased. This is the only role of central venous pressure monitoring. The currently popular practices of using a low central venous pressure reading as an indication for fluid therapy or insisting upon increasing the central venous pressure above normal, indicating fluid overload, before slowing the rate of fluid administration should be avoided. The central venous pressure monitoring device is not a volume gauge; it does not indicate when a patient is a quarter full or three-quarters full! It indicates to the physician only when the patient is *too* full and warns him against additional fluid administration.

Vasopressors. Although vasopressors have been used extensively in the treatment of hypovolemic shock, convincing evidence of their clinical efficacy is lacking. Studies on anesthetized animals have shown the detrimental effect of hypotension on coronary artery[16,19,29-32] and renal artery[30,26-64] flow and the salutary effects of the artificial elevation of arterial blood pressure by vasopressors in this setting.[11,29,31,32,63-65] Our results from the use of metaraminol in the anesthetized pig in hemorrhagic shock support these findings.[24]

Unfortunately, some authors have assumed that vasopressors have a similar effect in *nonanesthetized humans* and have advocated their use in the treatment of clinical shock. This assumption fails to take into consideration the variables introduced by anesthesia, the reports of the detrimental effects of vasopressors,[66-73] the role of catecholamines in preventing reexpansion of the blood volume after hemorrhage,[70] and the evidence that plasma catecholamine levels are already increased in shock.[9,42-75] Our studies indicate that a hemorrhage of 40% of blood volume does *not* adversely affect myocardial perfusion,[12] and that therapeutic amounts of metaraminol given after hemorrhage *decrease* myocardial perfusion and renal capillary blood flow in the nonanesthetized animal.[24] We are not aware of evidence that vasopressors improve capillary perfusion in nonanesthetized humans.

The ischemic insult of acute hypovolemia with pronounced hypotension frequently has its most serious and lasting effects on the central nervous system. Vasopressors may have an important role in maintaining cerebral perfusion following acute, massive hemorrhage in the few moments before blood volume replacement can be begun. Similarly, vasopressors help overcome the loss of peripheral vascular tone that accompanies acute cardiac arrest, thereby shortening the period of pronounced hypotension. Although logical, these popular hypotheses are unsubstantiated. We must know the effect of graded hypotension and vasopressors on cerebral *perfusion* before the usefulness of vasopressors in pronounced hypotension is accepted.

Alkalinizing and Buffering Solutions. The cellular anoxia of hypovolemic shock invariably interferes with aerobic metabolism and causes peripheral metabolic acidosis. If severe, this acidosis may interfere with cardiovascular function and, by lowering the 2,3-diphosphoglycerate level, impair peripheral oxygenation. Whether or not the acidosis requires specific therapy, however, is debatable. Collins and co-workers have summarized the published data on the role of acidosis in shock and have confirmed it in their clinical studies.[34] In most patients whose hypovolemic shock responds to fluid replacement, the metabolic acidosis, regardless of magnitude, rapidly reverses without specific therapy. Furthermore, most patients experience no difficulty from the infused acid load of stored blood.

Patients who demonstrate persistent metabolic acidosis and lactic acidemia after treatment usually have continued hemorrhage and shock or have had such extensive ischemic damage that survival is unlikely. Administration of alkali to such patients is usually without effect, even when the acidosis is reversed.

Metabolic defenses against acidosis are less efficient during hypothermia, in the newborn, and in patients with impaired hepatic function or preexisting myocardial disease. The normal defense mechanisms may be overwhelmed by sustained transfusion therapy exceeding 1 unit of banked blood every 4 to 6 minutes. Under any circumstances, it is unlikely that clinical acidosis alone significantly affects cardiovascular function or that patients responding favorably to transfusion therapy will require pharmacologic manipulation of their acid-base balance.[33-35] Routine administration of alkalinizing solutions during rapid or sustained blood transfusions may cause hypocalcemia, ventilatory depression, increased urinary potassium losses, and impaired oxygen transport.[34] If alkalinizing or buffering solutions are considered in patients who are not responding well to transfusion therapy, their use should be based on objective measurements of the acid-base status and should be accompanied by the cautious administration of calcium.

Surgical Intervention

Occasionally, it becomes evident that the patient is losing blood as rapidly as it is being administered and that reestablishment of normal circulatory dynamics by rapid fluid administration is not going to be successful. If so, immediate operation is necessary for hemostasis. Once the bleeding organ is exposed, hemostasis should be accomplished as expeditiously as possible. The splenic pedicle usually can be rapidly controlled, but injuries to organs such as the liver and vena cava are best controlled by firm packing until the blood volume can be restored and definitive surgical correction can be carried out with the patient normovolemic.

With profound hypovolemic shock, the aorta should be occluded to allow ventricular filling and perfusion of the brain. Some surgeons have advised against opening the abdomen in such patients for fear of losing the tamponade effect of the abdominal wall. This is probably more myth than wisdom, since the tamponade effect can be replaced by much more effective aortic occlusion within seconds. If a potentially salvageable patient undergoes cardiac arrests from hypovolemia, the chest should be opened immediately, the aorta cross-clamped, and open heart massage instituted. To avoid mortality and morbidity, which is certain to accrue with undue delays in this type of patient, it is imperative that resuscitation of badly injured patients be performed near an operating room.

References

1. Baue, A. E. 1968. Recent developments in the study and treatment of shock: collective review. *Surg. Gynec. Obstet.,* 127:849–878.
2. Clauss, R. N., and Ray, J. F. 1968. Pharmacologic assistance to the failing circulation: collective review. *Surg. Gynec. Obstet.,* 126:611–631.
3. Hamit, H. F. 1965. Current trends of therapy and research in shock: collective review. *Surg. Gynec. Obstet.,* 120:835–854.
4. Mills, L. C., and Moyer, J. H. 1965. "Shock and hypotension: pathogenesis and treatment," The Twelfth Hahnemann Symposium. New York, Grune & Stratton.
5. Wilson, C. B., Vidrine, A., and Rives, J. D. 1965. Unrecognized abdominal trauma in patients with head injuries. *Ann. Surg.,* 161:608–613.
6. Mellander, S. 1960. Comparative studies on the adrenergic neurohormonal control of resistance and capacitance blood vessels in the cat. *Acta Physiol. Scand.,* 50(suppl. 176):1–85.
7. Dow, R. W., and Fry, W. J. 1967. Venous compensatory mechanisms in acute hypovolemia. *Surg. Gynec. Obstet.,* 125:511–515.
8. Cloutier, C. T., Lowery, B. D., and Carey, L. C. 1969. The effect of hemodilutional resuscitation on serum protein levels in humans in hemorrhagic shock. *J. Trauma,* 9:514–521.
9. Moore, F. D. 1965. Annual discourse: the effects of hemorrhage on body composition. *New Eng. J. Med.,* 273:567–577.
10. Skillman, J. J., Awwad, H. K., and Moore, F. D. 1967. Plasma protein kinetics in the earl transcapillary refill after hemorrhage in man. *Surg. Gynec. Obstet.,* 125:983–996.
11. Catchpole, B. N., Hackel, D. B., and Simeone, F. A. 1955. Coronary and peripheral blood flow in experimental hemorrhagic hypotension treated with L-nor-epinephrine. *Ann. Surg.,* 142:372–381.
12. Simon, M. A., and Olsen, W. R. 1969. Capillary flow in hemorrhagic shock. I: Hemorrhage in the nonanesthetized pig. *Arch. Surg.,* 99:631–633.
13. Cohn, H. E., and Ballinger, W. F. 1964. *Research Methods in Surgery,* W. F. Ballinger (ed.). Boston, Little, Brown & Co., p. 202.
14. Beaconsfield, P., and Messent, D. 1955. Blood flow after general anesthesia in sympathectomized limbs. *Anesthesiology,* 16:428–433.
15. Greisheimer, E. M. 1965. The circulatory effects of anesthesia, in *Handbook of Physiology,* Vol. III, Sec. 2. Washington, D.C., American Physiologic Society, pp. 2477–2510.
16. Hackel, D. B., and Goodale, W. T. 1965. Effects of hemorrhagic shock on the heart and circulation of intact dogs. *Circulation,* 11:628–634.
17. Heilbrunn, A., and Allbritten, F. F. 1960. Cardiac output during and following surgical operations. *Ann. Surg.,* 152:197–210.
18. Nash, C. B., Davis, F., and Woodbury, R. A. 1956. Cardiovascular effects of anesthetic doses of pentobarbital sodium. *Amer. J. Physiol.,* 185:107–112.
19. Olsen, W. R., and Simon, M. A. 1969. Capillary flow in hemorrhagic shock. II: Hemorrhage in the anesthetized pig. *Arch. Surg.,* 99:634–636.
20. Price, H. L. 1960. General anesthesia and circulatory homeostasis. *Physiol. Rev.,* 40:187–218.
21. Barclay, A. E., and Bentley, F. H. 1949. The vascularization of the human stomach: a preliminary note on the shunting effect of trauma. *Gastroenterology,* 12:177–183.

22. Suzuki, M., and Penn, I. 1965. A reappraisal of the microcirculation during general hypothermia. *Surgery,* 58:1049–1060.
23. Olsen, W. R. 1968. A new research technique to determine changes in blood capillary flow. *Arch. Surg.,* 97:831–835.
24. Olsen, W. R. 1969. Capillary flow in hemorrhagic shock. III: Metaraminol and capillary flow in the nonanesthetized and anesthetized pig. *Arch. Surg.,* 99:637–640.
25. Sapirstein, L. A. 1956. Fractionation of the cardiac output of rats with isotopic potassium. *Circ. Res.,* 4:689–692.
26. Sapirstein, L. A. 1958. Regional blood flow by fraction distribution of indicators. *Amer. J. Physiol.,* 193:161–168.
27. Beecher, H. K., et al. 1947. The internal state of the severely wounded man on entry to the most forward hospital. *Surgery,* 22:672–711.
28. Shenkin, H. A., et al. 1944. On the diagnosis of hemorrhage in man: a study of volunteers bled large amounts. *Amer. J. Med. Sci.,* 208:421–436.
29. Corday, E., et al. 1959. Effect of systemic blood pressure and vasopressor drugs on coronary blood flow and the electrocardiogram. *Amer. J. Cardiol.,* 3:626–637.
30. Sapirstein, L. A., Sapirstein, E. H., and Bredemeyer, A. 1960. Effect of hemorrhage on the cardiac output and its distribution in the rat. *Circ. Res.,* 8:135–348.
31. Sarnoff, S. J., et al. 1954. Insufficient coronary flow and myocardial failure as a complicating factor in late hemorrhagic shock. *Amer. J. Physiol.,* 176:439–444.
32. Vowles, K. D. J., Couves, C. M., and Howard, J. M. 1957. Coronary and peripheral blood flow following hemorrhagic shock, tranfusion, and norepinephrine. *Circulation,* 18:946.
33. Clowes, G. H. A., et al. 1961. Effects of acidosis on cardiovascular function in surgical patients. *Ann. Surg.,* 154:524–555.
34. Collins, J. A., et al. 1971. Acid-base status of seriously wounded combat casualties: II: Resuscitation with stored blood. *Ann. Surg.,* 173:6–18.
35. Feins, N. R., and DelGuercio, L. R. M. 1966. Increased cardiovascular function in clinical metabolic acidosis, *Surg. Forum,* 17:39–40.
36. Swan, H. J. C., et al. 1970. Catheterization of the heart in man with use of a flow-directed balloon-tipped catheter. *New Eng. J. Med.,* 283:447.
37. Dudrick, S. J., et al. 1969. Can intravenous feeding as the sole means of nutrition support growth in a child and return weight loss in an adult? An affirmative answer. *Ann. Surg.,* 169:974–984.
38. Longerbeam, J. K., et al. 1965. Venous pressure monitoring: a useful guide to fluid therapy during shock and other forms of cardiovascular stress. *Amer. J. Surg.,* 110:220–230.
39. Mogil, R. A., Delaurentis, D. A., and Rosemond, G. P. 1967. The Intraclavicular venipuncture: value in various clinical situations including central venous pressure monitoring. *Arch. Surg.,* 95:320–324.
40. Wilson, J. N., et al. 1962. Central venous pressure in optimal blood volume maintenance. *Arch. Surg.,* 85:563–578.
41. Geis, P. W., et al. 1970. Extrapericardial (mediastinal) cardiac tamponade. *Arch. Surg.,* 100:305–306.
42. Lawton, R. W., Rossi, N. P., and Funk, D. C. 1969. Intracardiac perforation. *Arch. Surg.,* 98:213–216.
43. Thomas, C. S., Carter, J. W., and Lowder, S. C. 1969. Pericardial tamponade from central venous catheters. *Arch. Surg.,* 98:217–218.
44. Collins, R. N., et al. 1968. Risk of local and systemic infection with polyethylene intravenous catheters. A prospective study of 213 catheterizations. *New Eng. J. Med.,* 279:340–343.

45. Glover, J. L., O'Byrne, S. A., and Jolly, L. 1971. Infusion catheter sepsis: an increasing threat. *Ann. Surg.,* 173:148–151.
46. Smits, H., and Freedman, L. R. 1967. Prolonged venous catheterization as a cause of sepsis. *New Eng. J. Med.,* 276:1229–1233.
47. Smith, B. E., et al. 1965. Complications of subclavian vein catheterization. *Arch. Surg.,* 90:228–229.
48. Doering, R. B., Stemmer, E. A., and Connolly, J. E. 1967. Complications of indwelling venous catheters with particular reference to catheter embolus. *Amer. J. Surg.,* 114:259–266.
49. Bloomfield, D. A. 1971. Technique of nonsurgical retrieval of iatrogenic foreign bodies from the heart. *Amer. J. Cardiol.,* 27:538–545.
50. Atik, M. 1967. Dextran 40 and Dextran 70: a review. *Arch. Surg.,* 94:664–672.
51. Thompson, W. L., et al. 1970. Intravascular persistence, tissue storage, and excretion of hydroxyethyl starch. *Surg. Gynec. Obstet.,* 131:965–972.
52. Metcalf, W., et al. 1970. A clinical physiologic study of hydroxyethyl starch. *Surg. Gynec. Obstet.,* 131:255–567.
53. Carey, L. C., Lowery, B. D., and Cloutier, C. T. 1971. Hemorrhagic shock, *Curr. Probl. Surg.,* pp. 31–33.
54. Dillon, J., et al. 1966. The bioassay of treatment of hemorrhagic shock. *Arch. Surg.,* 93:537–555.
55. Dillon J., et al. 1966. The treatment of hemorrhagic shock. *Surg. Gynec. Obstet.,* 122:967–978.
56. Rush, B. F., et al. 1969. Limitation of blood replacement with electrolyte solutions. A controlled clinical study. *Arch. Surg.,* 98:49–52.
57. Marty, A. T. 1974. Hyperoncotic albumin therapy. *Surg. Gynec. Obstet.,* 139:105–109.
58. Moore, F. D., et al. 1966. Hemorrhage in normal man: I. Distribution and dispersal of saline following acute blood loss: clinical kinetics of blood volume support. *Ann. Surg.,* 163:485–504.
59. Carey, L. C., Lowery, D. B., and Cloutier, C. T. 1971. Hemorrhagic shock. *Curr. Probl. Surg.,* pp. 36–37.
60. Allen, J. G. 1970. Commercially obtained blood and serum hepatitis. *Surg. Gynec. Obstet.,* 131:277.
61. Silver, D. 1972. Blood transfusion and disorder of surgical bleeding, Chapter 6 in *Davis-Christopher Textbook of Surgery,* D. C. Sabiston (ed.). Philadelphia, W. B. Saunders, pp. 131–146.
62. Dow, R., and Fry, W. J. 1967. Hemorrhagic shock; changes in renal blood flow and vascular resistance. *Arch. Surg.,* 94:190–194.
63. Mills, L. C., and Moyer, J. H. 1960. The effects of various catecholamines on specific vascular hemodynamics in hypotensive and normotensive subjects. *Amer. J. Cardiol.,* 5:652–659.
64. Mills, L. C., Moyer, J. H., and Handley, C. A. 1960. Effects of various sympathicomimetic drugs on renal hemodynamics in normotensive and hypotensive dogs. *Amer. J. Physiol.,* 198:1279–1283.
65. West, J. W., Guzman, S. V., and Bellet, S. 1957. Comparative cardiac effects of various sympathomimetic amines. *Circulation,* 16:950.
66. Close, A. S., et al. 1957. The effect of norepinephrine on survival in experimental acute hemorrhagic hypotension. *Surg. Forum,* 8:22–26.
67. Drucker, W. R., Kingsbury, B., and Graham, L. 1962. Metabolic effect of vasopressors in hemorrhagic shock. *Surg. Forum,* 13:16–18.
68. Finnerty, F. A., Jr., Buchholz, J. H., and Guillaudeu, R. L. 1958. The blood volumes and plasma protein during levarterenol-induced hypertension. *J. Clin. Invest.,* 37:425–429.
69. Jackson, A. J., and Webb, W. R. 1962. Effects of norepinephrine on differential blood flow in graded hemorrhage. *Surg. Forum,* 13:14–15.

70. Lister, J., et al. 1963. Transcapillary refilling after hemorrhage in normal man: basal rates and volumes; effect of norepinephrine. *Ann. Surg.,* 158:698–712.
71. Longerbeam, J. K., Lillebei, R. C., and Scott, W. R. 1962. The nature of irreversible shock: a hemodynamic study. *Surg. Forum,* 13:1–3.
72. Morris, R. E., Jr., Graff, T. D., and Robinson, P. 1966. Metabolic effects of vasopressor agents, *Bull. N.Y. Acad. Med.,* 42:1007–1022.
73. Schmutzer, K. J., Raschke, E., and Maloney, J. V., Jr. 1961. Intravenous l-norepinephrine as a cause of reduced plasma volume. *Surgery,* 50:452–457.
74. Rosenberg, J. C., et al. 1961. Studies on hemorrhagic and endotoxin shock in relation to vasomotor changes and endogenous circulating epinephrine, norepinephrine and serotonin. *Ann. Surg.,* 154:611–628.
75. Walker, W. F., et al. 1959. Adrenal medullary secretion in hemorrhagic shock. *Amer. J. Physiol.,* 197:773–780.

6

Emergency Coronary Care

Condon R. Vander Ark

Coronary heart disease is the most common cause of death in the United States. More than 1 million people experience acute myocardial infarction or sudden coronary death each year, with approximately 650,000 cardiovascular deaths due to coronary heart disease, of which 360,000 are due to acute myocardial infarction. Sudden death outside the hospital accounts for 60 to 70% of deaths due to acute infarction and claims more lives each year than does any other single cause.[1]

Over the past 14 years the hospital coronary care unit has become the focal point of treatment of the patient with an acute myocardial infarction. These units are designed to place the patient under constant electronic monitoring and the care of highly trained medical and paramedical personnel. The mortality rate in hospitals before coronary care units were instituted was about 35%. Mortality rates in effective coronary care units have been reduced by as much as 50% with a current overall mortality rate of 15 to 20%. This significant reduction is clearly due to early detection, prevention, and treatment of life-threatening cardiac arrhythmias. Treatment of congestive heart failure and cardiogenic shock in these units has been less rewarding.

Although these units have resulted in a significant saving of human life, it must be remembered that less than half the patients with acute myocardial infarcts live long enough to benefit from this specialized cardiac care. Furthermore, the mortality rate in well run coronary care units has reached a plateau, and a further reduction in the mortality rate will be difficult to achieve and will require a great deal of expensive research. Even if it were possible to eliminate in-hospital deaths due to coronary artery disease, approximately 250,000 deaths each year would still occur before the victims of acute myocardial infarction reached the hospital.

The Problems of Delay

It seems clear that if a further significant reduction in the mortality rate of acute myocardial infarction is to be made, we must direct our attention to the time period between the onset of the acute coronary event and arrival in the coronary care unit. The usual cause of sudden death in a patient with an acute myocardial infarction is a cardiac arrhythmia, resulting in the heart being an ineffective pump. Effective treatment of these arrhythmias is possible, and when the disturbance is adequately controlled, the prognosis for the patient's return to normal life is not significantly different from that for the patient who has had a similar myocardial infarction without a disturbance of rhythm. Since we have the knowledge and the technology required to treat these patients effectively, the problem is in effectively delivering these skills to patients needing them.

A careful look at this critical period of time indicates the major problems that must be solved. The average time between onset of the initial symptoms and arrival at the hospital varies in reported series from four to more than eight hours.[2-4] The importance of this relatively long delay is apparent when one realizes that 40 to 60% of sudden deaths occur within the first hour after onset of symptoms.

Most of the time lost in getting to the hospital is due to the patient's delay. The patient may deny the presence of significant symptoms and displace them from the heart to other organ systems, such as the lungs, stomach, gallbladder, or esophagus. Patients who are convinced from the outset that their symptoms are of cardiac origin seek medical help most promptly. Delay is often the result of self-medication with either previously prescribed medications or home remedies. Delay is shortest in patients who decide to seek help because of the severity of their symptoms or prior education. Consultation with co-workers or friends is the next most effective means of decreasing this delay; a spouse appears to be least effective in reducing delay in seeking help.

The only effective way to reduce the time lost in deciding to seek help is to educate the public about the signs and symptoms of acute myocardial infarction and the necessity of seeking immediate medical care. Because the only symptom may be chest pain and waiting for additional symptoms may be fatal, one can easily envision some of the problems associated with this educational program. Physicians, of course, must refer these patients, without delay, directly to the emergency department of the hospital. If the patient does not have a physician, he should go directly to the emergency department by private or emergency vehicle for evaluation. The American Heart Association is beginning an educational program of this type. If the program is effective, it will bring many more patients to emergency departments, many with false alarms but many with acute infarction. This will require changes in the operating procedures of many emergency departments.

Once the patient has called for help, he encounters the next period of delay, which is frequently referred to as the transportation delay. This involves waiting for a friend to come pick him up, for his wife to come home with the car, or for an emergency medical team to arrive. Unfortunately, the call for emergency service may not bring an emergency medical team ready to deliver emergency care but only an ill-equipped ambulance with a chauffeur. The total time involved in transportation is usually relatively small (usually less than 30 minutes) but is, of course, highly variable, depending on the community setting. If the emergency medical team that arrives is not able to provide emergency care, however, this time may be wasted time.

The Mobile Coronary Care Unit

There are no set answers to the problem of delivering the required emergency care to the victim of a heart attack. It seems apparent that the solutions found in one community may be totally impractical in others. The initial work of Pantridge and co-workers in Belfast, Ireland, where a mobile coronary care unit was designed and staffed, has aroused great interest in this technique as a possible solution.[5,6]

Pantridge and co-workers equipped an ambulance, which is sufficiently large to allow at least limited movement of personnel about the patient, with all the routinely available monitoring and resuscitation equipment that one would find in a hospital coronary care unit. The ambulance is staffed by a physician and nurse who are experienced in all phases of in-patient coronary care. This unit is dispatched through the use of a special telephone number that can be called by any local physician or by a patient. These calls are screened by the cardiac care staff who then dispatch the ambulance. In the first six months of this service, 20% of patients were reached within 15 minutes of the call for help; with additional experience, 78% of patients were reached in 15 minutes and 50% within 10 minutes. When the ambulance arrives, the patient is immediately under intensive care. He is monitored, and any evident disturbance of cardiac rhythm is dealt with and stabilized before the patient is transported to the hospital. The trip to the hospital is carried out with no unusual haste. Upon arrival at the hospital, the patient is transferred directly from the ambulance to the coronary care unit under constant surveillance, with no time spent in the emergency room.

In this study, 48% of patients came under intensive care within two hours and 73% within four hours. As the study has progressed and community education improved, there has been a progressive increase in the number of patients placed under intensive care early. The major goal of the unit is to prevent cardiac arrest by treating cardiac arrhythmias that often precede ventricular fibrillation. There is, of course, no way to know how many cardiac arrests have been prevented. During the three years of the study, 126 patients with cardiac arrest outside the hospital were encountered. In 71 patients, no resuscitation had been attempted within four minutes of the arrest and none survived. In 55 patients, resuscitation was attempted within four minutes but was inadequate in 22. Of 33 patients in whom adequate resuscitation procedures were instituted within four minutes, 28 survived. This clearly demonstrates the effectiveness of adequate resuscitation procedures in patients with cardiac arrest if instituted early.

Limitations. The excellent results obtained by Pantridge and co-workers have presented a challenge to others to do as well. Grace and co-workers at St. Vincent's Hospital in New York City have been successful with a mobile coronary care unit patterned after the Pantridge experience.[7] There are, however, significant limitations to mobile coronary care units of this design. First, use of a trained physician and nurse to staff these vehicles in a country already short of medical personnel seems to be an inefficient use of this talent in our overall distribution of medical care. Second, use of a special emergency vehicle to pick up patients with a specific disease creates major problems in screening calls for assistance, and the number of emergency runs is necessarily limited. The third problem is one of evaluating cost-effectiveness. It has been estimated that in a community of 100,000 people, the cost of saving one life via the mobile coronary care unit is $4,600.[8] Additional problems are encountered if one attempts to estimate the value to the community of the lives saved. It may be that the large sums of money required would be more appropriately spent in other types of medical care programs.

A Training Program for Emergency Medical Technicians

Several solutions to the problems of emergency care for victims of acute myocardial infarction have been instituted. Several communities have developed special training programs for emergency medical technicians as a paramedical group. These groups then staff emergency vehicles that are equipped to deal with cardiac arrhythmias. The patient's electrocardiogram can be monitored both in the vehicle and by telemetry in a local hospital's coronary care unit. A two-way radio allows physicians to advise the emergency technicians on diagnosis and appropriate treatment. These units are effective in saving lives that would otherwise be lost and at less cost than the full mobile coronary care unit as described earlier.[9,10]

Perhaps the most effective approach to this problem is to assemble a professional paramedical group of emergency medical technicians and train them in all aspects of emergency care of patients. The importance of such professionals to the health care of a community can hardly be overestimated and should therefore be of broad community concern. This approach eliminates the need for separate teams and vehicles for special emergency situations and the need for telephone screening and triage of emergency calls. This group would be prepared to answer all calls for help and to deal effectively with whatever emergency situation was presented to them based on their own firsthand evaluation of the patient.

Some idea of the type of coronary care training required of these individuals may be gained by briefly considering what would be expected of them in the care of a patient with an acute myocardial infarction.

First, they would be expected to be able to recognize the signs and symptoms of acute myocardial infarction and be aware of the possible complications. Patients with acute myocardial infarction usually note the abrupt onset of a crushing precordial chest pain, which may radiate to the neck, shoulders, and arms. This is a catastrophic event that is usually associated with marked anxiety, fear, and a peculiar sense of impending doom. Other symptoms that may suggest complications include anorexia, nausea, vomiting, extreme weakness, dyspnea, and signs of impaired cerebral blood flow, such as mental confusion, agitation, convulsive seizures, and syncope. Cardiac arrhythmia may be associated with or be the cause of any of these findings.

The initial responsibility to the patient is to reassure him that effective help is available by explaining what is to be done and doing it efficiently. The patient should be promptly placed on an appropriate stretcher with his head and shoulders elevated 30 to 45 degrees. He should be secured so that in the event of cardiac arrest or syncope he cannot fall. All previously prescribed medication should be kept with the patient. Oxygen should be administered to all patients, and they should never be left unattended.

The patient should be attached as soon as possible to an oscilloscope for monitoring the electrocardiogram. The patient's blood pressure should be recorded, and a slow intravenous infusion of 5% glucose in water should be started. Any cardiac arrhythmia should be accurately diagnosed, and atropine should be administered for bradyarrhythmias. In the event of nodal or ventricular tachycardia, or frequent ventricular premature beats, the intravenous administration of lidocaine is indicated. In the event of cardiac arrest with asystole or ventricular fibrillation, cardiopulmonary resuscitation techniques, incuding defibrillation of the heart, should be immediately applied.

Acute pulmonary edema may develop in some patients and is manifested by severe dyspnea with noisy respirations, cyanosis, and agitation. This should be promptly treated with positive pressure oxygen administration and proper application of rotating tourniquets to pool blood in the extremities.

To develop competence in the application of the diagnostic and therapeutic procedures that have been outlined requires a major educational effort by the medical community. This cannot be accomplished with lectures and demonstrations alone but must be accompanied by the practical experience of working in emergency departments and coronary care units. It is also necessary in many instances to change laws so that paramedical personnel are permitted to give medication and carry out these procedures.

A Stratified System of Coronary Care

The fact that emergency coronary care is a community problem has been stressed recently by the American Heart Association's Inter-Society Commission report.[11] This commission recommends a stratified system of coronary care that must be based on community-wide planning. Stratified coronary care involves the organization of medical facilities within a community on three levels of capability.

The first level would be life support units consisting of emergency transportation in the form of mobile coronary care units or, perhaps, all-purpose emergency vehicles staffed and equipped as previously discussed. Also included at this level of care would be stationary life support units set up in all hospital emergency rooms and in areas of large concentrations of people, such as major sports stadiums and first-aid rooms of large companies. These units would triage patients with chest pain, institute immediate monitoring, and stabilize the patient who is being kept under continuous surveillance until a professional decision is made regarding further care or transfer to a hospital coronary care unit. Transfers should be carried out utilizing mobile life support units.

The second level of coronary care would be the fully equipped and properly staffed coronary care unit in the hospital, which would have the expertise to handle most victims of acute myocardial infarction. These units would have available to them the full range of services of a large community hospital with radiology, anesthesiology, laboratory, and social services. They should have the capability of installing cardiac pacemakers at least on a temporary basis.

The third level of coronary care would be regional reference centers. These centers, in addition to the capacity for life support and full coronary care, would also have a full-time staff of cardiologists, cardiac surgeons, and training programs in coronary care for physicians, nurses, and allied paramedical personnel. They should be able to offer the full range of specialized diagnostic studies and therapeutic procedures.

Individual communities must assess their available coronary care resources and determine the levels of coronary care they can effectively support. This must then be integrated into the larger community with higher levels of capability. Central to all of this planning is the development of a public and professional educational program to decrease the time between the onset of symptoms and the decision to seek medical help and the development of effective methods to facilitate prompt entry into the coronary care system. It cannot be overemphasized that coronary care is a community as well as a medical problem.

References

1. U.S. Department of Health, Education and Welfare. 1970. *Provisional Statistics, Annual Summary for the United States, 1969*. Washington, D.C., National Center for Health Statistics, Public Health Service.
2. McNeilly, R. H., and Pemberton, J. 1968. Duration of last attack in 998 fatal cases of coronary artery disease and its relation to possible cardiac resuscitation. *Brit. Med. J.,* 3:139.
3. Hackett, T. P., and Cassem, N. H. 1969. Factors contributing to delay in responding to the signs and symptoms of acute myocardial infarction. *Amer. J. Cardiol.,* 24:651.
4. Moss, A. J., Wynar, B., and Goldstein, S. 1969. Delay in hospitalization during the acute coronary period. *Amer. J. Cardiol.,* 24:659.
5. Pantridge, J. F., and Geddes, J. S. 1967. A mobile intensive care unit in the management of myocardial infarction. *Lancet,* 2:271.
6. Pantridge, J. F., and Adgey, A. A. J. 1969. Pre-hospital coronary care: the mobile coronary care unit. *Amer. J. Cardiol.,* 24:666.
7. Grace, W. J., and Chadbourn, J. A. 1969. The mobile coronary care unit. *Dis. Chest.,* 55:452.
8. Sidel, V. W., Acton, J., and Lown, B. 1969. Models for the evaluation of pre-hospital coronary care. *Amer. J. Cardiol.,* 24:674.
9. Rose, L. B., and Press, E. 1972. Cardiac defibrillation by ambulance attendants. *JAMA,* 219:63.
10. Yu, P. N. 1972. Prehospital care of acute myocardial infarction. *Circulation,* 45:189.
11. Study Group on Coronary Heart Disease, P. N. Yu, Chairman. Resources for the optimal care of patients with acute myocardial infarction. *Circulation,* 43:A–171.

7

Cardiopulmonary Resuscitation

Marvin M. Kirsh and Herbert Sloan

Because violence on our highways and in our cities is escalating, increasing numbers of patients are sustaining serious and potentially lethal visceral injuries. As a result of improved on-site resuscitation techniques and swifter transport to the hospital, a larger number of severely injured patients reach the emergency department alive. Cardiac arrest, however, may occur en route to the hospital or any time after arrival. The condition is most likely to develop in patients with penetrating and blunt intrathoracic injuries, massive bleeding, or severe tissue damage complicated by generalized tissue hypoxia. Cardiac arrest may result from respiratory or circulatory abnormalities. If it is the result of a respiratory complication, hypoxia is the principal cause. It may result from upper airway obstruction, tension pneumothorax, flail chest, pulmonary aspiration, massive intrapulmonary hemorrhage, rupture of the tracheobronchial tree, and central nervous system depression caused by a closed head injury or overzealous administration of sedatives.

Cardiac causes of circulatory arrest include ventricular fibrillation, ventricular asystole, pericardial tamponade, myocardial contusion, heart block, cardiac rupture, and hypovolemia. Cardiopulmonary resuscitation should be attempted on the victim who sustains a cardiac arrest at the scene of injury or during transport *but who is warm* on arrival in the emergency department.[5]

Diagnosis

Cardiac arrest may be defined as the clinical picture of cessation of circulation (unconsciousness; no pulse in large arteries; apnea) in a person who is not expected to die at the time. The diagnosis of cardiac arrest is made on clinical grounds. The cardinal sign is absence of palpable peripheral pulses in major arteries. This is the simplest and the most accurate, reliable, and universally applicable diagnostic feature of this catastrophe. The carotid, femoral, and brachial arteries are usually inaccessible in any patient. (The carotid is the easiest of these vessels to palpate under normal circumstances.)

The diagnosis of cardiac arrest can be made with a reasonable degree of assurance if, in addition to the absence of peripheral pulses, there is no blood pressure. The pupils begin to dilate within 45 seconds after cardiac arrest, although they may fail to do so if large doses of morphine have been administered. Absence of heart sounds in a quiet room is a useful sign of cardiac arrest, although not necessarily cardiac standstill. If the patient is obese, has a barrel chest, or the emergency department is a bedlam of noise, however, auscultation is unreliable. Prolonged auscultation with a stethoscope should not be carried out. Not only is it time-consuming, but it also seldom provides additional evidence of heart action in the absence of peripheral pulse or blood pressure.

Loss of consciousness usually occurs within one minute of arrest. Soon after the cardiac arrest has taken place, respirations cease or gasping respiratory efforts may occur for a short period of time. Although the skin has a grayish white appearance because of cessation of peripheral circulation, it is not necessarily a dependable diagnostic sign of cardiac arrest. Within a minute or two of cardiac arrest segmentation of retinal venous columns occurs and the retinal arterial patterns disappear. Since other physical findings are more easily available, the value of funduscopic examination as a diagnostic tool is limited. These signs are summarized in Table 7-1.

Electrocardiographic evaluation should be undertaken as early as possible, but cardiopulmonary resuscitation *should not be delayed* for the electrocardiographic studies to be conducted. The electrocardiogram can be used to distinguish among asystole, ventricular fibrillation, and electrical-mechanical dissociation after resuscitation has been started.

Table 7-1. Clinical Signs of Cardiac Arrest

1. ABSENCE OF PERIPHERAL PULSES
2. NO BLOOD PRESSURE
3. Absence of heart tones
4. Dilatation of pupils
5. No respiration or gasping respiration
6. Loss of consciousness in a previously conscious patient
7. Segmentation of retinal venous columns and absence of retinal arterial pattern on ophthalmologic examination

Treatment in the Hospital

There should be no delay in treatment of cardiac arrest because cerebral function is affected after three or four minutes. The immediate objective in cardiac resuscitation is to establish as quickly as possible a flow of oxygenated blood to the central nervous system and maintain its viability, and to reestablish functional circulation so that the patient can sustain his own circulation and respiration.[1,2,8]

These objectives are accomplished by initiating artificial ventilation and either open or closed chest massage. If possible, attention should be given to ventilation and circulation simultaneously. First priority, however, goes to ventilatory support. Restoration of blood flow to the vital organs (heart, brain, and kidneys) serves no purpose unless the blood circulated is well oxygenated. With the establishment of adequate ventilation and circulation, a large bore venous catheter should be inserted for the administration of intravenous fluids, blood, or medication, and the monitoring of central venous pressure. Percutaneous placement in the subclavian vein is the preferred method. Leads for the electrocardiogram should be placed on the patient but should not interfere with the resuscitative efforts.

Artificial Respiration. Before respiratory resuscitation is initiated, loose foreign bodies, mucus, blood, or vomitus should be removed from the patient's mouth and oropharynx with the fingers. Dentures should also be extracted. Insertion of a cuffed endotracheal tube is the most satisfactory and preferred method of controlling the patient's airway. Before this is done, however, the patient should be hyperventilated with 100% oxygen for 60 seconds by the bag and mask technique, which is described in detail later. To avoid additional hypoxia, intubation should be accomplished as quickly as possible with assisted ventilation interposed between attempts. Intubation is mandatory because it allows absolute control of ventilation, protects against the aspiration of gastric contents, and provides a means for easy removal of tracheobronchial secretions.

The patient should be ventilated at a rate of 10 to 15 times per minute. After the endotracheal tube is in place, both right and left sides of the chest should be auscultated to make sure that both lungs are equally ventilated. Uneven ventilation may indicate the presence of an associated hemothorax or pneumothorax, which should be treated by closed tube thoracostomy. It may also indicate that the endotracheal tube has been inserted into either of the mainstem bronchi and should be withdrawn into the trachea. A nasogastric tube should be inserted to avoid gastric distention. Initially the patient should always be ventilated manually and never placed on a respirator while undergoing external cardiac massage. Since these respirators are often cycled by the procedure of external cardiac massage, they cannot provide adequate oxygenation. If open cardiac massage is being carried out, these respirators may be used.

The endotracheal tube can usually be inserted with ease because the vocal cords will be relaxed. If difficulty is encountered during intubation, further attempts should be abandoned while trained personnel are being summoned. Cardiopulmonary resuscitation should *not* be delayed, however, while awaiting their arrival. An efficient and relatively simple way to accomplish artificial ventilation is by the Ambu bag and mask technique, in which a self-filling balloon is attached to an anesthetic face mask through a nonreturn valve. Before respiratory resuscitation with this technique is started, it is essential to insure an adequate airway by removing blood, mucus, and vomitus from the mouth and oropharynx. If an oropharyngeal airway is available, it may be inserted to assist in maintaining a clear airway. The patient's head should be fully extended, and the resuscitator should maintain an upward pull on the lower jaw with his fourth and fifth fingers. The mask is first applied at the bridge of the patient's nose and then over his mouth so that the edge of the mask rests on his chin. The mask should be held in place by firm downward pressure with the thumb and index finger. The opposite hand is used to compress the bag at a rate of 10 to 15 times per minute. A nasogastric tube should be inserted to decompress the stomach and prevent gastric dilatation.

If the equipment for this method of ventilation is not available, mouth-to-mouth resuscitation should be started immediately and continued until proper help or equipment arrives. In this technique, after a clear airway is obtained, the oropharynx is held open by hyperextension of the head and anterior displacement of the mandible. The resuscitator takes as large a breath as possible, covers the patient's open mouth, and exhales with sufficient force to expand the patient's chest noticeably. Leakage through the nose is prevented by occluding the patient's nostrils. Following each inflation, the resuscitator withdraws his mouth to allow for passive expiration by the patient. The initial inflations should be rapid. After the patient's lungs are reoxygenated, the rate should average 10 to 15 inflations per minute. This technique of resuscitation is more effective if the resuscitator hyperventilates between inflations. Gastric distention invariably occurs with this technique and a nasogastric tube should be inserted. Because this method is not as effective as either of the preceding ones, it should be utilized only if the others cannot be instituted. Tracheostomy is indicated when associated facial injuries are present and prevent the establishment of an adequate airway by the previously described measures.

Maintenance of Effective Circulation. In contradistinction to other conditions or situations in which cardiac arrest occurs, this catastrophic situation in association with trauma is best managed by open cardiac massage. There are several reasons for this. (1) Hypovolemia is frequently present in these patients, and open cardiac massage is more effective in maintaining circulation in an empty heart than is closed chest massage. (2) In a patient with pericardial tamponade or injury of the heart or great vessels secondary to blunt or penetrating trauma, closed chest massage is contraindicated because it may increase the bleeding or tamponade. Open cardiac massage enables one to control the cardiac or great vessel injury, relieve the tamponade, and, at the same time, provide an adequate cardiac output. (3) The condition of the patient whose cardiac arrest is due to a tension pneumothorax and subsequent hypoxia is worsened by closed chest massage. (4) Direct visualization of the heart provides for an accurate and repeated estimation of the heart's activity. Drugs may be injected under direct vision without lacerating coronary vessels or adjacent pulmonary parenchyma. (5) Coronary and cerebral circulation can be augmented by manual compression of the aorta. (6) Electrical defibrillation is more readily performed. (7) The procedure can be accomplished within a matter of seconds with minimal surgical skills. (8) Closed chest massage is contraindicated in the presence of a flail chest. Not only is it ineffective, but it may also produce a puncture injury of the lung or other vital intrathoracic structures.

In patients with the conditions just mentioned, or those who do not respond to closed cardiac massage within two minutes, open cardiac massage should be instituted. It should be attempted *only* in the emergency department where there are adequate facilities for mechanical ventilation and control of hemorrhage. Open chest massage should always be performed by a physician. Prior to the institution of open cardiac massage, adequate ventilation must be insured with either an endotracheal tube or the mask and bag technique. No time should be wasted in scrubbing the hands, preparing the patient's skin, or draping the area with towels. With the operator working from the patient's left side, an anterolateral incision is made as quickly as possible in the fourth or fifth intercostal space, extending from the lateral border of the sternum to the midaxillary line. Once the pleural cavity is entered, the rib spreader should be inserted. If additional exposure is needed, the incision can be extended across the midline by transection of the sternum.

The pericardium is opened widely in a vertical manner anterior to the phrenic nerve. In this way the physician can determine whether the heart is contracting weakly, in asystole, or in ventricular fibrillation. An asystolic heart appears motionless, soft, and bluish. A fibrillating heart shows fine or coarse twitching; upon palpation it feels like a bag of worms.[7]

First priority should be given to control of any obvious major cardiac or great vessel bleeding. Arterial blood indicates that attention must be directed to the left side of the heart, the coronary arteries, or the pulmonary veins, whereas venous blood should direct attention to the right side of the heart, the venae cavae, or the pulmonary arteries. Wounds of the heart and great vessels can be temporarily controlled by digital pressure or tamponade. As soon as bleeding is under control, cardiac massage must be started. Simultaneously, the blood volume should be restored. If circulation is reestablished, the patient can be transported to the operating room for definitive treatment of these wounds.[7]

Regardless of whether or not the heart is in asystole or in ventricular fibrillation, cardiac massage should be instituted first. If electrical defibrillation is to be successful, the myocardium must be well oxygenated and have good tone.

To perform internal cardiac massage, as much of the hand as possible is placed around the heart; fingertip pressure must be avoided because it may bruise or even rupture the heart. The left hand is placed over the heart so that the index, middle, and ring fingers are over the right atrium and posterior wall of the heart. The palm should be over the right and left ventricles and the thumb over the left ventricle. Compression begins in the palm and, with contraction of the little finger, moves toward the index finger. This compression lasts one-third to one-half second and is followed by abrupt relaxation. Rhythmic compression of the heart is maintained at a rate of 60 to 70 times per minute. If the heart is unusually large, two hands may be used for resuscitation. The right hand is placed behind the heart and the left hand anteriorly, and the heart is squeezed. The pressure is applied first over the apex and then rolled toward the base of the heart.

Intermittent occlusion of the descending aorta increases coronary perfusion and is of value in cardiopulmonary resuscitation.[4] A new method employing alternate manual compression of the heart and ascending aorta increases coronary perfusion even more. The left hand is positioned as described in the preceding technique. The index and middle fingers of the right hand are placed transversely across the posterior wall of the ascending aorta, 7 cm. or more above the aortic valve. The right thumb is positioned across the anterior wall of the vessel. Sequential compression of the heart and aorta should be maintained at a rate of one per second. These techniques are appropriate when there is difficulty in obtaining adequate oxygenation of the myocardium.

External Cardiac Compression. In closed cardiac massage, the heart is compressed between the sternum and the vertebral column; lateral movement of the heart is restricted by the pericardium. In order for closed cardiac massage to be effective, the patient must be in a supine position on a hard surface. If possible, the legs should be elevated to increase the venous return to the heart. Only the lower one-third of the sternum should be compressed. The heel of one hand should be placed directly over the lower third of the sternum, parallel with the long axis of the body. The heel of the other hand is placed on the dorsum of the first. The resuscitator should position himself well above the patient so that he will be able to use the weight of his body to apply pressure. The downward thrust must be forceful enough to depress the sternum 1½ to 2 inches and be directed directly posterior against the patient's vertebral column. The thrust is rapid and is held for approximately 0.5 second; then it is released instantly so that the patient's chest wall can recoil, producing negative intrathoracic pressure, which aids in venous return to the heart. The sternal compression should be at a rate of 60 times per minute. More rapid rates may not allow enough time for ventricular filling.[3]

It is important to remember that patients undergoing closed cardiac massage cannot be ventilated with pressure cycled respirators during resuscitation. These respirators are often cycled by this procedure and, therefore, are incapable of providing adequate oxygenation. The patient with an endotracheal tube should be ventilated by hand with 100% oxygen during external cardiac massage. Regardless of the artificial ventilation technique, the patient should be ventilated at a rate of 12 times a minute, whereas external cardiac massage is carried out at a rate of 60 times per minute. In general, it is best to interpose the ventilations between every fifth or sixth external cardiac compression.

Cardiac massage can be judged to be effective enough to produce adequate circulation on the basis of the following criteria: (1) return of palpable peripheral pulses, (2) constriction of previously dilated pupils, (3) a systolic blood pressure exceeding 70 mm. Hg, and (4) improvement in the patient's color.

In children and infants, it is sufficient to carry out closed chest resuscitation by applying pressure over the lower one-third of the sternum with the index and middle finger of one hand, with the thumbs of both hands, or with the palm of one hand only. Because of the flexibility of their bony skeleton, much less pressure is required to depress the sternum. The sternal compression rate should be 100 per minute.

Metabolic Acidosis. This is an inevitable complication of cardiac arrest and must be treated promptly and adequately. It results from the absence of peripheral perfusion during the period of arrest as well as from the marginal perfusion status of the resuscitative efforts. Acidosis prevents effective resuscitation because it depresses myocardial contractility, decreases cardiac and peripheral vascular responses to both endogenous and exogenous catecholamines, and renders the fibrillating heart refractory to electrical defibrillation.

The most convenient and effective drug for the treatment of metabolic acidosis is sodium bicarbonate. Initially 2 ampules (89.2 mEq.) are given intravenously as a bolus and 1 ampule (44.6 mEq.) is given every 5 to 8 minutes during resuscitation. If desirable after the initial dose, the sodium bicarbonate can be given by continuous intravenous infusion (500 ml. of 5% sodium bicarbonate containing 60 mEq.). An average of 150 to 250 mEq. of sodium bicarbonate is usually needed to correct the acidosis. Frequent determinations of arterial or venous pH are desirable as a guide to effectiveness of treatment.

Conversion of Ventricular Fibrillation. Electrical countershock with either AC or DC current is the method of defibrillation. If electrical defibrillation is to be successful, the myocardium must be well oxygenated and in good tone (vigorous or coarse fibrillation). The depressed myocardium (weak or fine fibrillation) is usually refractory to electrical defibrillation. The fibrillatory status or tone of the myocardium may be enhanced by intracardiac administration of cardiogenic agents, such as epinephrine (2 to 3 ml. of 1:10,000 dilution) or calcium chloride (2 to 3 ml. of 10% solution) prior to electrical defibrillation.

In addition, acidosis should be corrected (arterial pH at least 7.30) with sodium bicarbonate. Open chest electrical defibrillation is accomplished by placing two large paddle electrodes firmly over the ventricles. Before being applied, the paddles should be covered with saline-soaked gauze to avoid burning the epicardium. One paddle is then placed at the base of the heart, overlying the right atrium, and the second paddle is placed on the apex of the heart. The electric shock should be administered only when no one is in contact with the patient or the bed. Alternating current requires a shock of 110 to 180 volts; direct current requires a shock of 20 to 60 watt-seconds for defibrillation. If a single shock is ineffective, a series of two or three shocks in rapid succession should be given.[6]

In closed chest resuscitation, two large, well insulated electrodes should be used. For optimal results, one electrode should be placed in the region of the first and second interspace parasternally while the other electrode is placed over the apex of the heart. Prior to their application, the electrodes should be coated with electrode paste to insure good contact with the skin. Either alternating or direct current may be used. The alternating current shock should be 440 to 880 volts delivered for 0.25 second. The dose of direct current shock is 200 to 400 watt-seconds delivered for 4 to 6 milliseconds. If a single shock is ineffective, a series of two or three shocks in rapid succession should be given.

If a state of refractory ventricular fibrillation exists, measures that should be tried besides repeat injections of epinephrine or calcium chloride or both include intracardiac administration of procainamide (100 to 200 mg.) or lidocaine (100 mg.), or intravenous administration of propranolol (3 to 5 mg.) and additional sodium bicarbonate.

Even if closed cardiac massage is used, these drugs can be injected directly into the heart. The needle can be inserted into an intracardiac chamber either from the subxiphoid approach or from the fourth or fifth intercostal space at the left midclavicular line. A long, thin-walled, 18-gauge needle should be used. Following an injection into the arrested heart, cardiac massage is necessary to achieve coronary circulation.

Not infrequently ventricular irritability in the form of ventricular tachycardia, multifocal ventricular premature beats, or recurrent ventricular fibrillation occurs after successful conversion. This is best treated with drugs that depress ventricular rhythmicity. Lidocaine (Xylocaine) is the drug of choice. After an intravenous bolus of 75 to 100 mg. is given, it should be administered as a continuous intravenous infusion of 1 to 4 mg. per minute. Other drugs of value under such circumstances are quinidine sulfate (100 mg.) and procainamide (200 mg.) intramuscularly every 4 to 6 hours.

Ventricular Asystole and Bradycardia. If the heart is in asystole, an intracardiac injection of epinephrine (0.5 to 1.0 ml. of a 1:10,000 solution) should be given, followed by cardiac massage. This may convert asystole to ventricular fibrillation, which then may be terminated with electrical defibrillation. If the heart remains in asystole in spite of one or more injections of epinephrine, other drugs should be used. Calcium chloride (5 to 10 ml. of a 10% solution) can initiate a heartbeat and improve myocardial contraction. If beneficial action occurs, this dose may be repeated every 8 to 10 minutes as long as it prompts a response.

Isoproterenol (0.02 to 0.04 mg. every 3 to 5 minutes) is another valuable drug for myocardial stimulation. It also may be given as a continuous intravenous infusion of 1 to 4 μg. per minute. As with ventricular fibrillation, sodium bicarbonate (44.6 mEq. every 5 to 8 minutes) should be given during the resuscitative efforts.

If marked bradycardia is present, and there has been no response from the previously mentioned drugs, atropine (0.4 to 0.6 mg.) may be of value. If the drug is beneficial, the dose can be repeated after 10 to 15 minutes.

If all these measures fail to produce an effective heart rate and beat, the physician should consider artificial pacing of the heart. With the chest open, an epicardial pacemaker wire can be sutured onto the surface of the right ventricle in an area free of coronary arteries. The pacemaker should be set for a rate of 70 to 80 beats per minute.

With closed chest massage, cardiac pacing may be accomplished transthoracically by passing a thin-walled, 18-gauge needle through the anterior chest wall into the cavity of the right or left ventricle. A unipolar pacing wire is inserted through the needle into the ventricular cavity. The needle is then withdrawn over the wire, allowing the wire to remain in the heart through the anterior chest wall. The wire electrode is then attached to a pacemaker, and endocardial pacing is established at a rate of 70 to 80 beats per minute.

If effective pacing of the heart is not obtained initially with either technique, the amplitude of the electrical energy level should be increased until effective pacing is obtained.

If these measures produce an adequate heart rate but the patient remains hypotensive in the absence of hypovolemia, additional inotropic support is needed. A continuous infusion of isoproterenol at a rate of 1 to 4 μg. per minute is of value in augmenting myocardial contractility and thereby increasing the cardiac output and arterial blood pressure. Other inotropic agents that may be of value are glucagon (4 mg. intravenously as a bolus or continuous infusion per hour) or levarterenol and phentolamine (2 ampules of levarterenol and 10 mg. of phentolamine added to a 250-ml. bottle of 5% dextrose and water). The drugs chosen should be infused at a rate adequate to maintain arterial blood pressure between 90 and 100 mm. Hg.

If these measures produce an adequate heart rate but cardiac output remains ineffective, even after full doses of inotropic agents and vasopressors, a state referred to as electrical-mechanical dissociation exists. The situation is almost always fatal; there is no effective treatment. Intraaortic balloon counterpulsation is of value in patients with otherwise hopeless cardiogenic shock. Prolonged circulatory assistance with these devices may be of value in patients who are dying of electrical-mechanical dissociation from trauma.

If open chest resuscitation restores circulation, careful hemostasis is established. The thoracic cavity is then irrigated with a copious amount of saline solution containing antibiotics. The pericardium is left open, and a drainage tube is placed in the posterolateral gutter of the chest and connected to a waterseal suction system. The thoracotomy wound is closed using catgut sutures for both pericostal approximation and soft tissue layer closure. Broad-spectrum antibiotics should be administered intravenously in large doses for seven to ten days. If the chest is closed carefully, infection rarely occurs even though the procedure was performed in an unsterile manner.

Other Therapeutic Measures. Hyperkalemia is a frequent occurrence in cardiac arrest. Because it poses a significant threat to a successful outcome, it must be recognized promptly and treated aggressively. Hyperkalemia may result from rapid infusion of the cold bank blood that is usually necessary in these severely injured patients, in whom the level of circulating epinephrine is increased. This results in glycogenolysis by the liver with release of the potassium stored there. Acidosis, which invariably accompanies cardiac arrest, causes the release of potassium into the extracellular fluid from its intracellular site.

As soon as possible, a blood specimen should be obtained for analysis of arterial blood gases and serum potassium. Hyperkalemia can often be detected from the electrocardiogram. When the potassium level exceeds 6.4 mEq. per liter, there are tall, steep, and symmetrical T waves with a narrow base. In addition, the QRS complex is prolonged, the S–T segments are depressed, and the P–R interval is prolonged.

When the serum potassium exceeds 6.5 mEq. per liter or the previously described electrocardiographic findings are present (especially a widened QRS complex), immediate therapeutic measures are required. Rapid-acting agents that can be used to counteract the hyperkalemia are sodium bicarbonate (2 ampules of a 7.5% hypertonic solution), calcium chloride (10 to 20 ml. of a 10% solution), and hypertonic glucose and insulin (50 ml. of 50% glucose with 10 units of regular insulin). These agents may be used individually or, preferably, in combination.

After these agents have been given intravenously as a bolus, a mixture of 1 liter of 10% glucose, 2 ampules of 7.5% sodium bicarbonate, and 10 to 20 units of insulin should be infused continuously. Frequent monitoring of the serum potassium and electrocardiogram for evidence of recurrent hyperkalemia is mandatory.

Renal Function. Regional blood flows are approximately 50% of normal during external or internal cardiac massage. In an attempt to increase renal blood flow during the resuscitative period, mannitol (25 gm.) or furosemide (50 to 100 mg.) should be given as an intravenous bolus. It is uncertain whether these agents help to prevent renal failure.

Indications for Discontinuing Cardiopulmonary Resuscitation. It is difficult to state categorically when to abandon resuscitative efforts. As long as massage appears to be adequate, a good peripheral pulse is maintained, and the pupils remain constricted, resuscitation should continue. If effective heart action cannot be restored after 60 minutes of intensive and adequate resuscitative efforts, cardiopulmonary resuscitation should be discontinued. Definitive signs of central nervous system death are difficult to determine without an electroencephalogram. Dilated pupils that remain fixed for 15 to 30 minutes despite adequate resuscitation are indicative of brain death. Funduscopic evidence of brain death is fragmentation and random movement of blood within the retinal vessels. Unconsciousness, absence of reflexes, and lack of spontaneous respirations also reflect central nervous system death. When these signs are observed, resuscitative efforts should be discontinued.

Postresuscitative Care. Patients who have been successfully resuscitated require specialized observation in an intensive or coronary care unit for at least 72 hours. The endotracheal tube should be left in place and respiratory support provided until the patient is able to breathe spontaneously. To avoid the potential danger of high partial pressure of oxygen in the inspired gas, the lowest possible inspired oxygen concentration that will achieve approximately 90% oxygen saturation of the arterial hemoglobin should be used. Blood gas studies should be performed frequently to evaluate the effectiveness of therapy and to avoid the undesirable sequela of hypoxia or alkalosis or both. This phase of therapy is extremely important because recurrence of hypoxia, no matter how slight, may prove fatal.

The blood pressure must be monitored closely because persistent hypotension is a common occurrence following resuscitation, especially if the resuscitative effort was prolonged. Circulatory support with the inotropic agents previously discussed may have to be continued in the postresuscitative period. Continuous electrocardiographic monitoring with rapid correction of arrhythmias is mandatory. Ventricular arrhythmias, such as ventricular tachycardia or frequent premature ventricular contractions, are best treated with a continuous infusion of lidocaine at a rate of 1 to 4 mg. per minute. Marked bradycardias are usually best treated by electronic pacing. Supraventricular tachycardias are usually best treated with digitalis and quinidine. The central venous pressure should be monitored constantly and hypovolemia or hypervolemia treated accordingly. Serum electrolytes, especially potassium, blood urea nitrogen, and serum creatinine should be followed closely. If hyperkalemia and renal failure develop, they should be treated promptly and aggressively.

If neurologic changes are present, measures to prevent or decrease cerebral edema must be instituted. These include limitation of fluid intake to 600 ml. per square meter of body surface per day, generalized hypothermia to 32° C, osmotic diuresis with urea (1 gm. of 20% urea per kilogram of body weight every 8 hours), and glucosteroids (dexamethasone, 8 mg. intramuscularly initially followed by 4 mg. every 6 hours). The dosage of dexamethasone may be gradually decreased after three or four days. Ten percent low molecular weight dextran is of value for cerebral edema and should be used, if necessary, in the postresuscitative period.

Long-term studies of changes in physical ability and mental and occupational status have been made in a large number of patients who were successfully resuscitated and were well enough to leave the hospital. There were no significant changes in the mental status of any of the survivors. Persistence of any severe physical disability was uncommon.

Cardiopulmonary Resuscitation at the Scene of Injury

The diagnosis of cardiac arrest at the scene of the injury should be assumed in an unconscious patient when breathing is absent and a peripheral pulse cannot be felt. Resuscitative measures should be initiated immediately, even if the diagnosis is uncertain, because the chance for recovery is often lost during the critical period between diagnosis and institution of cardiopulmonary resuscitation.

Artificial ventilation is accomplished by mouth-to-mouth breathing or by the bag and mask technique if available. Circulation is maintained by closed chest cardiac massage. Open chest cardiac massage should *never* be used.

Prior to the institution of artificial ventilation, the resuscitator must insure that the airway is patent by removing mucus, blood, or vomitus from the patient's mouth and oropharynx with his finger. The patient should be placed flat on a firm surface. If only one person is available for the resuscitative efforts, he may employ a sequence of ventilating the lungs two or three times (mouth-to-mouth) followed by external cardiac massage at the rate of 60 times per minute. After each series of 10 to 15 compressions, the resuscitator reventilates the lungs rapidly two or three times, taking no more than 5 seconds to do so, following which he returns to external cardiac compression and repeats the cycle until spontaneous breathing is resumed and an effective heartbeat is present or until additional help arrives and other facilities for artificial ventilation become available. If two persons are available for resuscitation, one can continually compress the sternum at a rate of 60 times per minute while the other ventilates the lungs at the rate of 12 times per minute. The patient should be transported as quickly as possible to the nearest hospital. During transit, resuscitative efforts should continue.

Artificial ventilation by the bag and mask technique with 100% oxygen is the preferred method during transport. Intravenous or intracardiac injections of drugs should *not* be administered by anyone other than a physician.

References

1. Feldman, S., and Ellis, H. 1967. *Principles of Resuscitation.* New York, Oxford University Press.

2. Holmes, J. C. 1970. Cardiac resuscitation. *Mod. Treat.,* 7:209.
3. Jude, J. R., and Elam, J. O. 1965. *Fundamentals of Cardiopulmonary Resuscitation.* Philadelphia, F. A. Davis Co.
4. Molokhia, F. A., et al. 1972. A method of augmenting coronary perfusion during internal cardiac massage. *Chest,* 62:610–613.
5. Naclerio, E. A. 1971. *Emergency Treatment of Chest Trauma.* New York: Grune & Stratton.
6. Spitzer, S., and Oaks, W. W. 1971. *Emergency Medical Management; the Twenty-First Hahnemann Symposium.* New York, Grune & Stratton, pp. 206–233.
7. Steichen, F. M., et al. 1971. A graded approach to the management of penetrating wounds of the heart. *Arch. Surg.,* 103:574–580.
8. Stephenson, H. E., Jr. 1969. *Cardiac Arrest and Resuscitation, 3rd ed.* St. Louis, C. V. Mosby Co.

8

The Unconscious (Comatose) Patient

Roland G. Hiss and Earl R. Feringa

Unconsciousness is generally defined as unresponsiveness and loss of awareness of the environment. This includes nonresponsiveness to verbal and visual commands as well as lack of response to and perception of all stimuli except those causing deep pain. Consciousness is one of the higher functions of the brain; unconsciousness is therefore a lack of normal brain function. This may result from derangement of the brain itself or a problem in the general system supplying the brain with necessary nutrients.

Unconsciousness, or coma, is the end state of a sequence of deteriorations of higher mental functions. Less severe dysfunctions appear as acute confusional states, in which the conscious function is impaired but not absent. The causes, detection, and management of these states are the same as for fully manifest unconsciousness, and the discussion provided in this chapter is applicable to these conditions of partial consciousness. Patients' behavior during complete unconsciousness is uniform; manifest behavior during acute confusion may vary depending upon the endogenous characteristics of the patient. Some patients in acute confusion are somnolent and passive; others are agitated and combative. The degree of energy being expended in a confused state is not a function of the cause, nor is it related to severity. Behavioral differences from one patient to another are particularly noticeable in confusional states secondary to drugs. Suppressant drugs, such as the barbiturates, may induce passive sleep in some patients and agitation in others; similarly, a given dose of a phenothiazine may have little effect on an agitated alcoholic patient, but induce an anesthetic state in a patient with degenerative brain disease.

5

Although loss of consciousness is much more frequent in brainstem disease than in the more common lesions of the cerebral hemispheres, unconsciousness can occur after supratentorial or infratentorial disease. A general principle applies to lesions that cause loss of consciousness— loss of consciousness is the result of bilateral cerebral disease. Because the brainstem is compact and its blood supply comes from a single vessel, the basilar artery, bilateral disease is much more common in brainstem disease than in lesions elsewhere in the nervous system. Lesions above the tentorium, however, can also cause loss of consciousness. This is true particularly when the lesion causes bilateral disease because of its distribution, as in the case of meningitis, subarachnoid hemorrhage, or bilateral cerebral infarction, or when the lesion causes increased intracranial pressure, as in the case of a brain tumor or subdural or intracerebral hematoma.

Generally speaking, unilateral cerebral infarction is *not* followed by unconsciousness. In some cases, after a large cerebral infarction occurs, cerebral edema develops, causing increased pressure and loss of consciousness after several hours or days. Any noxious substance, poison, metabolic abnormality, endocrinopathy, or other process that involves both sides of the brain may be associated with loss of consciousness. Focal epileptic seizures frequently are not accompanied by loss of consciousness, but when seizure activity is bilateral, it is almost always accompanied or followed by at least brief loss of consciousness.

Causes for Unconsciousness

A classification of the causes of unconsciousness is provided in Table 8-1. Four of the seven headings are related to organ systems in which dysfunction can lead to unconsciousness. The other three headings are physiological or functional groups unrelated to anatomic structure. This lengthy categorization of the etiology of unconsciousness is provided as a review to the reader and is intended to organize the detection process into an orderly and systematic approach. The outline can form the basis of a flow sheet for the diagnosis of the cause of unconsciousness for a specific patient.

Assessment and Management of the Unconscious Patient in the Field

Unconsciousness of unknown cause is a serious medical problem and requires definitive medical attention. For this reason, the approach to an unconscious patient discovered in the field should be institution of life-saving measures (if needed) and transportation to a medical facility. Even the most highly trained physician is unable to conduct an appropriate investigation of unconsciousness without bringing the patient to an emergency department or similar facility. Time and effort spent trying to rouse the patient may be directly harmful when the cause is not known and waste valuable time.

The steps listed here are recommended for anyone called to assist an unconscious patient found in the field. They can be used by all rescue workers (ambulance attendants, policemen, firemen, and ski patrol) as well as by formally trained health professionals (nurses and physicians). The personal qualifications of the rescue worker are no reason for varying the procedure.

The steps to be followed in attending to a person found unconscious in the field are as follows:

1. An Eight-Second Appraisal. Upon arriving at the side of a patient unconscious for unknown causes, the would-be rescue worker has a vital need for certain critical pieces of information. The need for this information is greater than the need to *do something,* at least for a few seconds. During an eight-second interval, the rescuer can determine the approximate pulse rate, quality and rate of respiration, skin color, size and symmetry of pupils, and immediate danger if present, and gather several important clues as to possible cause. This information is worth an eight-second delay in institution of any supportive measures that might be started blindly without such information.

2. Removal From Immediate Danger, if Present. This step covers the obvious need to remove both patient and rescuer from serious immediate danger if present, such as fire, smoke, impending explosion, noxious fumes, or electrical wires.

3. Cardiopulmonary Resuscitation. If the eight-second appraisal has revealed that cardiac arrest, respiratory arrest, or both have occurred, there is an immediate need to institute cardiopulmonary resuscitation in accordance with the procedures listed in Chapter 7. If the patient has been removed from immediate environmental danger, this step holds a greater priority by many orders of magnitude than any other. Part of this step is determination of the adequacy of the airway. The patient's mouth should be searched for a bolus of food or other foreign body, and false teeth, if present, should be removed.

4. Standard Management of Serious Injuries. Arterial or other significant bleeding and obvious fractures need first aid attention as described elsewhere in this text. The cause for unconsciousness, if not cardiopulmonary arrest, does not obviate the need to attend to these other matters first. If the cause for unconsciousness is serious enough ultimately to cause death, the few minutes saved by immediate trans-

Table 8-1. Classification of the Causes of Unconsciousness

Exposure to foreign substances
  Inhalants, *e.g.,* carbon monoxide and other poisonous gases, and anesthetic
    agents
  Drowning
  Ingestion of poisons, *e.g.,* arsenic, methyl alcohol, lead, and mercury
  Drug ingestion, *e.g.,* barbiturates, tranquilizers, and opiates
  Alcoholic intoxication

Metabolic derangements
  Hypoglycemia
  Uremia
  Hepatic failure
  Diabetic ketoacidosis
  Electrolyte imbalance
  Hyperventilation
  Anemia (severe)

Cardiac malfunctions
  Arrest
  Arrhythmia other than arrest, *e.g.,* Stokes-Adams syndrome, ventricular fibril-
    lation, and occasionally severe bradycardia or other types of tachycardia
  Failure
  Trauma

Respiratory compromise
  Asphyxiation
  Acute respiratory disease
    Infection
    Obstruction by foreign body or secretions
    Bronchospasm
    Paralysis of respiratory muscles, *e.g.,* myasthenia gravis, Guillain-Barré
      syndrome, and tick paralysis
  Chronic respiratory disease
    Progressive disease
    Superimposed infection

Peripheral vascular abnormalities
  Trauma
  Vascular disease
  Hypotension (regardless of cause)
  Hypertensive encephalopathy

Disturbances of brain proper
  Trauma
    Closed head injury
    Concussion
    Epidural hematoma
    Acute or chronic subdural hematoma
    Cerebral contusion or laceration
  Infection
    Meningitis
    Encephalitis
  Cerebrovascular disease
    Ruptured aneurysm or arteriovenous malformation
    Intracerebral hematoma
    Bilateral cerebral infarction
    Brainstem infarction or hemorrhage

Table 8-1—cont.

Nutritional disorder, *i.e.,* Wernicke's encephalopathy
Functional disorder, *i.e.,* postictal state
New growths
   Primary glioma or meningioma
   Secondary growths—most commonly from lungs in males and from breast
     in females
Cerebral edema due to any of the foregoing causes
Psychogenic disturbances
  Hysteria
  Catatonic schizophrenia

portation to medical care will not prevent death, but transportation without appropriate first aid measures may threaten a patient in whom the cause for unconsciousness is reversible.

5. Management of Seizures. A seizure state, if present, should be managed in accordance with the steps recommended in Table 8-2. With very rare exception, a patient does not die in a seizure.

6. Collection of All Possible Information. An unconscious patient is unable to communicate, by definition. For this reason, the most important tool in the medical diagnostic process, the patient's history, is not available from the usual source, the patient. Any witnesses should be questioned concerning the circumstances leading to the unconsciousness, its duration, the identity of the patient, and medical information perti-

Table 8-2.   First Aid for Epileptic Convulsions*

Keep calm. You cannot stop a seizure once it has started. Do not try to revive the patient. Let the seizure run its course.

Try to prevent the patient from striking his head or body against any hard, sharp, or hot objects, but do not interfere with his movements.

Do not force anything between the patient's teeth.

Place something soft, such as a rolled-up coat, beneath the person's head.

Carefully observe the seizure for a later report to medical personnel.

When he stops jerking, turn the patient's face to the side and make sure his breathing is not obstructed. Loosen tight clothing.

On very rare occasions, when a patient seems to pass from one seizure to another without regaining consciousness, call the patient's doctor for instructions.

Do not be frightened if the person having a seizure stops breathing momentarily.

A seizure is not contagious. Ordinarily it is over in a few minutes.

When the patient regains consciousness, let him rest if he wishes.

* Reproduced through the courtesy of the Epilepsy Center of Michigan, 10 Peterboro Street, Detroit, Michigan 48201.

nent to the patient. If it is apparent that a witness has considerable information, bring him with the patient to the medical facility so that he can supply it directly to the attending physician. In this way, the time for field interview is avoided and more direct information is available to the physician. Related conditions, such as the setting in which the patient was found, the patient's position, apparent trauma, fumes, electric wires, drugs, and alcohol on the patient's breath may also provide clues.

7. Transportation to Definitive Medical Facility, Assuming Multiple Injuries. All unconscious patients should be transported directly and promptly to a definitive medical care facility. Unless it is clear that the patient has not sustained trauma, he should be transported with the assumption that injury to the neck or back may have occurred. This requires standard stretcher management or use of the full-length backboard, which prevents motion of the entire vertebral column (see chapter on trauma to the central nervous system).

8. Staying With the Patient. The rescue workers who discover and manage the emergency involving an unconscious patient should stay with him until he has been brought to definitive medical care. Their information is valuable to the attending physician who is at the same disadvantage they were concerning information about an unconscious patient. Changes in level of consciousness en route should be noted and reported.

Assessment in an Emergency Care Facility

The management of an unconscious patient who is brought to an emergency care facility can be divided into three phases: (1) appraisal of the cardiopulmonary status, detection of shock, major hemorrhage, or severe hypoglycemia, and immediate institution of appropriate corrective measures if necessary, (2) evaluation of the patient concerning the cause of his unconsciousness and other possible injuries or illnesses, and (3) treatment of the patient, which often involves hospital admission after obtaining baseline studies.

Phase I—Immediate Action. The emergency department physician should perform the eight-second appraisal advocated for the rescue worker in the field to determine the approximate heart rate, respiratory rate, quality of respiration, color of skin or mucous membrane (to assess arterial oxygenation), and size and asymmetry of pupils. If this immediate first-line appraisal indicates that cardiac arrest, respiratory arrest, or respiratory obstruction is present, immediate corrective steps are necessary as outlined in the appropriate chapters. Cardiac and pulmonary difficulties are not necessarily coincident. Cardiac status may be adequate with labored or obstructed breathing requiring an oral airway, suction, or endotracheal intubation.

If the cardiopulmonary status, as determined by pulse and respiration, is not immediately life-threatening, the situation should be more definitively determined by taking the blood pressure, making a more accurate assessment of cardiac rate and rhythm, and conducting a standard physical examination of the heart and lungs. If shock is present, measures directed toward its alleviation should be instituted (see Chapter 5). The control of significant hemorrhage should be included in this immediate action phase as well.

Hypoglycemia severe enough to produce unconsciousness is also an immediate action problem. The diagnosis of severe hypoglycemia and a caution about its treatment are discussed in Phase III. Asymmetry of pupillary size, particularly the presence of a dilating pupil, accompanied by a contralateral hemiparesis and a deepening level of coma requires prompt action. These signs indicate the presence of serious intracranial pathology, the management of which is discussed in Chapter 16.

An important part of this phase of assessment of the patient is the removal of all clothing for a quick evaluation of other possible injuries or other obvious medical problems. If trauma to the spinal column has not been excluded, the clothing should be cut away to avoid unnecessary movement of the patient until the nature of the problem is further defined.

Phase II—Definitive Assessment of the Patient's Condition. Following attention to first order problems (such as cardiac and respiratory function, control of bleeding, and correction of shock), an orderly evaluation of the patient's unconsciousness can begin. The first step in this process should be a comprehensive attempt to obtain all background medical information about the patient and the circumstances surrounding his discovery in the field. The persons who discovered the patient and brought him to medical attention should be questioned about the items discussed in the section on management of the unconscious patient in the field. Any witnesses, family members, or other companions should be included in this query, and if none is available, the patient's family should be contacted by phone to provide any information they can about previous medical conditions, recent circumstances, and medications being taken. The name of the patient's physician should be sought, and he should be contacted for any information he can provide.

The patient's wallet and other personal effects should be searched to determine his identity and to discover if there are any cards bearing medical information. Contact with the hospital record room may disclose previous admissions, in which case the medical records of treatment should be reviewed. Through this collective process, previous diagnosis of heart disease, neurologic disease, diabetes, drug information, and similar relevant matters can be obtained.

The next step is to draw blood for a panel of laboratory tests. The time required to draw the blood is brief and does not significantly delay institution of other measures. These studies can be sent to the laboratory for processing while the remaining phases of the evaluation are being carried out. If there is still no clue to the cause of the unconsciousness, a broad selection of studies is necessary to avoid missing a significant condition. The recommended studies, *assuming there is no available information about the patient,* are as follows:

1. Hematocrit, white cell count, and differential if the white cell count exceeds 10,000.
2. Typing and cross-matching of blood for transfusion if signs of significant hemorrhage are present.
3. Blood glucose. (If hypoglycemia severe enough to produce unconsciousness is suspected, *i.e.,* blood glucose levels of 30 mg.% or less, quick confirmation can be obtained using a Dextrostix applied to a drop of blood obtained by finger puncture.)
4. Serum electrolytes.
5. Creatinine or blood urea nitrogen.
6. Serum drug and toxicology studies available on an emergency basis in the hospital. (This varies with the hospital laboratory but usually includes barbiturate, alcohol, bromide, and gluteth-amide levels.)
7. Coma screen. Some regional reference laboratories provide analysis of serum that includes a broad range of pharmacologic and toxicologic substances known to produce coma. One such laboratory is the Poisonlab in Denver, Colorado. Others may be available locally or regionally.
8. Two tubes of serum frozen and stored for potential future use. These may be invaluable for toxicologic study or acute phase viral antibody titer as the patient's story unfolds. A sample of blood drawn during the emergency situation prior to the institution of therapy may be more definitive than subsequent samples.
9. Complete urinalysis with particular attention to sugar and acetone.* A ferric chloride test for phenothiazines is also useful.
10. Blood gases (pO_2, pCO_2, and arterial pH) if the patient is cyanotic, if there is any question about the adequacy of respiratory function, or if fat embolism is a possibility even though respiration appears to be adequate.
11. Other tests as indicated by the information to this point. This may include liver function studies (including serum ammonia

---

* The acetone test may be positive in aspirin intoxication. In this case the test with boiled urine will also be positive, whereas true acetone boils away.

levels) if the patient is jaundiced or has a large liver, or serum calcium studies if information suggests a history of bony disease or parathyroid disease.

12. Skull films are needed if either increased intracranial pressure or head trauma is a possibility.

Following initiation of laboratory studies, the remainder of the physical examination should be performed. The temperature must be obtained rectally. The general physical examination should include an evaluation of the abdomen for masses, guarding, or changes in bowel sounds. There should be special observation of the extremities, particularly for cyanosis, signs of petechia, which might indicate fat embolism, or evidence of broken bones. Especially in cases of traumatic injury it is very important not to focus all one's attention on the brain to the exclusion of serious injury to bones or soft tissues.

The neurologic examination involves an evaluation of the patient's mental status, cranial nerves, motor function, sensory apparatus, and reflexes. Examination of the mental status of the unconscious patient can be very brief if there is no response, but if the patient makes any response to any stimulus, it is important that it be noted. It may be necessary to use painful stimuli to detect residual awareness. Moderate sternal pressure or supraorbital pressure may be sufficiently painful to awaken a patient who is excessively drowsy and not truly comatose. Evaluation of response to pain and to questions should be recorded objectively for future evaluation.

Examination of the cranial nerves in the unconscious patient is *not* impossible and, in fact, is very important. The first cranial nerve usually cannot be tested. Although visual acuity and visual fields cannot be tested, one should assess the response of the pupils to light and record their size. A funduscopic examination is necessary to detect papilledema, hemorrhages, or evidence of hypertension or diabetes. Extraocular movements can be tested in the unconscious patient. Doll's eye movements (rotation of the head rapidly from side to side while the eyes are held open) may demonstrate that the third and sixth cranial nerves, the interconnections between these two nerves, and the connections from these nerves to the vestibular apparatus are all operational. *If there is a question of a fractured cervical spine, this test should not be done.*

The fifth cranial nerve can usually be evaluated by testing the corneal reflex, by tickling the nose with a piece of cotton lightly twisted in the nares, or by applying a painful stimulus to the supraorbital ridge. As the fifth cranial nerve is tested, the response may demonstrate an intact seventh cranial nerve. If nasal tickling initiates a facial grimace, the seventh nerve is functional. Similarly, a blink response requires at least some seventh nerve function.

The eighth cranial nerve is difficult to test in comatose patients, but the response to cold caloric stimulation can be evaluated. Caution should be used in this test because it is uncomfortable to the patient and it can cause nausea and vomiting with the possibility of accompanying aspiration. When appropriate, this test probably should be done after the patient is admitted to the hospital and by someone competent to interpret its results.

The ninth and tenth cranial nerves are best evaluated by observing the way in which the patient handles secretions. If these nerves are paralyzed, either unilaterally or bilaterally, and particularly if paralysis is acute, the patient may have a tendency to choke on saliva. If the mouth can be opened without undue effort, one can test the gag response by placing a tongue blade against the lateral pharyngeal wall first on one side and then on the other. An intact gag response probably indicates that the ninth and perhaps the 10th cranial nerves are working appropriately. Neither the sternocleidomastoid strength nor any other reasonable measure of the eleventh cranial nerve can be evaluated. Similarly, in an unconscious patient, it is impossible to test the power of the twelfth cranial nerve, but the presence of tongue fasciculations in some patients might indicate lower motor neuron disease.

Throughout the examination the motor system should be observed for movements that are spontaneous or in response to stimulation. When they occur in response to stimulation (*e.g.,* pressing on the sternum) the presence or absence of ataxia in these movements and preferential use of one limb should be noted. Even when a patient makes no movements it is important to evaluate muscle tone and bulk. Tone can be evaluated in all patients as the limb is moved through a rapid passive range of motions. Observation for fasciculations may occasionally be helpful.

Sensory examination is usually not possible. Occasionally the unconscious patient responds to painful stimuli, but if he responds to other stimuli, he cannot be considered unconscious.

Reflex examination is possible in all patients. The presence of a jaw jerk, a suck response, a snout response, or a rooting response can be considered to be evidence of bilateral cerebral disease, at least in the cortical bulbar motor system. Deep tendon reflexes should be evaluated carefully and observed for symmetry and briskness of response. In every case one should attempt to elicit the Babinski sign, and occasionally information is obtained by attempting to elicit the Hoffmann or Trömner reflex.

The most important thing to do in the assessment of the central nervous system in the emergency department is to test the functions that can be evaluated. Changes in the neurologic examination in the ensuing

24 hours are extremely important in the evaluation of the patient. A good baseline examination in the emergency department is invaluable to the clinician responsible for subsequent care.

If the patient has a stiff neck (a sign of meningeal irritation), it is always necessary to differentiate infection of the meninges from inflammation of the meninges secondary to subarachnoid hemorrhage. In these cases a spinal tap should be done. This diagnostic test, however, should *never* be performed prior to careful examination of the optic fundi for evidence of increased intracranial pressure and a careful review of skull films to be sure there is no evidence of increased intracranial pressure, mass lesion, or skull fracture. If either fundi or skull films suggests the possibility of a mass lesion, emergent neurologic *consultation* should be sought before a lumbar puncture is performed.

Not every unconscious patient should undergo a spinal tap. This test has some danger and very little value except when subarachnoid bleeding or meningitis is suspected. Because the only sign of meningitis or subdural hematoma in the very young, the very old, or the very debilitated may be simply failure to thrive, after one has looked for evidence of increased intracranial pressure, lumbar puncture may be an important emergency diagnostic procedure in such patients.

If a spinal tap is done, the spinal fluid pressure should be determined. If the patient is not fully relaxed when the pressure is recorded, it should be noted on the chart. If the fluid obtained is bloody, a red cell count should be obtained in the first and fourth tubes of fluid removed. (When the fluid is very bloody, an hematocrit may be substituted for a red cell count.) A white cell count should always be done. In addition, a tube of fluid should be spun down in a centrifuge and the supernatant compared against a white background to a tube of clear water for evidence of yellow coloration (xanthochromia). All spinal fluid, even that which is bloody, should be sent to the laboratory for culture. Bloody fluid is sometimes seen in meningitis, particularly that caused by *Haemophilus influenzae*. Spinal fluid protein and sugar should always be determined and the concomitant blood sugar assessed.

If the spinal fluid is turbid, it is necessary to take only enough fluid for culture, a sugar analysis, a cell count, a gram stain of a smear, and a protein evaluation. In every case a gram stain of the spinal fluid should be done in an effort to identify the organisms, which might help direct initial therapy.

When a spinal tap is done because of signs of meningeal irritation and the fluid obtained is crystal clear with normal or mildly increased intracranial pressure, there is a particular need to obtain enough fluid for multiple evaluations. In such cases, the entire spectrum of chronic meningitis should be considered. Cell counts, protein and sugar analyses, cultures for tuberculosis and fungi (with at least 5 ml. of fluid), a colloidal gold curve, and a serologic test for syphilis on the spinal fluid are all needed. It is also often desirable to do a cell block to look for evidence of carcinomatous meningitis or other involvement of the meninges by tumor. The total amount of fluid required is nearly 35 ml. Marked increase in intracranial pressure may make it inadvisable to remove this much, but if such a contraindication does not exist, all studies should be done from the first spinal tap. Great care should be exercised to be sure that all these tests are accomplished and that the fluid is not lost in transport to the laboratory.

Additional studies in the emergency department may be appropriate. An electrocardiogram is necessary if the physical examination raises a question of significant cardiac arrhythmia. The patient should be taken to the x-ray department for skull films and views of the cervical spine unless the information obtained to this point has definitely excluded trauma to these areas. Other radiographic examinations might be indicated by the findings in the emergency department.

Phase III—Therapeutic Management of the Unconscious Patient in the Emergency Department. Definitive therapeutic steps depend entirely on individual findings for a given patient. No treatment scheme is applicable to all patients who are unconscious, although, as a general rule, in any patient who has been seriously injured, or who has any abnormality of the vital signs (pulse, blood pressure, respiratory rate, and temperature) a large caliber intravenous route should be established. Many physicians believe that a plastic intravenous cannula is appropriate in this circumstance to maintain the route while the patient is being examined, moved, and transferred from examining tables to stretchers.

Most patients brought unconscious to the emergency department have a condition that requires hospitalization for definitive treatment. For this reason, the extent of therapy attempted in the emergency department and that delegated to in-patient care is a matter of individual logistics, circumstance, and the physician's judgment as to what would be most practical and expeditious.

Only a few patients brought to the emergency department unconscious can be definitively treated there and released. These include the diabetic patient in insulin shock whose hypoglycemia (and unconsciousness) are corrected by intravenous glucose. (See discussion of this subject later in the chapter.) Another is the epileptic patient who is in a postictal state when he arrives at the emergency department and recovers there. If the cause of the convulsive episode was related to a lapse in medication, the patient can be released after the appropriate dosage schedule has been reviewed with him. A patient convulsing for the first time, however, should be admitted for evaluation and institution of an appropriate treatment program. A patient with status epilepticus should also be admitted.

The general rules applicable to admission of patients from the emergency department to the general hospital are also relevant to the unconscious patient. Before transport, however, his vital signs should be stabilized and necessary resuscitative procedures instituted. Baseline studies, including x-rays, which will be needed by the in-patient attending staff, should be obtained in the emergency department to facilitate and expedite the overall management of the patient.

In the following section, a series of specific conditions are noted and recommendations for appropriate emergency room treatment outlined. These should be instituted following the Phase II evaluation. Some are of sufficient urgency that they should be instituted as soon as their need is discovered, even if the orderly sequence of evaluation has to be interrupted. The decision to proceed with therapeutic steps before completion of the full diagnostic evaluation is a matter of clinical judgment and experience. Generally, however, urgency is defined in terms of threat to vital signs. In each case, the treatment program is recommended for a patient who is unconscious due to the condition listed; *i.e.,* the condition is *very* severe. Less severe forms of these same conditions might be managed differently.

If the patient is hypotensive, institute the measures outlined for the management of shock in Chapter 5.

If cardiac arrhythmia is present, electrocardiographic identification of the exact arrhythmia is the mandatory first step. (The timing for the performance of the electrocardiogram must fit other priorities, depending upon the situation.) The treatment is specific, and therapy for one patient might be contraindicated for another. There are only two cardiac arrhythmias with sufficient impact on cardiac output to produce unconsciousness from the arrhythmia only. The first of these is ventricular fibrillation. The second is a high degree of atrioventricular block with a slow idioventricular rhythm. Ventricular fibrillation is handled as a cardiac arrest and has already been discussed.

When severe atrioventricular block is present, bradycardia is so pronounced that cardiac output is below the level required to maintain full cerebral function. Whether there is a variable second degree or a third degree (complete) atrioventricular block is not as critical as the ventricular rate that results. A patient with bradycardia of less than 40 beats per minute, regardless of cause, runs the risk of insufficient blood flow to the brain to maintain consciousness. In addition to the slow pulse, there may be noticeable cannon waves in the neck.

The treatment for severe atrioventricular block with pronounced bradycardia is intravenous isoproterenol (Isuprel). A 5-ml. vial, which contains 1 mg. of the drug, should be diluted in 500 ml. of a 5% glucose solution and the resulting mixture given at a rate of 10 to 15 ml. per minute initially. After reasonable control of the ventricular rate is effected, the rate of administration should be slowed so that the patient does not receive more than 100 ml. of the solution during the initial phase of treatment. The intravenous apparatus should be left in place so that additional amounts can be given as needed in the next several hours.

Many episodes of severe atrioventricular block are precipitated by hyperkalemia; for this reason a molar sodium lactate solution should be given after blood has been drawn for serum electrolyte determinations. Similarly, diuretics that induce a potassium diuresis, such as the thiazides, should also be administered when the potassium level is known. All of these measures represent a means for *emergency* treatment of a life-threatening situation and should be employed to stabilize the patient while more permanent modalities of treatment are arranged.

For symptomatic atrioventricular block, the primary *definitive* treatment is the use of demand pacemakers. These are placed through the intravenous route during the emergency situation and implanted for long-term therapy. It may be appropriate to insert a transvenous pacemaker while the patient is in the emergency department, if hospital logistics are appropriate, but placement of a permanent pacemaker is not an emergency department procedure. When the cardiac rhythm is stabilized, the patient should be admitted to the hospital, preferably to a cardiac unit, for further observation, testing, and treatment.

There are other cardiac arrhythmias that affect cardiac output sufficiently to disturb mental function without creating complete unconsciousness. Patients may act confused and irrational, yet still not meet the strict criteria for unconsciousness. Arrhythmias in this category include ventricular tachycardia, atrial flutter or fibrillation with a fast ventricular response, and occasionally atrial tachycardia. Although these arrhythmias are not as threatening to life as are the two previously described, they are serious, deserve immediate attention, and in almost all instances warrant hospitalization of the patient.

If intracranial pressure is increased, causing unconsciousness, particularly when associated with trauma, it can frequently be improved with early steroid treatment. This is described elsewhere in this volume.

If meningitis is present, it is always necessary to begin therapy immediately after spinal tap and appropriate cultures of the spinal fluid and blood have been obtained. When the spinal fluid is turbid and shows a high white cell count, particularly polymorphonuclear leukocytes, the patient should be given ampicillin in doses up to 400 mg. per kilogram of body weight per day intravenously. This treatment is appropriate for all patients over 2 months of age. Very young children, the very elderly, and debilitated or immunosuppressed patients have gram-negative meningitis more frequently and therefore require coverage with antibiotics that have a more specific effect on these organisms. All patients with meningitis should be admitted to the hospital at once and receive careful and constant monitoring.

If the patient is apneic, hypoventilating, or cyanotic, he should receive immediate attention in the form of mouth-to-mouth resuscitation until a mask and breathing bag has been brought to the bedside. (Presumably this equipment is immediately available in the emergency department.) Adequate temporary respiratory support for the apneic patient can usually be provided with a bag and mask supplied with 100% oxygen. This should suffice during the time necessary for preliminary review of the patient's problem, at which time endotracheal intubation should be accomplished if impairment of natural respiration persists. The exact order of events is dictated by the circumstances, but the need for adequate oxygen flow to the lungs can never be ignored.

If bronchospasm is present, it should be handled in the same manner as described for apnea and hypoventilation. If the unconsciousness is attributable totally to the bronchospasm, the patient must be managed as if he were in respiratory arrest, because bronchospasm severe enough to produce unconsciousness is, functionally, a form of respiratory arrest. Endotracheal intubation and respiratory support with a bag and mask is mandatory. When this is accomplished, other measures directed to the cause of the bronchospasm should also be instituted promptly. These almost always include administration of epinephrine (0.3 ml. of a 1:1,000 solution) and institution of an intravenous drip with aminophylline. If assisted respiration with a mechanical device is needed, the apparatus should be of the volume type. Caution should be employed to avoid cycling the machine too rapidly for the obstructed lung to decompress between cycles. Rapid cycling can produce gross overinflation of the lung and life-threatening respiratory insufficiency.

When the patient has a severe respiratory problem, there is a temptation to request a chest x-ray as part of the admitting procedure. This study is undoubtedly useful in some cases, but the risk of respiratory compromise during the filming procedure in the x-ray unit must be kept in mind. A patient whose ventilation is being supported is probably not a candidate for a routine chest x-ray, and the status of his chest might be better evaluated by routine physical examination. A portable chest x-ray machine on the ward may contribute additional information and is an appropriate compromise in this situation.

If the patient is hypoglycemic, intravenous administration of 50 ml. of a 50% glucose solution given by syringe should promptly restore consciousness. It is mandatory to confirm the diagnosis of hypoglycemia before administering hypertonic glucose. This can be done by using Dextrostix to approximate the blood glucose level of fingertip blood or by obtaining a reliable description of the conditions of hyperinsulinism from the patient's companions.

When the patient is responsive, a full history of the circumstances surrounding the episode can be obtained and an appropriate decision made for disposition. An occasional patient does not respond immediately to rapid intravenous administration of glucose. This is apparently related to cerebral changes during hypoglycemia that are slow to correct. These patients deserve hospitalization for further observation.

Some patients with unconsciousness due to increased intracranial pressure awaken upon administration of concentrated sugar solutions. This is due to temporary reduction in cerebral edema because of the osmotic effect of the hypertonic solution. The physician should not misinterpret these events by hastily concluding that hypoglycemia was the cause of the unconsciousness. When glucose restores awareness in a patient with increased intracranial pressure, a serious emergency is present. There is always a rebound *increase* in intracranial pressure following glucose decompression and it requires very prompt neurosurgical or neurologic assistance. Awareness of the possibility of there being two causes for unconsciousness that *both* respond, at least temporarily, to hypertonic glucose is helpful in avoiding a serious diagnostic error. The problem can be *avoided* by pretreatment estimation of the blood glucose level.

If heavy alcoholic intake or chronic alcoholism is evident, it is important that the physician be reluctant to consider this to be the patient's total disability. The incidence of subdural hematoma, head trauma, Wernicke's encephalopathy, bleeding disorders, and other acute complications of alcohol abuse is much too high to risk blaming unconsciousness on alcohol *per se.* It is essential that all such patients be admitted to the hospital for at least 24 hours of observation. Each patient should be covered with adequate doses of thiamine to prevent (or arrest) Wernicke's hemorrhagic encephalopathy. This diagnosis can sometimes be made in the emergency department based on the presence of ophthalmoplegia, ataxia, and confusion. When the confusion is so severe that the patient is rendered unconscious, the other signs may not be readily observable. Under such conditions, the administration of thiamine to a known alcoholic may be life-saving and should be considered emergent. Skull films should be taken of all alcoholics who are unconscious to consider the possibility of subdural hematoma, skull fracture, or other serious intracranial disease.

Alcoholism is a very common entity, and it may be a mere coincidence in a patient unconscious from an *unrelated* cause. This is reason for further caution in not ascribing unconsciousness automatically to alcohol intake and being aware of alcohol-related diseases or injuries.

If unconsciousness is secondary to drug ingestion, admission to the hospital is necessary for supportive care and consideration of dialysis if the drug involved is dialyzable. Drugs inducing unconsciousness are by nature sedatives, unless the unconsciousness is caused by drug-induced cardiovascular or metabolic derangements. Sedative overdose often leads to respiratory suppression and to the need for immediate institution of respiratory support measures (assisted respiration with a bag and mask and then endotracheal intubation and use of a mechanical respirator.)

A major effort that can be made in the emergency department for a patient with a drug overdose (or accidental poisoning) is an attempt to identify the responsible substance. The patient's family or living companions as well as any physician the patient has seen in recent months should be telephoned. Available medical records should be searched for information concerning medications prescribed for the patient. If a prescription bottle is brought with the patient and identifies him and the pharmacy, but not the drug, the police can be asked to contact the pharmacist and request that he review his records to identify the prescription. Most pharmacists are willing to provide this service regardless of the hour of day or night, and they usually can do so faster than the physician who prescribed the drug.

A note of caution deserves repetition. Gastric intubation for any purpose should not be undertaken in an unconscious patient without first protecting the airway with an endotracheal tube. Vomiting induced by the intubation procedure carries the high risk of aspiration in an unconscious patient. The results are disastrous.

If the patient is delirious, one should look for the metabolic or toxic cause. Delirium is a state characterized by hyperactivity, increased heart rate, increased respiratory rate, and, frequently, severe anxiety. The most common cause is delirium tremens associated with alcoholic withdrawal, but similar pictures can be seen in many metabolic states, such as uremia and drug intoxication, and as a result of simple causes, such as absorption of atropine used in an ophthalmologic examination.

The hyperactive, anxious patient responds most readily to administration of chlordiazepoxide (Librium). Because there is a cross-tolerance between alcohol and chlordiazepoxide, large doses may be required to induce a calming effect. The initial dose for the alcoholic may be as large as 50 mg. intramuscularly, and if a response is not obtained, 100 mg. can be administered hourly intramuscularly until the patient responds. The dose of the drug should be sufficient to make the patient drowsy, but not unconscious, and render him arousable for meals, but somnolent if undisturbed. This may occasionally require doses as large as 2,400 mg. in the first 24 hours. Once the desired level of sedation is attained, the physician must carefully decrease the dose, giving only enough to keep the patient in the desired somnolent, nonhyperactive state. Usually this requires approximately 50 to 100 mg. every 6 to 8 hours. The patient should be kept in a somnolent state for approximately 72 hours and then allowed to emerge slowly from the sedative program. Chlordiazepoxide is far preferable to paraldehyde or diazepam (Valium) for delirium tremens because its prolonged effect and slow excretion prevent the withdrawal problems associated with the other two drugs.

Before therapy is begun, it is extremely important that a correct diagnosis be firmly established. Delirium tremens is a state of acute anxiety with multiple sympathetic effects, including changes in blood pressure, heart rate, and breathing. It should not be confused with alcoholic "shakes," or with alcoholic hallucinosis in which the patient has visions and hears voices but is not truly in an acute anxiety state. These other conditions associated with alcoholic withdrawal are best treated with good food, sufficient hydration, and good nursing care; a sedative program is not needed. Deliria due to other metabolic disturbances also respond to chlordiazepoxide, but smaller than average doses rather than large doses are required. Uremic delirium, for instance, should be treated with chlordiazepoxide in the dosage range of 10 to 25 mg. three or four times a day.

If the patient is convulsing, it is not essential that the seizure be stopped promptly. First aid for convulsive disorders has been previously discussed and is as appropriate in the emergency department as it is in the field. Status epilepticus is present *only* when the patient has repeated seizures and does not regain consciousness between seizures. This is a medical emergency and should be treated promptly by a qualified physician. The therapeutic objective is not to stop a seizure in progress but to prevent its recurrence after a brief lapse of time. It is not, however, necessary to stop the seizures at once.

The treatment of choice is phenobarbital and diphenylhydantoin (Dilantin) administered until a sufficient level of the anticonvulsant is established to last 12 to 24 hours. Phenobarbital should be administered intramuscularly unless the patient is in shock (in which case slow intravenous administration is appropriate) in a dose appropriate for the patient's muscle mass. The dose of phenobarbital for a 150-lb. adult with normal muscle mass is 120 mg. intramuscularly. The dosage should be increased or decreased depending on the patient's muscle mass. If the patient is still convulsing 20 minutes later, an additional 60 mg. of phenobarbital should be administered intramuscularly. This dose should be repeated every 20 minutes until the seizures stop or until the total dose of phenobarbital reaches 300 mg. for a 150-lb. adult (also increased or decreased depending on the patient's muscle mass).

Only a few patients continue to have seizures following maximal phenobarbital administration. If seizures do persist, diphenylhydantoin should be administered very slowly into the tubing of a well placed intravenous line. Initially, 200 mg. should be administered over a period of five to seven minutes. If the patient continues to have seizures 20 minutes later, an additional 100 mg. should be given intravenously over a period of five minutes. This dose may be repeated every 20 minutes until a total of 600 mg. has been administered. In almost every case, this therapy successfully controls status epilepticus and keeps the patient seizure-free for the next 24 hours.

Patients whose seizures are not controlled by the preceding regimen should be seen by a competent neurologic consultant. If a consultant is not available, a trial of short-acting anticonvulsants should be employed. These include diazepam (5 to 10 mg. intramuscularly or intravenously), paraldehyde (7 ml. intramuscularly in each buttock), or general anesthesia. All patients with status epilepticus should be admitted to the hospital for therapy.

If the patient is in a postictal state following a generalized motor seizure and is confused or unconscious, it is inappropriate to administer sedative medication. The dosage of anticonvulsants should be adjusted only if the patient has been taking his medications regularly, and if no unusual stress or illness has been associated with the current seizure.

It is inappropriate to make changes in basic anticonvulsant medication in the emergency department. Sedatives such as diazepam, chlordiazepoxide, paraldehyde, amobarbital (Amytal), or narcotics are contraindicated. The best treatment is *no* medication. If the postictal state persists beyond two hours, the patient should be admitted to the hospital for 24 hours of observation. If the patient becomes alert within two hours of the seizure and has a history of similar episodes, he should not be admitted but sent to his regular physician for adjustment of medications as indicated.

If uremic or hepatic failure is the cause for unconsciousness, hospitalization is required. These situations are not usually emergent in terms of need for life-saving measures in the emergency department. Furthermore, it is not equipped to provide the treatment programs required to manage patients with uremic or hepatic failure properly. The emergency department personnel can provide service by drawing specimens for initial hematologic and biochemical studies and then arranging expeditious admission.

Summary

This chapter provides a resumé of the causes of unconsciousness and a suggested plan of approach for the rescue worker in the field and the physician of first contact in the emergency care facility. Emergent treatment programs for conditions that, in our opinion, *should* be treated in an emergency department are also provided.

A final note merits specific attention. This is the importance of an accurate recording of the examination and findings in the emergency department for the benefit of the health care team who will provide subsequent care. A carefully performed and recorded examination, particularly the neurologic examination, can later be interpreted and used by any competent clinician, but a superficial examination, or one that is incompletely recorded, is of value to no one.

Further comment on the subject of the unconscious patient can be found in the references cited.[1,2,3]

References

1. Plum, F., and Posner, J. B. 1972. *The Diagnosis of Stupor and Coma,* 2nd ed. Philadelphia, F. A. Davis Co.
2. Sabin, T. B. 1974. Current concepts: The differential diagnosis of coma. *New Eng. J. Med.,* 290:1062.
3. Adams, R. D. 1970. Coma and related disturbances of consciousness, in *Principles of Internal Medicine,* 6th ed., Wintrobe, M. M., *et al.* (eds.). New York, McGraw-Hill.

9

Accidental Poisoning

George H. Lowrey

For three decades, in the United States, accidents have been the leading cause of death between the ages of 1 and 16 years. Poisoning is one of the most important of these accidents. Recent statistics indicate that more than 2,400 deaths from poisoning occur annually in the United States, and the estimated number of nonfatal poisonings is approximately 1,000,000 a year. Most of these accidental poisonings, both fatal and nonfatal, occur in the preschool age group.[1,2]

Several hundred poison information and therapy centers (poison control centers) have been opened in the United States and Canada within the past 15 years. Their primary purpose is to aid physicians in the identification of toxic ingredients in common household products, medicinal agents, plants, and a host of miscellaneous items. In some centers, teams have been formed to give emergency treatment for poisoning.

Through the information furnished by the poison control centers, particularly the National Clearinghouse for Poison Control Centers in Washington, D.C., an improved method of attack is available. In poisoning, as in infectious diseases, prevention rather than treatment is the preferred method of control. Much of the following discussion is concerned with the epidemiology of poisoning in childhood. Use of this knowledge can be as effective in "immunizing" children against accidental poisoning as the current methods of immunization are in protecting them from poliomyelitis and tetanus. All physicians must constantly attack the problem by proper and repeated instruction of families. Obviously, general practitioners and pediatricians will assume the principal roles, but public health nurses and physicians, school physicians, and other personnel in the health sciences can play important parts.

135

The Problem

Who is poisoned, and what are the circumstances surrounding these accidents? The answers to these questions are not complicated or difficult to understand. Table 9-1, summarizing four years of experience at the University of Michigan Poison Information and Therapy Center, clearly indicates who is poisoned. These data are typical of those compiled at other centers. Approximately 80% of poisonings occur in children less than 6 years of age, with the largest number between the ages of 1 and 3 years. Education at this age is most difficult because of immaturity. This is also the group that is the most uncritically inquisitive; youngsters at this age examine things by sight, by touch, and instinctively by taste. It is important to remember that the best way to prevent poisoning in this age group is to remove potential poisons from the environment of the child.

Statistics from all poison control centers are in agreement that medications, both internal and external, are responsible for the greatest number of accidental poisonings in childhood. Aspirin, accounting for approximately 25% of all poisonings, is responsible for the largest number of deaths by a single agent. Sedatives and tranquilizers rank second among the offending medications. Barbiturates were the most

Table 9-1. Summary of Consultations and Treatments for a Four-Year Period at the Poison Information and Therapy Center, University of Michigan Medical Center

	Distribution of Cases by Age Group					
Substances	<1 Year	1–3 Years	3–6 Years	6–15 Years	Adult	Total*
Medications	24	359	65	9	66	561
Cleansing and polishing agents	33	186	23	3	15	276
Cosmetics	19	122	15	7	7	177
Pesticides	6	66	18	5	11	114
Hydrocarbons and related products†	10	64	12	4	15	116
Plants	5	66	21	4	7	108
Miscellaneous	42	179	43	15	74	382
	139	1,042	197	47	195	1,734

* Age was not indicated in a few instances; the total therefore is greater than the sum of the separate age groups.
† This category excludes some hydrocarbons found in cleansing agents, *e.g.*, waxes and floor cleaners.

common of these substances, but in the past few years tranquilizers have overtaken this unenviable position. The fact is a rather sad commentary on the American way of life. Most commonly the toddler finds a bottle of medicine on the table of his parents' bedroom and ingests the contents. In second place among locations of medicinal agents involved in poisoning is the medicine cabinet or counter top in the bathroom.

Most parents do not realize the potential danger of common household cleansing and polishing agents. Recent legislation has resulted in improvement of the warning labels on containers for these products but, human nature being what it is, most people will not read labels regardless of the color of the ink or the size of the type. The number of potentially toxic ingredients in cleansing and polishing agents, as well as in substances comprising the other categories in Table 9-1, is multitudinous.

Gleason, Gosselin, and Hodges[3] list more than 20,000 household and farm products that contain toxic ingredients, and the listing does not include medications, plants, and other miscellaneous substances having toxic potential. The products involved in poisoning are carelessly placed by adults where they can easily be reached by children. The storage area under the kitchen sink is a favorite place for exploration by the young child and, unfortunately, a place where many toxic substances are kept. An example of a hazard overlooked by many people, including physicians, is the all-purpose metal polishes, a large number of which still contain cyanide.

Pesticides are often kept in an unlocked workroom, garage, or tool shed. This is a dangerous practice even if there are no young children in the home, because children in the neighborhood may find them.

Transferring potentially dangerous materials to food or beverage containers is a near-homicidal practice if children are around. There are few stronger enticements to youngsters to taste or drink the contents.

In most areas of the United States the incidence of accidental poisoning is higher among persons in the lower socioeconomic class than among the general population. Poor housing, overcrowding, and inadequate storage space plus lack of information increase the hazard.[4] Furthermore, there is strong evidence that this type of accident is likely to be repeated in such a home situation.[5] A striking exception is the increased frequency of accidental poisoning in the homes of physicians, dentists, and pharmacists, which is attributed to the presence of professional samples. Readers, take note.

Federal law requires that potentially dangerous substances be designated as such on the container's label. This legislation is a great improvement but unfortunately is not the entire answer to the problem. Many products that are compounded, packaged, and sold within a small locality do not bear labels. Such products are a real hindrance to the work of the poison control centers because it is often difficult or impossible to trace the source of the substances.

Although relatively few accidental poisonings are the result of ingestion of dangerous plants, the number of fatalities resulting therefrom is disproportionately high. Our experience indicates that the proportion of children requiring hospitalization for ingestion of poisonous plants is higher than in any other category. The first death in our series resulted from ingestion of a poisonous mushroom. House plants as well as those found outdoors may be toxic.

In 76% of the cases of accidental poisoning in childhood recorded at the New York City Poison Control Center, the mother was in the home at the time.[5] This observation reemphasizes the importance of keeping poisonous substances away from children, because constant vigilance is almost impossible.

Emergency and Follow-up Treatment

Certainly every physician should know the geographic location of and the fastest means of communication with the nearest poison control center, which can supply all the information necessary for proper care of the potentially poisoned patient. About 8% of the calls received by such centers cannot be answered directly because of lack of information. In most of these instances a call is placed to the manufacturer of the product to obtain further information about the ingredients.

Maintaining an airway is of utmost importance in the comatose or semicomatose patient. This may require the use of an endotracheal tube. Proper positioning of the patient during emesis or gavage to prevent aspiration is essential.

Emetics. An immediate step that may be taken in the home is removal of the offending agent. Since most accidental poisonings involve ingestion of toxic substances, induction of vomiting is desirable except when extremely caustic agents (acids and alkalies) or volatile oils have been swallowed. Syrup of ipecac (15 ml. as an initial dose) is suggested as an emetic agent for both the home and the hospital emergency department. It is highly effective, and a single dose induces vomiting in about 80% of patients. If this does not occur within 30 minutes, the dose may be repeated one time. A glass of water given a few minutes following the ipecac will increase the chance of vomiting if the stomach is empty. Studies of both animals and humans have revealed that vomiting is a more efficient method of emptying the stomach than is gastric lavage. If the patient is unconscious, however, vomiting should not be induced.

Apomorphine hydrochloride (0.1 mg./kg. for adults, 0.06 mg./kg. for children) given subcutaneously will usually produce emesis within a few minutes of administration. This means of emptying the stomach is finding an increasing acceptance in many poison centers and seldom causes narcotic effects in the doses recommended.[10]

Other agents that have been used to induce vomiting include salt water, mustard, and weak copper sulfate solution. These agents are less effective and more difficult to administer, however, and some have potentially toxic side effects.

Gastric Lavage. Only if emesis does not take place or if it is ascertained that the stomach contents are not completely removed should gastric lavage be used. The largest tube that can be passed through the nose should be obtained. After one has made sure that the tube is in the stomach, copious amounts of saline solution or water are used to wash out all materials. Only small amounts are administered at any one time followed by repeated aspiration. If there is a specific antidote for the toxic substance ingested, it can be administered through the tube before withdrawal. Care should be taken to avoid bronchial aspiration. Strong acids, alkalies, and hydrocarbons, such as kerosene, probably should not be removed by lavage or vomiting unless very large quantities have been ingested. (There is still some debate over the value of either emesis or lavage in treating poisoning due to kerosene, gasoline, and similar volatile agents.)

For ingested products, it is advisable to use one of the preceding procedures within the first four hours. Beyond that time, these methods are increasingly less effective.

Activated Charcoal. This substance reduces gastrointestinal absorption of certain groups of poisons. The charcoal should not be administered at the same time as or before the syrup of ipecac is given, because the syrup will be absorbed by the charcoal. The recommended amount of charcoal is 5 to 10 gm. thoroughly blended with a sufficient amount of water to make it easily ingestible. It is important to recognize that ordinary, or unactivated, charcoal has essentially no absorptive powers and is therefore useless in the treatment of poisoning. Most authorities have not advocated the use of charcoal alone in the treatment of potentially toxic accidents but have suggested its use following administration of syrup of ipecac by approximately 15 to 20 minutes.

Among the more common substances effectively absorbed by activated charcoal are amphetamines, barbiturates, nicotine, Parathion, phenol, digitalis, morphine, salicylates, and sulfonamides. The material is much less effective against ethyl and methyl alcohols, most caustic alkalies and mineral acids, boric acid, and the heavy metals, including iron.

Table 9-2. Antidotes

Substance	Antidotes
Organic phosphate insecticides	Pralidoxime chloride (Protopam chloride), atropine sulfate
Inorganic cations	
Mercury	Dimercaprol (BAL)
Arsenic	Dimercaprol (BAL)
Lead	Versene, penicillamine, dimercaprol (BAL)
Iron	Deferoxamine
Cyanides	Nitrite, thiosulfite
Narcotics	Naloxone, levallorphan tartrate
Warfarin	Vitamin K
Dicumarol	Vitamin K

Antidotes. Specific antidotes are available for only a few of the common poisoning agents, some of which are included in Table 9-2. The details of their use should be obtained from one of the standard texts on toxicology.[3,6,7,10]

Peritoneal Lavage and Renal Dialysis. Removal of a toxin by either of these methods may be life-saving in a number of instances, but they are formidable procedures and not to be taken lightly. Substances for which these techniques may be indicated include the following:

Amanita phalloides mushrooms

Antifreezes (glycol type)

Heavy metals in soluble compounds

Heavy metals after therapy with chelating agents (acute)

Methanol

Other substances, when the poisoning is severe, may be similarly treated.

Forced Diuresis. This procedure is frequently indicated in severe poisoning with long-acting barbiturates, amphetamines, alcohols, salicylates, strychnine, isoniazid, bromides, and a few other drugs that are excreted primarily by the kidneys. This requires the use of ample fluids and an adequate osmotic load to increase the proximal tubular excretion of drugs. When indicated, an alkaline pH should be maintained using sodium bicarbonate or THAM (tris [hydroxymethyl] aminomethane) when treating acid drugs, such as barbiturates and salicylates. An acid pH may be maintained through the use of intravenous ascorbic acid or administration of ammonium chloride and is indicated for amphetamine and strychnine poisoning.

Exchange Transfusion. Successful use of exchange transfusion in treatment of poisoning with a number of different agents has been reported. Compared with peritoneal or renal dialysis, exchange transfusion is technically more difficult and potentially more dangerous. It would appear to be wise to employ this procedure only when the toxic ingredient is not water soluble or easily removed from the blood by dialysis or diuresis.[8]

Ancillary Procedures. If the identity of the offending agent is not known or if the quantity absorbed is questionable, chemical analysis of suitable biologic specimens may be helpful. Since this is time consuming even under optimal conditions, the patient must be treated in the interim period. Often it is wise to collect such specimens for analysis even though the results will not be available for consideration in making therapeutic decisions. These results are necessary for medicolegal aspects of many cases. It is important to emphasize that therapy usually is supportive only, and in most instances no specific antidote will be available.

The removal of a patient from an environment in which he is inhaling air containing a toxic substance or his body is being exposed to one is seldom a problem faced in the hospital emergency department. Both of these sources should be kept in mind, however, in all puzzling medical cases presented to the physician. If the patient's clothing is soaked with a potentially toxic substance, it must be removed promptly and the surface of his body cleansed of the material. Examination of the eyes for possible exposure to toxic substances should always be a part of the initial examination when the possibilities of exposure exist. Although a few toxic agents are extremely potent and work very rapidly, as a general rule it is safe to take the time to obtain an accurate history and, if possible, to identify the source of the material. This may involve a brief search of the premises. Although this extra precaution may appear to delay therapy, it often proves to be of benefit to the patient because a specific antidote may then be utilized.

Prevention by Education

Poisoning is one of the common accidents of childhood. In many instances the parents are unaware that the agent ingested is toxic, and often the label on the container, even if read, does not convey the potential danger. If we are to prevent accidental poisoning, we must be fully informed of the circumstances surrounding these events and must bring to the attention of the public the important preventive measures implicit in the statistics gathered by the poison control centers.

Pediatricians, emergency department physicians, and general practitioners who care for preschool children are in an advantageous position to act as educators of parents. Repeated instruction concerning the ways to prevent accidental poisoning is as important a part of medical care as immunization against the preventable infectious diseases and should start at the same time. Some of the more important points to be made are as follows.[2,9]

1. Keep all drugs, known poisons, and other chemicals out of reach of children or, better yet, under lock and key.
2. Make periodic inventories of medicines and other chemicals and discard the old ones in such a way they cannot be reached by children (or pets).
3. Read all labels and follow instructions carefully.
4. Do not store potentially poisonous substances in containers for food or beverages.
5. Give medications only as directed by the physician and make sure that specific instructions are obtained from him.
6. When using cleaning fluids, make sure that ventilation is adequate. When using pesticides, be careful to avoid contamination of food, inhalation, and excessive contact with the skin.
7. Instruct children not to eat any plant or other vegetation inside or outside the home without first obtaining adult approval.
8. If there's a possibility that a child may have been exposed to a poisonous substance, keep the container and its label and call the physician.
9. Physicians should prescribe only enough of a medicine for a single course of treatment.

References

1. Poison Control Statistics. 1974. National Clearinghouse for Poison Control Centers, Washington, D.C.
2. Lowrey, G. H. 1965. Accidental poisoning in childhood. *Postgrad. Med.,* 38:78.
3. Gleason, M. N., Gosselin, R. E., and Hodges, H. C. 1975. *Clinical Toxicology of Commercial Products, Acute Poisoning (Home and Farm),* 4th ed. Baltimore, The Williams & Wilkins Co.
4. Mellins, R. B., Christian, J. R., and Bundesen, H. N. 1956. The natural history of poisoning in childhood. Pediatrics, 17:314.
5. Wehrle, P. F., et al. 1961. The epidemiology of accidental poisoning in an urban population. III. The repeater problem in accidental poisoning. Pediatrics, 27:614–620.
6. Dreisbach, R. H. 1974. *Handbook of Poisoning: Diagnosis and Treatment,* 8th ed. Los Altos, Calif., Lange Medical Publications.
7. Goodman, L. S., and Gilman, A. 1975. *The Pharmacological Basis of Therapeutics,* 5th ed. New York, The Macmillan Co.
8. Lowrey, G. H. 1965. The most common household poisons: Signs, symptoms, and treatment. *Univ. Mich. Med. Cen. J.,* 31:71.
9. Coleman, A. B., and Alpert, J. J. (eds.). 1970. Poisoning in children. *Pediat. Clin. N. Amer.,* 17:471–753.
10. Arena, J. M. 1975. Poisoning—treatment and prevention. JAMA, 232:1272–1275.

10

The Emergency Treatment of Adolescent Drug Abuse

Derek Miller, M.D.

Acute drug toxicity has always been a problem in emergency medicine. For many years medical students were warned not to send home from the emergency department of the hospital an alcoholic who might possibly have a concussion. More recently, physicians in these areas have recognized that they have a medicolegal responsibility not to let such drug toxic persons leave the hospital while they are intoxicated and a possible danger to themselves or others, particularly if the patient arrived in an automobile.

The drug scene that has developed during the last two decades has lowered the age and increased the number of drug toxic persons who appear in emergency room situations. Nowadays, young people often arrive having abused either alcohol or other drugs, and commonly urgent treatment is required.

To some extent, formal emergency medicine was slow to respond to the challenge of the increase in drug intoxication among young people. As a result, a wide-spread use of paramedical treatment settings, *e.g.,* drop-in centers, drug help services, storefronts, and free clinics, have been created. As so often happens, these centers may develop a vested interest, with a variety of rationalizations about the establishment, in keeping their clients away from physicians. This response may partially have been due to orthodox medical attitudes, but it can mean that effective therapeutic aid is not made available early to patients. As a result, sometimes adolescents who arrive in emergency departments from such services have been exposed to a variety of superficial approaches to treatment that have turned out to be inadequate or represent a misdiagnosis. Only when this has been apparent has the emergency service been called upon for assistance. Acute schizophrenic reactions are likely to be misdiagnosed as being due to hallucinogens; abuse with heroin-barbiturate mixtures may be treated by giving the victim coffee and trying to keep him awake.

Paramedical clinics, particularly because of the reluctance of many young people to go to an emergency department, provide a necessary service, and emergency medicine personnel should attempt to work with them. One difficulty has been that often those in the emergency system see themselves as providing only for trauma rather than acute medico-psychological care. Paramedical centers often help runaway adolescents get in touch with their families; young people who are being exploited, sexually or otherwise, by their more aggressive peers, may find a haven in them. Furthermore, the centers provide food, shelter, and immediate care for drug toxic youths, often facilities that cannot be provided with ease in hospital areas. They may also provide the only human contact that is not drug toxic that can demonstrate caring for those drug abusing young people who normally are not motivated to seek medical help.

To some extent, providing social workers and nursing specialists with more experience in the psychological care of young people allows similar assistance to be given in the more usual hospital setting.

Therapeutic and Legal Problems

Many adolescents say that they do not want help, and thus they are often misunderstood by physicians and other caring adults. It is a mistaken belief that adolescents necessarily mean what they say. This is a particular problem therapeutically and legally. In so far as the therapeutic aspect is concerned, the verbal expression of wishing to be separate from adults is often taken at face value. The refusal to accept treatment is taken literally, whereas the firm expectation from physicians that the patients will allow themselves to be examined and treated is usually accepted without demur. If adults withdraw on the basis of having listened to the adolescent's words rather than his actions, at best this increases alienation between the generations; at worst, a sick young person is not treated. The attitude of the 17-year-old who denies that he wishes to communicate with adults is the same as that of a younger adolescent who in the midst of a family quarrel rushes to his room and slams the door. The technique of refusal may represent a request for further assistance, even if this is implicit rather than explicit. Drug intoxication, as any other psychophysiological symptom, represents both an attempt to escape from intolerable psychic tension and a request for help for personality difficulties. As with so many symptoms of adolescent disturbance, the severity of the symptoms does not necessarily indicate the intensity of the personality conflict.

In delivering emergency care, there are three necessary approaches to treatment:

1. The drug toxic patient must be medically managed.
2. The psychological significance of the toxicity should be recognized. The alcoholic may be seriously depressed. The adolescent who overuses phencyclidine (sold on the streets as PCP or THC) might also be suffering from a schizophrenic reaction. On the other hand, an adolescent who takes a cocktail of drugs, including heroin, may be suffering from an acute identity problem without a fundamental personality disturbance.
3. The adolescent may need help with an acute conflict, and if the presentation is acutely toxic, it may be a way of trying to get help for both problems.

The physician's plan for disposition of the patient should be based on the following criteria:

1. The maturational age of the patient. With equivalent psychological difficulties, early adolescents who abuse drugs are less likely to exercise good judgment than are persons in the middle and later stages of this age period.
2. The conscious motivation and reliability of the patient and the family. Many parents unconsciously abet their child's drug abuse. Not noticing the smell of marijuana in a closed automobile, failing to see needle track marks, and doing household tasks with a person who is hallucinating on lysergic acid diethylamide (LSD) without broaching the subject all demonstrate an unwillingness to intervene in a helpful way.
3. The extent of the underlying disturbance. One should look for the following situations:
   a. Isolation of the nuclear family from a meaningful emotional network of relatives and friends. Adolescents without these relationships are vulnerable to disturbances.
   b. Whether the adolescent as a child before the age of 2 experienced consistent adult handling in a relatively stress-free environment. Distress inflicted at an early age is likely to produce emotional disturbances at puberty.
   c. Acute adolescent stress, in particular, separation from meaningful loved adults by separation, divorce, or death, or from peers because of moving to a new home or school. Drug abuse is a common response to mourning.
4. Whether the adolescent has a capacity to value the self and avoid chemical regression by abstaining from drugs, without external controls.

The negative attitude of adolescents to accepting the need for help, an acceptance that threatens their tenuous sense of autonomy, means that a young person who is obviously drug toxic, or in some other way suffering from an acute psychological syndrome, may refuse treatment. If the adolescent is in danger of hurting himself or others, emergency treatment must be instituted, regardless of what the adolescent may say. In states in which the basis for legal commitment is a person's inability to care for the self, that concept can also apply. If emergency treatment must be instituted without the informed consent of the patient or his parents, the reason must be clearly documented by the physician.

In some states the issue is being argued as to whether parents have the right to insist that their children over the age of 13 receive treatment. If possible, parents should sign an informed consent document for children who are minors, even in emergency situations. Children have the right to an attorney and, depending on local statutes, may appeal to the probate court if parents insist on treatment. As soon as they are out of immediate danger, they should be informed of this right. In reverse, if parents insist on withdrawing their child from treatment and the physician considers that such an action would jeopardize the child's life, the physician may (and in some states must) seek protective services from the probate court for the young person.

When an adolescent is thought not to be in immediate danger and treatment is verbally refused, the problem is complex. In states that adopt the attitude that only dangerousness to the self or others, whatever the legal definition of that might be, is indication for commitment, adolescents who can be significantly helped by treatment may not get it. Even commitment, however, does not nullify a patient's right to refuse treatment. An adult or adolescent, even if legally committed to a hospital for treatment, may refuse to allow a physician to undertake a treatment procedure.

In some states an adolescent who appears in the emergency department and then declines treatment can refuse to allow the hospital staff to tell his parents of his appearance. This is the case with the so-called emancipated minor and may also be true for an adolescent suffering from venereal disease or drug intoxication. Specific laws have been passed that no longer make it obligatory to inform parents of these syndromes; this presumably means that the adolescents can refuse to let their parents be informed of their difficulties. Emergency department staff may be maneuvered by the adolescent to behave in a way that is implicitly hostile to parents. An adolescent's refusal to tell his father or mother of difficulties with which they might be helpful is an explicit attack because by withholding information he is preventing that parent from fulfilling his or her role.

When an adolescent is thought to be either in immediate danger or imminently dangerous, emergency treatment with nondangerous drugs must be undertaken for both legal and moral reasons. If, in the opinion of the physician, treatment is needed but not of extreme urgency, the proper step would appear to be to have a guardian *ad litem* appointed by the juvenile court. The problem is that the need to protect the rights of the individual carries with it two assumptions. The first is that all patients are competent to make a decision about the need for treatment. Denial is a way for all people to cope with anxiety-provoking situations. An understanding physician who properly and firmly insists that there is a need for intervention may implicitly reassure a patient about the justification for this step. Unfortunately, telling an anxious patient, filled with the need to deny difficulties, that he may seek legal assistance, an attitude that the law requires, can carry with it the assumption to the patient that the doctor is unsure of his position with respect to the necessity for treatment. This reinforces both anxiety and denial.

The second assumption is that if refusal is greeted with an invitation to seek legal advice, the young person will hear the rejection he has invited but does not want. The law assumes that an adolescent means what he says. It is almost abnormal for an adolescent under the age of 16 (two years postpubertal) to admit verbally that treatment is needed. To do so would be to admit that the striving for autonomy has been abandoned. Adolescents, like 2-year-olds, therefore are likely to say "no." The issue is that help is requested in action and not words, a concept that is not legally understood.

The issue of informed consent is significant in the treatment of acutely toxic adolescents. It is doubtful that any anxious patient with a problem remembers after 24 hours the discussions that took place in obtaining informed consent for an intervention. Legal authorities probably do not understand that explanations to those who are acutely anxious may lead to a whole discussion not really being heard. Persons who are just being admitted to a hospital, or who are arriving in an emergency department, are likely to be so anxious that there is very little awareness of what they have signed or what a consent undertaking is about. It would hardly seem to be appropriate to try to explain the risks of any intervention to an adolescent who is suffering from an acute anxiety reaction. Under those circumstances, the physician must use his judgmet. Legal liability for a refusal to tell an adolescent or parents of possible risks is always present. If a decision is made that it is not in the patient's interests to do so, it can cause difficulty in any type of practice, and the reason for the action should be documented. Hospital insurance carriers have to indicate whether or not they will support the staff in such a situation.

A real difficulty with adolescents, particularly with those who abuse drugs, is that whatever the underlying syndrome, they experience iden-

6

tity problems. Beneath the experience of toxicity, a common basic complaint is, "I feel nothing," "I am dead inside," or "I don't know who I am." Adolescents in such situations are all too willing to adopt the identity that society gives them, whether it be unofficial (a freak) or official (a delinquent or mentally ill person). Because of the self-labeling propensity of adolescents as a result of society's expressed attitudes, many professionals are understandably and properly reluctant to label young people as mentally ill by taking action before a judge. When the issue is one of emergency care, perhaps lasting only a day or two, this reluctance is increased. A balance has to be drawn between the needs of the adolescent for treatment and possible long-term difficulties.

Differential Diagnosis of Drug Reactions

Society is particularly preoccupied with the issue of heroin abuse. In its acute stage, such drug abuse is less usual in adolescents than is acute toxicity due to abuse of sedatives, such as barbiturates, and especially alcohol. The abuse of hallucinogens, such as LSD, or stimulants, such as the amphetamine derivatives, is also common, although it appears that the incidence of hallucinogen abuse is declining.

Adolescents who seek emergency assistance often do not know what drug has been taken. The differential diagnosis of the drug response requiring emergency treatment is not helped much by a patient's or friend's statement as to what has been ingested. Overdosage with a single or combined drugs may be manifested in a wide variety of symptoms. These include a variety of behavioral disturbances, exacerbations of previous physical or psychological illness, central nervous system depression, or excitement. If a drug has been injected, there are likely to be the complications of either nonsterile drug administration or intraarterial instead of intravenous injection. One drug may potentiate the after effects of others. Marijuana, for example, may precipitate an acute hallucinatory response in a person who has previously taken LSD.

The diagnosis of the type of drug abused may require laboratory analysis of blood or body fluids. Even if the type of drug is known, its dose and purity are uncertain if it has been obtained on the street. The problem with laboratory analysis is often the time required to obtain it. Often emergency supportive treatment has to be undertaken with no certainty of the drug's identity. The study of symptoms helps differentiate the drugs used, although alcohol may be a complication of any one symptom, particularly in adolescents. In addition to the vital signs listed in Table 10-1, cerebral vascular accidents have been reported with the overuse of amphetamines.

Abuse of opiates is more usual among deprived ethnic minorities than in less depressed neighborhoods, particularly with adolescents and young adults. Generally, the greater the social pathology to which a heroin abuser has been exposed, the more likely is the response to rehabilitation to be positive. Young people who have not been exposed to severe social conflict and deprivation and who abuse the opiates are likely to suffer from very severe psychopathology. Their prognosis is therefore considerably less satisfactory. In either situation, emergency medicine is likely to be concerned with the management of acute toxicity. The emergency staff, however, still has a responsibility to direct the patient, or his family, toward appropriate longer term help.

The differential diagnosis of the etiology of opiate abuse is not always made in centers in which methadone maintenance is used. Sometimes adolescents are sent to such centers and essentially given the label of addicts by being inappropriately placed on this type of regimen. In general, the younger the addict, the more appropriate it is to seek sophisticated psychosocial consultation in order that some attempt might be made to deal with the etiology of the syndrome rather than to adopt a symptomatic approach alone. This concept is appropriate for all drugs that are abused, particularly alcohol.

Adolescents should be helped with the pathology underlying the drug abuse. Any treatment in which the individual's psychopathology is ignored is likely to have many expensive failures. Programs for drug-dependent adolescents, such as Synanon, Lexington, and Daytop, in which the etiology of drug dependence is often inadequately diagnosed, do not help those who suffer from personal psychopathology, which is neither diagnosed nor treated.

As with any drug of abuse, the treatment of the young heroin addict ultimately consists of the treatment of the basic character problem and the social pathology that helped create it. At present it appears that society has neither the resources nor the will to undertake such a task. The now declared illegal testing of the urine of young soldiers to determine whether they had recently abused opiates is not the equivalent of undertaking the complete treatment that would be needed to help young addicts with severe personality problems. Although the severity of the drug dependence is not usually a measure of the severity of the personality problem, it is rare to find adolescents in whom only an adolescent identity problem is involved in heroin abuse. When this does occur, it is more likely in areas of society in which severe social pathology exists. Thus, a number of young soldiers who abused drugs in Vietnam ceased to do so on return to urban life.

Table 10-1. Differential Diagnosis in Drug Abuse

System	Possible drug abused	Possible drug withdrawn
General appearance		
Restless, agitated appearance	Amphetamines Hallucinogens Alcohol	Heroin Barbiturates
Quiet, withdrawn appearance	Heroin Barbiturates Hallucinogens	Amphetamines
Vital signs		
Blood pressure		
Elevated	Amphetamines Hallucinogens	
Orthostatic hypotension	Phenothiazines Marijuana	Barbiturates
Pulse		
Tachycardia	Nonspecific	
Irregularity	Amphetamines	
Temperature		
Fever	Hallucinogens	Heroin Barbiturates
Respiration		
Suppression	Methaqualone (in large doses) Barbiturates Narcotics Minor tranquilizers Glutethimide (Doriden)	
Apnea, acute laryngospasm	Glutethimide	
Skin		
Perspiration	Most acute toxicities	Most acute withdrawals
Dry	Anticholinergic drugs and hallucinogens	
Goose flesh	Hallucinogens	Heroin
Malar flush	Marijuana (particularly in pubertal adolescents)	
Eyes		
Conjunctival injection	Marijuana	
Lacrimation		Heroin
Acute glaucoma	Anticholinergic drugs Amyl nitrite inhalation	
Extraocular movements		
Lateral nystagmus	Barbiturates Marijuana	Barbiturates
Exaggerated blink reflex		Barbiturates
Pupils		
Pinpoint	Heroin	
Dilated-reactive	Amphetamines	
Dilated-nonreactive	Anticholinergic drugs	

Table 10-1—cont.

System	Possible drug abused	Possible drug withdrawn
Nose		
Rhinorrhea		Heroin
Injected, ulcerated, or perforated septum	Cocaine (sniffing) Marijuana	
Chest		
Pulmonary edema or fibrosis	Dextropropoxyphene (Darvon) intoxication Intravenous use of heroin or other opiates or their talc contaminants	
Bronchial constriction	Heroin	
Abdomen		
Cramps		Heroin
Hepatic failure	Toluene and chloroform	
Psychological state		
Disorientation	Hallucinogens Amphetamines Cocaine Marijuana Anticholinergic drugs Cocaine in large doses Barbiturates Alcohol	Barbiturates Alcohol
Aggressive behavior	Alcohol Barbiturates	
Paranoid psychosis	Amphetamines	
Stupor, stroke, coma (Needle marks may be present)	Barbiturates (Erythematous plaques, vesicles, or bullae may be present at the site of a lesion) Heroin	
Motor patterns		
Speech		
Thick and slurred	Alcohol Barbiturates	
Slow and clear	Heroin	
Muscular movements		
Resting, tremors	Amphetamines Hallucinogens	Heroin
Gross tremors		Barbiturates
Seizures	Codeine Propoxyphene Strychnine Hallucinogens Amphetamines Methylphenidate Methaqualone	Barbiturates Alcohol
Reflex response		
Increased	Amphetamines	
Decreased (superficial reflexes)	Barbiturates	

Acute Heroin Overdosage

Recognition of the syndrome is essential, but general management of severe shock may precede it. Death due to respiratory failure is common in heroin overdosage. The management of respiratory failure includes the maintenance of respiration and circulation; positive pressure respiration and defibrillation may be required. Adequate oxygenation is crucial. Typically, a combination of needle track marks, coma, pinpoint pupils, and depressed respiration to two to four breaths per minute, with consequent cyanosis, makes the diagnosis.

Apart from taking appropriate measures to support circulation and respiration, heroin antagonists should be used. Nalorphine (3 to 5 mg. intravenously) is an effective antagonist, but it causes a fairly serious respiratory depression. If, as is likely, the heroin has been used in combination with barbiturates, this side effect can be serious. Naloxone (Narcan) is a heroin antagonist that does not have this effect and is therefore the drug of choice. In unconscious victims, it should by preference be given intravenously. If no veins are accessible because of previous drug injections, it may be given intramuscularly or subcutaneously. The usual initial adult dose is 0.4 mg. This may be repeated at two or three minute intervals if respiration does not improve.

If there is no improvement in the patient's condition, it is almost certainly due to drug mixture of barbiturates or other narcotics or possible trauma or disease. Cardiopulmonary resuscitation is vital, and if naloxone is not available, nalorphine may be given intravenously at 10 to 20 minute intervals. The patient must not be left unattended when full responsiveness occurs because methadone as well as heroin may have been abused.[1] In this case the patient may relapse into coma. After the patient has recovered from the acute attack, hospitalization to ensure against the development of pneumonia and to pinpoint the medical diagnosis is indicated.

Heroin overdosage may occur because of the variation in the amount of heroin present in the street drug. Dealers tend to vary either the amount of adulterant present or its contents (with barbiturates, for example), depending on the supply-and-demand situation of the market. Some deaths from heroin are due to an allergy to the drug or an adulterant (quinine, for example) or to injection while intoxicated with alcohol. Most deaths, however, are probably due to injection of more potent heroin than that to which the addict has become accustomed. In England, where only pure heroin is used, the death rate is considerably greater than in the United States.[2]

One side effect of the use of heroin antagonists is that the patient may recover from the acute respiratory and circulatory distress only to develop symptoms of acute withdrawal, such as abdominal pain, lacrimation, yawning, and painful muscle spasms. Since both naloxone and nalorphine are short-acting drugs, the victim of a heroin overdose must be continuously observed because he may relapse into coma even though only heroin has been abused.

Methadone substitution is not normally a procedure carried out in the emergency area. Typically, an initial dose of 15 to 20 mg. of methadone is given orally, and then 1 mg. is substituted for 2 mg. of heroin. Since the exact dose of heroin is rarely known, the initial dose of methadone will probably be slightly larger than necessary.

Sometimes adolescents appear in the emergency department complaining that they are dependent on heroin and seeking admission to a hospital for drug withdrawal treatment. If hospitalization is contraindicated, out-patient withdrawal treatment is not impossible for adolescents. Sometimes very little needs to be done. On occasion, chlordiazepoxide in doses of 25 to 50 mg. orally three or four times daily makes withdrawal a smooth process. If chlorpromazine is going to be given to minimize acute withdrawal symptoms, liver function tests are necessary. Adolescents may be withdrawn from apparently large doses of heroin, however, with very little symptomatic disturbance, providing the medical staff does not suggest to the patient that symptoms are likely to occur. Prepubertal children and adults are more likely than adolescents to experience acute withdrawal symptoms.

Barbiturate Intoxication

Persons who suffer from acute barbiturate intoxication may appear in the emergency department in two typical situations. Sometimes young people may require emergency treatment because of an acute overdose resulting from a suicide attempt. Accidental overdose due to experimentation is also common. Sometimes adolescents attempt to withdraw themselves from barbiturates, suffer a central nervous system catastrophe as a result, and appear as a neurologic emergency. Some adolescents walk into emergency areas because they are dependent on barbiturates and methaqualone (Quaalude) to ask for help with withdrawal. Many young people know that withdrawal from dependence on barbiturates is hazardous.

The treatment of the coma of acute barbiturate intoxication requires a clear airway. The patient should be adequately ventilated, if necessary by using a positive pressure ventilator and compressor. There is no indication for a high oxygen content, and air should be used at a rate of 10 to 12 respirations per minute. If an acutely intoxicated patient is dehydrated, an intravenous infusion of dextrose and water, or saline, is indicated. Adequate physical and neurologic examinations are necessary in any type of coma; assessment of the level of coma is essential,[3] and for this to be meaningful in terms of possible recovery, a record of the time the examination was performed should be kept. The progression of the patient through various stages of coma indicates the progress of therapy. Basically, the classification for the levels of coma is the same as that for those of anesthesia.

Withdrawal from chronic barbiturate intoxication requires in-patient hospitalization, although the use of withdrawal through out-patient therapy has been reported.[4] The withdrawal of the patient from chronic barbiturate dependence requires skilled management. A switch from a short-acting drug to phenobarbital is necessary. Desirably, 30 mg. of phenobarbital should be substituted for each 100 mg. of short-acting barbiturate the patient reports having used. Normally, this process takes about two days. Sometimes patients grossly overstate the amount of drugs they have been taking. If an excessive amount of phenobarbital therefore is given, toxic symptoms, *i.e.,* slurred speech, nystagmus, or ataxia, will appear during the first day or so of treatment.

In the event that the drug is being withdrawn too rapidly, as indicated by tremors, muscular weakness, hyperreflexia, or postural hypertension, 200 mg. of phenobarbital can be given by intramuscular injection. These are the symptoms seen when patients appear in the emergency department because they have started to withdraw themselves from barbiturates. After the patient has been stabilized on phenobarbital, the total daily dosage is decreased by 30 mg. a day as long as the withdrawal is proceeding smoothly. The phenobarbital is generally given in divided doses.

A number of young people die each year in status epilepticus from the acute withdrawal of "downers." Because of the confusion caused by barbiturates, adolescents who inject themselves or their friends with barbiturates may inadvertently pierce an artery and cause severe arterial spasm. The "high" of barbiturates is the equivalent of alcoholic intoxication; judgment therefore is not at its best. Adolescents who have been injecting barbiturates may also have liver disease as a result of syringe hepatitis.

A significant number of adolescents appear in emergency departments with severe poisoning due to nonbarbiturate sedative overdosage. Generally, such patients should be appropriately managed medically and treated conservatively until the drug has been metabolized. As with barbiturates, proper therapy requires meticulous attention to the maintenance of adequate respiration and the avoidance of respiratory infection.

Acute Alcoholism

Commonly seen in combination with use of other drugs, acute alcoholism is becoming increasingly common among adolescents. The reason is that young adolescents conform to the norms of society and identify in particular with other adolescents and young adults. When it became legally possible to drink at the age of 18, two consequences were inevitable. Many 18-year-olds are still superficially negativistic to the explicit rules of society, and they are willing to buy liquor for early and middle stage adolescents who ask them. In addition, the permission given to late adolescents by society to use alcohol is also considered by the younger group as permission for them. Between 16 and 18 years, the maturational and chronological ages can still be very dissonant; this is less true by the age of 21. Despite the flurry in society about marijuana involvement, alcohol remains the drug of choice for adults and late adolescents.

The treatment of acute alcoholic intoxication in young people and older adults is essentially the same. There is no evidence that any of the traditional techniques of sobering people affect the rate at which alcohol disappears from the blood. If alcoholic stupor is present, no special therapeutic measures are called for if vital signs are normal. Alcoholic coma is extremely rare in adolescents and is a medical emergency. Emergency support of life functions is as essential in alcoholic coma as in acute barbiturate intoxication.

Physical withdrawal syndromes are relatively rare in adolescent alcoholics, and no cases in this age group appear to have been reported in the literature. Adolescents may become as psychologically dependent on a long-term alcohol intake as they do on marijuana and cigarettes. It is not unusual for a number of adolescents to drink every day regardless of whether they are in school or at work. Adolescents are as reluctant to admit that they have adopted alcoholism as a total lifestyle as are older adults. Marijuana, which many fantasize never causes emotional dependence, is sometimes used every day with alcohol added intermittently.

Psychological symptoms associated with withdrawal are seen in adolescents. Tremors, and on occasion hallucinosis, may be present. Nutritional deficiencies are common in adolescents because of their aberrant diets, but they are rare just because of association with alcohol abuse, although they may be present in those from deprived neighborhoods and those who are runaways. When adolescents suffering from acute alcoholism are seen for initial diagnosis and for treatment, the treatment includes replacement of deficient vitamins and attention to fluid balance. Antibiotics may be necessary. Cross-dependent drugs, such as phenobarbital (0.6 to 1.2 gm. daily) or chlordiazepoxide (300 to 500 gm. daily), may help to prevent toxic neurologic symptoms. Generally, chlordiazepoxide is the drug of choice in the adolescent age group, although giving mood-changing drugs to adolescents always carries the implication that drug taking is acceptable, providing adults prescribe them.

Adolescent Reactions to Hallucinogenic Drugs

General use of LSD seems to be declining; certainly fewer adolescents experiencing bad trips are appearing in emergency departments. The acute panic reaction due to LSD typically produces changes in perception, judgment, and the sense of time and of the body's position in space. Concentration, body image, and mood may all be affected. Sometimes when the hallucinations become painful, panic and a feeling of total helplessness ensue.

It is now generally agreed that tranquilizers should not be used for the acute hallucinosis caused by LSD or any other psychodelic drug because their use may mask the effects of other drugs, such as strychnine, which are commonly mixed with street drugs. Similarly, barbiturates, which are potentiated by the phenothiazines, may be mixed with LSD.

Adolescents on bad trips should preferably be under the care of physicians or paramedical personnel who are able to diagnose the influence of drugs other than hallucinogens. Within the context of the quickly diagnosed intoxication, vital signs should always be monitored. The optimal treatment of acute hallucinosis is to "talk down" the adolescent. In order for it to be done satisfactorily, adequate handling of the patient in a safe, comfortable, and nonfrightening environment is required. The more womblike this is, the better. Inevitably, the average emergency department, with its bustle and surgically oriented rooms full of instruments, is a frightening place for a drug toxic adolescent. Nevertheless, because of the toxicity of many street drugs, particularly phencyclidine, many adolescents on bad trips end up in hospital emergency departments in the course of adequate overall treatment. The street scene has, therefore, implications for the design of hospital emergency areas.

"Talking down" is done primarily by two techniques. The therapist accepts the attitudes, words, and feelings of the patient and, adopting a firm, gentle, supportive stance, makes clear to the patient that he exists apart from the effect of the drug. The individual's attempt to hurt himself needs to be contained by gentle, firm physical control by other people, not by physical restraints.

Often body image boundaries become highly fluid, and physical contact such as holding and stroking is needed. This may create anxiety in some patients because of a perceived sexual threat. Boys who are anxious about homosexuality may become frightened of either sexuality or aggression if they are touched during the "talking down" process. One boy who became wildly anxious when his best friend tried to be physically reassuring said, "I felt he was putting my arms and legs through a meat grinder, and I thought he was going to do that to my cock and balls. It's funny I felt all that because he's my best friend." This type of complication means that when adolescents are "talked down," people of both sexes should be involved in the process.

The acute hallucinosis may be over in about six hours, but particularly after a bad trip, episodes of acute flashbacks may occur intermittently for weeks or months. Often they occur spontaneously; sometimes they are precipitated by smoking marijuana. Sometimes patients with a flashback appear in the emergency department in a panic. The treatment of these acute anxiety attacks is general reassurance, rarely tranquilizers. Again, with adolescents such drugs should not be given as part of the reassuring technique; this is likely to be perceived by the patient as societal reinforcement for drug abuse.

In patients who regularly abuse hallucinogens, a chronic syndrome that includes perceptual disorders may be present for weeks. Commonly the world is perceived as flat, and binocular vision is temporarily lost. The anxiety produced by this may induce the victim to perpetuate the state of being "strung out" by repeatedly taking small doses of hallucinogens. The attempt is to control the helplessness associated with an inconsistently appearing painful experience by deliberately inducing its appearance; the unpleasant experience is at least felt as being within the individual's control.

The duration of an acute hallucinogenic episode varies, but it is always finite. Because of the time taken to talk a patient down from a bad drug experience, some physicians use this as justification for chemical intervention. Chlorpromazine (50 mg. orally) will end an episode of acute hallucinosis. Liver function tests are particularly important in a patient with a history of heroin usage, because previous syringe hepatitis may have caused liver damage. Diazepam (Valium) in small doses (5 mg. orally) relieves the associated tension and does not oversedate the patient. Many patients in an acute hallucinogenic and toxic confused state may be hyperanxious, if not paranoid, about any pill that may be offered them. Thus, they may refuse medication by mouth.

Phencyclidine is a relatively new drug of abuse that is sometimes sold as THC, the active principle of cannabis. Phencyclidine is an hallucinogenic compound that is used as a tranquilizer for animals. When given to humans in doses of 0.1 mg. per kilogram of body weight, the immediate effects of phencyclidine include thought disorganization, concreteness, prolongation and modification of time sense, depersonalization, impaired coordination, and proprioceptive and body image sensations. Numbness of the extremities and a fluctuating sense of body size seem to be especially common; these effects are especially attractive to some patients with character problems who enjoy this "warming" experience. In patients with chronic schizophrenia, the drug has intensified the thought disorder and stimulated a considerable negative effect.[5]

The patient on a bad trip with phencyclidine often feels he is dead. As with LSD, the reassuring technique is to separate the drug from the person. Even though only phencyclidine has been taken, because of a possible paradoxical effect, phenothiazines should not be used. In addition to respiratory difficulties, convulsions may occur with phencyclidine, and the seizures can become life threatening. A combination of medical support for vital functions and anticonvulsant medication is indicated.

Marijuana smokers may sometimes appear in an emergency area in a toxic psychosis. The incidence is rare, and the diagnosis is made on the basis of the history and then an acute delusional episode. Usually the reaction has been in evidence for more than five hours before the patient is brought in. The differential diagnosis is between a toxic psychosis and a schizophrenic syndrome. Hospitalization is probably indicated. Marijuana is likely to be dangerous in persons with diabetes because one of its side effects is elevation of the blood sugar level.[6]

Parents and Drug Abuse

Many adolescents who appear in emergency departments and are suffering from toxic drug reactions either are emancipated minors or have run away from their parents. In the emergency management of drug toxicity, the function of the emergency physician is to make an adequate diagnosis as soon as possible, support life functions, and treat complications. He should avoid measures that reinforce drug misuse. As at any other time in the treatment of adolescents, the physician should be aware of the significance of his relationship with the patient. As a significant extraparental adult,[7] his attitudes about giving additional drugs and the relationship he might have made with the patient's family may influence the successfulness of the patient's rehabilitation. Within the context of the emergency department situation, once the drug toxic adolescent has recovered, the relationship between the patient and the physician may determine whether or not additional out-patient care can be undertaken.

Threats should never be used to persuade adolescents to seek further help; their only effect is likely to be to stimulate death-defying behavior. Preferably, for adolescents who are able to leave the hospital, a psychiatrist should see them before they go. He should see the individual himself the next day; otherwise the chance for adequate assessment and treatment is likely to be lost.

Chronic drug abuse, whether it be regular or progressive, is a symptom, not a disease entity.[8] Significant emotional disturbances, including family and societal pathology, are in the etiology of the syndrome. The particular problem connected with adolescent drug abuse is that in this area of human functioning, collusive and unconsciously provocative parental behavior is likely. Drug abuse is a symptom similar to that seen in adolescents who are sexually disturbed or who show inappropriate symptomatic aggression directed either toward others as assaultive behavior or toward the self as suicide attempts. Two typical parental stances may be seen.

Some parents become overanxious at drug experimentation. They commonly do not understand that drug experimentation, as distinct from drug abuse, needs to be felt as secret and forbidden by early adolescents. "With it" parents, who state that they do not mind the "moderate use of grass," may destroy an adolescent's attempt at autonomy with permissiveness. They give the adolescent permission to use drugs and force him into a position in which more has to be used.

Some parents are so overcontrolling in response to adolescent experimentation with drugs or sex that they force on their young people a degree of destructive rebellion or isolated withdrawal. The emergency department staff should understand the role of the parents in the adolescent's drug abuse before assuming that they will help their child get assistance. The parents' answer to the question of whether they have ever noticed that their child takes drugs indicates a great deal about parent-child-drug interactions.

Hospitalization

The difficulty in diagnosing the etiology of drug abuse is often a justification for hospitalizing the early drug-dependent adolescent. Only when adolescents are free of drug use will they be able to achieve a meaningful emotional relationship with others. Only through positive emotional attachments to individuals who do not abuse drugs is it possible for young people to abandon the habit. These relationships cannot be made while the adolescent is drug toxic. Neither can the differential diagnosis be made among the adolescent drug abuser who is suffering from resolvable traumatic or situational anxiety, the abuser who has identity difficulties but an otherwise reasonably intact personality, and the abuser who has severe emotional illness, either characterologic or schizophrenic.

Some adolescents may have a sufficiently intact personality to work out their difficulties either in groups or through individual relationships that are healthy, but specifically psychotherapeutic. Others, without being able to use formal psychotherapy, may be able to use a network of human contacts. Some adolescents need more formal psychotherapy to help in resolving the conflict. The emergency department staff needs to decide whether or not a patient should be admitted to the psychiatric ward if medical admission is not indicated. Admission is justified if sophisticated psychiatric diagnosis is possible, and if competent adolescent treatment settings are available. There is justification for hospitalizing severely drug dependent adolescents for a brief period of four to six weeks to determine whether, when they are detoxified from drug use, they are able to achieve meaningful emotional relationships with others.

As adolescents progress into maturity, they may be able to ask for help in words rather than through action, but this depends on their social environment: the availability of persons able to help, the quality of care available, and how these are perceived by local youth. If magical solutions are offered, adolescents are quick to perceive them as pretentious and no better than the solutions they themselves try. "All you want to do is get us strung out on your thing rather than mine," said one angry late adolescent to a family practitioner who offered him tranquilizers for his drug dependence. The ability to ask for assistance in words also depends on an adolescent's perception of the value of helping adults as people and whether or not they are thought to be collusive in the drug scene.

In all the emotional problems of adolescence that require treatment, the motivation of the adolescent and his family is always a crucial issue in treatment. Before the drug scene had spread pervasively through society, the most difficult problems of adolescent treatment were those connected with sexual perversions and promiscuous behavior, because these activities seemed to offer a magical solution to difficulties and by infantile behavior helped in the flight from psychological tension. Now drugs provide this regressive and apparently magical solution to conflict and, therefore, motivation for therapy is adversely influenced. Furthermore, adolescents who were initially motivated to seek assistance and are in ongoing psychotherapy for problems unrelated to drugs may discover these and then become relatively inaccessible.

Usually only early adolescents who are in severe psychic pain—very depressed or psychologically disintegrating—are consciously motivated. It is not unusual, however, for family psychopathology to appear under the guise of adolescent maladjustment. The adolescent is the "ticket of admission" for the family to obtain help, although in these situations the motivation is not usually that of the young person.

Insofar as the problem of drug dependence is a problem of motivation, the physician is in a position similar to that in which he may have been in the past with an actively destructive or delinquent adolescent. The physician may have to be prepared to arrange for the protection of the young person directly with all the legal and therapeutic complications of assuming a magical, omnipotent role.

References

1. Dole, V. P. et al. 1971. Methadone poisoning. *N.Y. State J. Med.,* 71:541–563.
2. Chemlin, C. et al. 1972. The epidemiology of death in narcotic addicts. *Amer. J. Epidem.,* 96:11–22.
3. Reed, C. E., Diggs, M. F., and Foote C. C. 1952. Acute barbiturate intoxication: A study of 300 cases based on a physiologic system of classification of the severity of the intoxication. *Ann. Intern. Med.,* 37:290.
4. Gay, G. R., et al. 1971. A new method of out-patient treatment of barbiturate withdrawal. *J. Psychedel. Drugs,* 3(2):81–88.
5. Rosenbaum, G. et al. 1959. Comparison of Sernyl with other drugs. *Arch. Gen. Psychiat.,* 1:651–656.
6. Bier, M. M., and Steahly, L. P. 1974. Emergency treatment of marijuana complicating diabetes, in *A Treatment Manual for Acute Drug Emergencies,* P. G. Boune (ed.). Washington, D. C., NCDAT Pub., pp. 88–95.
7. Miller, D. 1974. *Adolescent Psychology, Psychopathology and Psychotherapy.* New York, Jason Aronson, pp. 52–56.
8. Miller, D. 1973. The drug dependent adolescent, in *Adolescent Psychiatry,* Vol. II, S. C. Feinstein and P. Giovacchini (eds.). New York, Basic Books, pp. 70–98.

11

Tetanus

F. Robert Fekety and Joseph Silva

Tetanus (lockjaw) is a disease of the neuromuscular system caused by an exotoxin produced by *Clostridium tetani* in infected wounds. Although the site of the infection is often insignificant, the disease has a high mortality rate and is characterized by intense stimulation of motor neurons and painful generalized muscle spasms.[1,3]

Historical Aspects. Tetanus was recognized by a number of ancient physicians, including Hippocrates, but its nature was unclear until 1884 when Nicolaier produced a similar disease in animals by inoculating them with garden soil. He also noticed long, thin bacilli in the wound pus and suggested that these organisms multiplied locally and produced a poison similar to strychnine. Kitasato isolated *Cl. tetani* in pure culture from pus in 1889, using anaerobic media and the technique of heating the exudate to 80° C for about one hour to destroy nonsporulating organisms. When pure cultures of the organism were inoculated into animals, the disease was reproduced. Injection of small amounts of a toxin produced by the organism was found to result in the production of protective antibodies in 1890, and Ramon developed tetanus toxoid in 1923. Total paralysis with curare became feasible as definitive therapy in 1953.[1]

Microbiological Aspects. *Clostridium tetani* is a large, gram-positive, nonencapsulated, motile, spore-forming anaerobic bacillus with a characteristic "drumstick" appearance. It is an obligate anaerobe. Spores of *Cl. tetani* are highly resistant to antiseptics and moderately resistant to heat. Boiling for four hours may be required to kill the spores, but autoclaving them for 10 minutes at 120° C is effective.

Clostridium tetani can be isolated from soil, street dust, the air of operating rooms, unsterile surgical supplies, clothing, vegetables, and animal and human feces.

The organism produces two exotoxins: tetanospasmin and tetanolysin. Although there are 10 antigenic types of the organism, their toxins are immunologically identical. Tetanospasmin is a potent neurotoxin that causes the muscle spasm of tetanus. A fraction of a milligram is lethal to man. Tetanolysin hemolyzes erythrocytes *in vitro*. Its relation to the disease is uncertain, although experimental evidence suggests it has severe cardiovascular effects.[5,24]

Pathogenesis of the Disease. Tetanus bacilli usually gain entrance to the body through wounds. Multiplication of the organism and production of the toxin depend on devitalized tissue and anaerobic conditions. In countries with good medical care, serious wounds are usually treated properly; an increasing proportion of tetanus is traced to minor or insignificant wounds that never receive treatment. The most common lesions responsible for tetanus are lacerations, splinters, compound fractures, infected abortions, gunshot wounds, cutaneous and decubitus ulcers, tooth extractions, burns, frost-bite wounds, nail or pitchfork puncture wounds, human or animal bites and narcotic injections.[11] Addicts who inject drugs subcutaneously ("skin-poppers") are especially prone to tetanus. This practice is particularly common in young women, whose immunity may have waned. Historically, tetanus has been a frequent complication of war wounds (Fig. 11-1), but immunization has practically eliminated this problem.

Ischemia, necrotic tissues, foreign bodies, and coexisting infections with aerobic organisms that decrease the tissue oxygen tension are the most important factors predisposing to the disease. Spores may persist dormant in the tissues for long periods and later produce tetanus when the proper conditions occur.

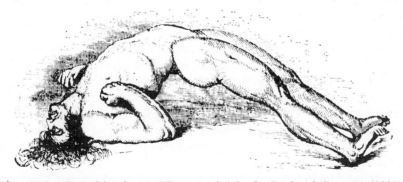

Fig. 11-1. Convulsion in a soldier wounded in the Battle of Corunna (1809). The original sketch by Sir Charles Bell is in the College of Surgeons in Edinburgh. The opisthotonos, alertness, and risus sardonicus are characteristic of tetanus. Bell, a surgeon, noted that "were the painter to represent every circumstance faithfully, the effect might be too painful, and something must be left to his taste and imagination."

The organism shows little tendency to invade tissues and produces few local pathologic changes. Even in fatal tetanus the toxin does not produce detectable histologic lesions in the neuromuscular system. The primary targets of the toxin are the anterior horn cells of the spinal cord, and centers in the medulla and other parts of the central nervous system. The toxin has a high affinity for nervous tissue and gangliosides, and is not neutralized or removed by antitoxin after combination with ganglioside receptor sites. The route by which the toxin travels from the wound to the nervous system is still controversial. Toxin can travel up nerves centripetally to the spinal cord and then throughout the central nervous system, and it also can spread to the nervous system via the blood. The biochemical action of the toxin has not been established, but it is believed that it interferes with the action of cholinesterase and inhibitory neurons governing motor impulses at synaptic junctions, thus inducing motor hyperactivity and spasticity. It seems to convert synaptic inhibition to excitation.[24]

Epidemiology. Tetanus occurs world-wide, but in the United States the incidence has declined markedly over the past 25 years, with about 200 to 300 cases now reported annually. Many mild cases are not reported. About three-fourths of cases in the northern hemisphere occur from April through September, and the disease is more common in warm climates. Rates are higher in the southern states and developing countries.[11]

Outdoor injuries contaminated with soil are frequently important in pathogenesis, and tetanus is more frequent in men who have agricultural or outdoor occupations. The disease is also more frequent in blacks, which is partly attributed to their lower frequency of immunization. Incidence and mortality rates are higher in persons over 50, narcotic addicts and neonates. Poverty, unavailability of good medical care, and a lack of education are associated with high rates of tetanus.

Neonatal tetanus is an important cause of infant mortality in developing countries. Neonatal tetanus in the United States occurs at a rate of about two cases per million live births, but in blacks the rate is 10 times higher. It is often related to the delivery of unimmunized mothers outside of hospitals by midwives who use unsterile techniques in managing the umbilical cord. In some primitive countries, animal dung is used as a dressing on the cord stump, a practice that frequently causes neonatal tetanus.

Clinical Manifestations. The incubation period of tetanus following the injury may be as short as two days or as long as several months. Ordinarily the illness begins 6 to 14 days after the injury. The usual prodrome consists only of restlessness, headache, and soreness calling attention to the rigidity of a muscle group. The muscles of the face and jaw are most frequently involved, but pain may be noted first in the back or neck. Low back pain is a common early symptom and may be ignored. Spasticity of the muscles of mastication causes trismus or the inability to open the mouth, thus accounting for the name *lockjaw*. Prolonged contraction of facial muscles along with clenched teeth may produce a distorted grin in severe cases (risus sardonicus). Rigidity may affect only the wounded limb (local tetanus), or the patient may have mild generalized spasticity. In severe cases, generalized rigidity and intermittent convulsions (reflex spasms) occur, and they are the most serious manifestations of the disease.[1,3,10]

It is important to appreciate the varying degrees of severity of tetanus. The *incubation period* is defined as the period between injury and the first sign of tetanus; the *onset period* is the period between the first sign of the disease and the first generalized spasm. Both are of use in estimating severity and in predicting prognosis. If the incubation period is less than seven days and the onset period is less than three days, the illness may be expected to be severe and have a high fatality rate (70%); if the incubation period is longer than two weeks, only 20% of victims die. The onset period is more reliable in estimating prognosis. If it exceeds five days, the mortality rate is only 10%, as contrasted to a fatality rate of 80% when signs of symptoms rapidly progress within the first 24 hours.

The *mild case* of tetanus is characterized primarily by rigidity and muscle pain. Muscle spasms are short and do not interfere with breathing. The mortality rate for mild tetanus is less than 10%, and the patient usually begins to improve after about five days.

The *moderate case* of tetanus is characterized by severe generalized rigidity and dysphagia. The mouth can hardly be opened, and muscle stiffness makes the patient lie rigidly in bed as if at attention. Opisthotonos may be observed during paroxysmal spasms. Reflex spasms or tonic seizures may occur spontaneously, but more frequently result from external stimuli such as cold air, noise, changes in lighting, moving or turning the patient, and ingestion of fluids. Paroxysms may also be precipitated by internal nervous stimuli from distention of bowel or bladder, or mucus plugs in bronchi and coughing. Improvement in moderate tetanus usually begins in the second week.

The most important difference between mild and moderate tetanus is the absence of dysphagia in mild tetanus, even though there may be pain on swallowing. Dysphagia is caused by pharyngeal muscle spasm and is important primarily because it predisposes to aspiration and pneumonia. Patients with tetanus involving the head and neck are usually placed in the moderate category. A tracheotomy is indicated in every patient with moderate tetanus. The patient with mild tetanus should be encouraged to drink some liquid every few hours under supervision so that one can detect the onset of dysphagia due to spasms of the pharyngeal muscles. Coughing or sputtering while drinking is an early characteristic sign of the moderate case.

The *severe case* of tetanus is characterized by opisthotonos, board-like abdominal rigidity, and paroxysmal spasms or convulsions, which are prolonged, frequent, and interfere with breathing. Spasms of the laryngeal muscles, diaphragm, and intercostal muscles prevent ventilation and cause asphyxia in severe tetanus and are its most important characteristic. Fractures and dislocations of vertebrae or long bones, ecchymoses, and muscle hematomas may occur during these violent spasms. Patients with severe tetanus may also have evidence of autonomic dysfunction as evidenced by paroxysmal hypertension, tachycardia, profuse sweating, hyperthermia, and peripheral vasoconstriction, either spontaneously or in response to stimuli known to precipitate spasms.[9] If the patient with severe tetanus survives, a gradual reduction in intensity and frequency of spasms usually begins in the second week of the illness, but complete recovery may take six weeks or more.

Although patients with moderate and severe tetanus may be mentally alert and tragically aware of their condition, most severely ill patients are actually stuporous or unconscious. The electroencephalogram may show a sleep pattern. It is surprising how little most patients remember of the details of the acute illness during convalescence.[8]

Neonatal tetanus is usually of the generalized or severe form and begins three to ten days after birth. The first sign is usually difficulty in sucking, which progresses to total inability to feed. Spasms and death soon ensue.

The *physical examination* in tetanus usually reveals only marked muscular hypertonicity, hyperactive deep tendon reflexes, and sustained clonus. There is no sensory involvement. There is usually only a low-grade fever unless the patient has other complicating infections or sympathetic hyperactivity. Peripheral vasoconstriction, tachycardia, and blood pressure alterations are frequent in severe tetanus.[9] Mentation is normal in early tetanus but may be clouded in severe tetanus.

Laboratory studies show a moderate leukocytosis and eventually anemia. The cerebrospinal fluid pressure may be slightly increased, but it is otherwise normal. Myoglobulinuria may be detected. Fewer than half of wound cultures in tetanus are positive for the etiologic agent, since other organisms frequently coexist in the wound and overgrow *Cl. tetani*. The electroencephalogram may be normal or show a sleep pattern.

An important factor in *differential diagnosis* is the history of immunization against tetanus. The disease is extremely uncommon in any person who has had a *complete* series of tetanus immunizations. The most common local condition that results in stiffness of the jaw and that is sometimes confused with tetanus is an alveolar (dental) abscess or local infection of the mouth. This is usually unilateral and readily detected on physical examination. Meningitis can be excluded if the spinal fluid is normal and not only the neck but all muscle groups are rigid.

All too frequently, patients with early tetanus are mistakenly thought to be psychoneurotic. Complaints of stiffness of the jaws or back are often ignored, particularly when the patient is an addict. Hysterical reactions and bizarre dystonic extrapyramidal neuromuscular reactions to phenothiazine drugs are also misleading. In these patients, the jaw usually can be opened completely, even though tremors and bizarre grimacing are frequent. The patient treated with phenothiazines may also have athetoid movements, tonic torticollis, and clonic twitching. An intravenous injection of 50 mg. of diphenhydramine (Benadryl) produces relief in about one-half of patients with phenothiazine reactions.

Although strychnine poisoning is very similar to tetanus, generalized muscular rigidity develops rapidly and trismus tends to appear late. Encephalitis occasionally may be confused with tetanus, but these patients have a clouded sensorium, they are febrile, and their cerebrospinal fluid reveals protein and cellular abnormalities. Animal bites are implicated in both rabies and tetanus. The most important feature distinguishing rabies is that trismus is not present and the spinal fluid may be abnormal.

Complications. Bronchopulmonary infections are important causes of morbidity and mortality, but they are less common following early and skillful use of tracheostomy and respirators. The frequency of pulmonary emboli in patients with tetanus requiring pharmacologic paralysis is high. In some series, cardiac arrhythmias and myocardial infarction are frequent, especially in patients over 50. These may be related to the intense muscular work and sympathetic hyperactivity that characterize severe tetanus. Acute gastric ulcers, fecal impaction, and urinary retention and infection often complicate severe tetanus. Death due to tetanus is most frequently related to asphyxiation during a generalized spasm or to a complicating pulmonary infection.

One of the most remarkable features of tetanus is that the disease produces no histopathologic lesions in the nervous system, and that when patients recover, even from the most severe forms of the disease, they usually recover completely. A recent retrospective analysis of 25 tetanus patients, however, revealed sequelae of sleep disturbances, seizures, myoclonus, decreased libido, postural hypotension, episodes of irritability, and electroencephalographic abnormalities persisting for several months to years after the disease resolved.[8]

Prognosis. The overall mortality rate in tetanus is 30 to 40%. The rates are higher in neonates, addicts, and the elderly.

Prevention of Tetanus

There is no doubt that huge strides have been made in the prophylaxis of tetanus in the past century. The basic principles are: (1) promotion of toxoid immunization before and after injury, (2) prompt and meticulous surgical care of wounds, (3) use of human tetanus immune globulin (TIG) in nonimmune persons, and (4) use of antibiotics as ancillary measures in tetanus-prone wounds. If these measures are correctly applied, tetanus can and should become a disease of historical significance only.

Active Immunization Before Injury. Tetanus toxoid is one of the most effective immunizing agents known. In fully immunized persons the failure rate is less than 4 per 100 million persons. Active immunization can be achieved safely and with virtual certainty unless the individual has a disease associated with deficient antibody production. Passive immunization after injury is much less efficacious. Furthermore, active immunization is the only way to prevent tetanus resulting from wounds so insignificant that the patient does not seek medical attention. Newborn infants of fully immunized mothers are immune to the disease, and active immunization of women is the only satisfactory way to prevent neonatal tetanus, especially in developing countries.

Most school children in the United States are adequately immunized against tetanus, and most adult men are given boosters at the time of military service. These two groups, therefore, are usually immune. In the United States the following groups are relatively underimmunized: (1) impoverished children or adults who have been denied adequate preventive medical care, (2) young adult women who have not received a booster since early childhood, and (3) elderly adults who have never been immunized or have not received a booster for more than 20 years.

There are two types of tetanus toxoids in general use: an alum-precipitated or adsorbed toxoid and a fluid toxoid. The alum-precipitated toxoid is effective and more satisfactory, and should be used for all primary immunization. Either toxoid may be used as a booster following wounding.[13]

The American Academy of Pediatrics recommends active immunization of infants with the diphtheria, tetanus, and pertussis vaccine (DPT) at two months of age, with boosters one and two months later. Another booster is given at 15 to 18 months of age, and again between 4 and 6 years of age prior to entry to school. A combined tetanus and diphtheria toxoid (Td) is recommended for those over six years of age. Plain tetanus toxoid may be used in adults.

The first dose of tetanus toxoid usually produces no more than transiently detectable and nonprotective levels of antibody. Protective levels are reached about 10 days after the first booster injection. Because these levels are not maintained, a second booster is needed, and it rapidly produces very high and long-lasting levels of protective antibody. Subsequent booster or reinforcing doses rapidly evoke protective levels of antibody. Immunity is estimated to last for at least 10 and probably 20 years.[14]

Routine boosters are recommended only every 10 years from the age of 12 to 14 on. Annual boosters or boosters at the time of going to summer camp, for examples, are unnecessary, and may result in needless adverse reactions to tetanus toxoid. Hypersensitivity reactions to toxoid are being recognized with increasing frequency, and are more frequent when antibody titers are high.[4] Frequent boosters thus tend to predispose to them. The usual manifestation is an urticarial rash or an inflamed injection site. Serum sickness and anaphylactic reactions to toxoid have been reported but are extremely rare.

Prevention of Tetanus After Injury. Regardless of the immunization status of the patient, immediate surgical treatment of the wound with removal of all necrotic tissue and foreign bodies should be provided. Debridement is the most important aspect of prophylaxis against tetanus. The following are high risk or tetanus-prone injuries, and patients with them should receive the best possible preventive measures: compound fractures, gunshot wounds, burns, crush injuries, wounds with retained foreign bodies, deep puncture wounds, wounds contaminated with soil or manure, wounds untended for more than 24 hours, wounds infected with other bacteria, wounds with necrotic and avascular tissue, and wounds following induced abortion.

A careful immunization history should be obtained from patients with tetanus-prone injuries. Immunized persons are urged to have a written record of their immunization status. A patient should be considered unimmunized if he has not received a complete series of tetanus immunizations with a booster dose within the past 10 years.

The American College of Surgeons has developed guidelines for immunoprophylaxis following wounding. With minor modifications, these recommendations are summarized as follows:

> *Immunized patients.* A toxoid booster is not needed if the patient has received a booster within the previous five years and the wound is relatively minor and easily debrided. On the other hand, if the wound is severe, neglected, tetanus-prone, or more than 24

hours old, a booster of 0.5 ml. of adsorbed tetanus toxoid should be given unless a booster was received within the previous year.

When the patient has been actively immunized, and the interval since the last reinforcing or booster dose is less than 10 years, a booster of 0.5 ml. of adsorbed tetanus toxoid is sufficient for the prophylaxis of tetanus. Administration of antitoxin or immune globulin is not necessary unless the wound is severe, neglected, tetanus-prone, or more than 24 hours old. It must be emphasized that a booster alone is sufficient only if the patient has received a complete immunizing series in the past.

To those who have not received a booster within 10 years (and those with severe, neglected wounds), a booster of 0.5 ml. of adsorbed toxoid should be administered, and 250 units of human tetanus immune globulin should also be given intramuscularly. Consideration should be given to treating such patients with penicillin or tetracycline for four or five days, but antibiotics are no substitute for immunization. The use of equine antitoxin is not recommended in such persons because of the high frequency of serious allergic responses to it.

Unimmunized patients. Patients who have not been *completely* immunized previously with tetanus toxoid should be given passive immunization with immune globulin unless the wound is clean and minor and the development of tetanus is unlikely. Active tetanus immunization should also be initiated with 0.5 ml. of adsorbed tetanus toxoid in susceptible patients, and they should be given instructions for completing the immunizing series. *In nonimmune persons, tetanus toxoid given at the time of treatment of a wound will provide no protection against tetanus from that wound. Passive immunization is needed instead.*

Nonimmunized persons at risk of developing tetanus need to be given no more than 250 units of human tetanus immune globulin. This is always given intramuscularly, never intravenously (because of the risk of anaphylactoid reactions). It is nonsensitizing, does not produce allergic reactions, does not require prior skin testing, and does not transmit serum hepatitis (hepatitis B, Australia antigen positive hepatitis). It is less expensive than equine antitoxin (TAT) when the costs of allergic reactions to the latter are taken into consideration. A dose of 250 units contains enough antitoxin to provide passive immunity for about one month, and should be repeated if the injury is still tetanus-prone one month later. If the wounds are massive, difficult to debride, and highly contaminated with material likely to contain tetanus spores, the dose of human tetanus immune globulin should be 500 units.

Human tetanus immune globulin may be given at the same time as toxoid, but it should be administered in a different extremity and in a different syringe. It probably should *not* be given more than an hour *before* tetanus toxoid, but should be given at the same time or an hour or two *after* toxoid in order to avoid competition or inactivation.[15]

If human tetanus immune globulin is not available, one should consider infusing 1 unit of plasma from a person who has been immunized against tetanus within the past year. If neither human tetanus immune globulin nor plasma is available, the use of equine antitoxin may be considered. This should be uncommon, and in the United States is not recommended. If human tetanus immune globulin can be obtained within 24 hours following treatment of the wound, equine antitoxin should not be given. All persons considered to be candidates for equine antitoxin because the immune globulin is not available should be questioned regarding possible sensitivity to horse serum. If the patient has a definite history of allergic reactions to equine serum, it should not be used, and prophylaxis with antibiotics until the wound is healed (along with active immunization) should be substituted. Desensitization with equine antitoxin probably is of little value in preventing severe reactions. A history of allergic disease of any type should be considered a warning of probable hypersensitivity reactions to equine antitoxin. The use of equine antitoxin must be based upon a decision that the possibility of tetanus outweighs the danger of serious reaction to heterologous serum.

Equine antitoxin is still used frequently outside of the United States. All persons selected to receive equine antitoxin should be tested for sensitivity to it by both skin and conjunctival tests. We suggest the following method:

1. The initial skin test should be an intradermal deposit of 0.02 to 0.03 ml. of a 1:100 dilution of normal horse serum or antitoxin. A positive skin reaction consists of an area of erythema no less than 1 cm. in diameter and a wheal at least 0.5 cm. in diameter within 30 minutes. Reactions of a lesser degree are negative.

2. Simultaneously with the preceding test, a single drop of a 1:10 dilution of the equine serum should be deposited in the conjunctival sac of one eye. Appearance of conjunctivitis within 30 minutes is a positive test.

3. After 30 minutes, if neither of the preceding tests is positive, 0.02 to 0.03 ml. of a 1:10 dilution of horse serum should be used as another intradermal test.

4. If none of the preceding tests is positive, the indicated dose of equine antitoxin may be administered. If the tests are positive, chemoprophylaxis may be used, because desensitization is probably of little value. An attempt should be made to obtain immune globulin or plasma.

5. Only specifically assigned and trained persons should be allowed to administer and interpret these tests. When questions arise about the advisability of utilizing equine antitoxin or the interpretation of the test, an experienced physician should be consulted.

6. There should be a one-half to one hour observation period following the skin test or the serum injection. Emergency medication such as adrenalin (1:1,000) should be readily available. The patient should be seen by a nurse or doctor before being discharged from the clinic.

7. When equine antitoxin is given, a dose of 5,000 units may be used for adults. In infants and children, an equivalent dosage based on body weight should be given, but not less than 3,000 units.

8. Equine antitoxin administration should be considered a once-in-a-lifetime procedure, and all patients receiving it should be actively immunized with toxoid so that equine antitoxin will never again be needed.

If a wounded patient has a disease associated with poor production of gamma globulin, he should be given tetanus immune globulin even though he has been actively immunized. These diseases include congenital hypogammaglobulinemia and related syndromes, chronic lymphocytic leukemia, multiple myeloma, macroglobulinemia of Waldenström, and malignant lymphoma. Patients with kidney or heart transplants, or who are receiving x-irradiation, immunosuppressive drugs, or adrenocorticosteroids are also often deficient in antibody-forming capacity and are best treated with tetanus immune globulin after receiving a tetanus-prone wound.

Chemoprophylaxis. Antimicrobial drugs may aid in preventing tetanus by inhibiting the multiplication of *Cl. tetani* and by killing the vegetative form of the organism. They probably do little to influence spores, which may persist in tissues in a dormant state until antibiotics are withdrawn, after which they may cause tetanus. Adequate surgical debridement is thus essential when antibiotics instead of passive immunization are used. Antibiotics may be beneficial because they inhibit co-infecting aerobic organisms, thus preventing the development of anaerobic conditions, but antibiotics have no effect on the tetanus toxin. Some physicians in the United Kingdom have recommended chemoprophylaxis with antibiotics as an alternative to using equine antitoxin.[21] Whether this is beneficial is not yet certain, but there seems to have been no increase in the frequency of tetanus in the United Kingdom since this practice became popular. Toxoid should also be administered, probably weekly for the first month after injury.

Clostridium tetani is susceptible to a variety of antimicrobial drugs, especially penicillin, tetracycline, erythromycin, ampicillin, and cephalothin; it therefore is not difficult to choose a suitable drug for a given patient. The organism is rarely susceptible to streptomycin. If chemoprophylaxis is to be given, it must be started early, probably within the first six hours after injury, if it is to be efficacious. Antibiotics should be continued for five days or longer, depending upon the healing of the wound. If these conditions cannot be met, some other form of prophylaxis should be used.

Treatment of Tetanus

The treatment of established tetanus involves consideration of four major areas: (1) optimal wound care, with elimination of *Cl. tetani* and termination of toxin production, (2) potential inactivation of toxin with antitoxin, (3) management of seizures, rigidity, respiratory distress, and other manifestations of the intoxication, and (4) provision of optimal supportive care. The rates of mortality and complications from tetanus are low in centers where tetanus is seen frequently and treated according to a routine, even though preferred regimens vary markedly among hospitals and countries.[2]

Wound Care. The site of *Cl. tetani* infection is frequently obvious when the wound is contaminated with soil or foreign bodies or contains inflamed or necrotic tissue. Such wounds should be extensively debrided or excised and may be irrigated with undiluted hydrogen peroxide (3%). The wound should be allowed to heal by secondary intention. Extremity amputation is rarely necessary because of tetanus and should be avoided. Repeated debridement may be necessary. When the site of infection is not apparent, foreign bodies (such as splinters) in the hands or feet, minute puncture wounds, dental abscesses, chronic mastoiditis, sinusitis, decubitus ulcers, or induced abortions are the likely factors. Cultures and gram stains of the wound exudate are helpful in guiding antibiotic therapy when mixed infection is present.

Procaine penicillin G (1.2 million units twice a day intramuscularly) is adequate for treatment of superficial wounds. If the wound is extensive and contains much necrotic tissue, 10 to 20 million units of intravenous penicillin G should be given daily. Gentamicin can be given if gram-negative bacteria are also present. Antibiotic therapy can be modified later according to the response and results of cultures. Tetracycline (250 mg. intravenously four times daily), cephalothin (2.0 gm. intravenously four times daily), or erythromycin (250 mg. intravenously four times daily) may be used for patients who are allergic to penicillin. Antibiotics should not be used as substitutes for surgical drainage unless the focus of infection cannot be identified.

Tetanus Antitoxin. Proof of the effectiveness of antitoxin or immune globulin in the treatment of tetanus is still not available. Once toxin has been bound to nervous tissue, there is no evidence that it can be inactivated or removed by antitoxin. Antitoxin is used primarily because it may neutralize toxin that is circulating or still unbound. Free tetanus toxin has been detected in wound margins, blood, and cerebrospinal fluid. There are reports that antitoxin is beneficial in treating humans with tetanus, but others believe it is of little value.[17,23] Most physicians give the patient the benefit of the doubt and use antitoxin.

Antitoxin derived from either humans (TIG) or immunized horses (TAT) has been used. Ample supplies of human tetanus immune globulin have obviated the need for equine tetanus antitoxin in the United States. Equine antitoxin has produced adverse reactions, such as serum sickness, polyneuritis, myocarditis, and anaphylaxis in 5 to 6% of adult recipients. Less serious reactions occur almost uniformly. Adverse reactions to human tetanus immune globulin are rare. There is a suggestion, however, that equine antitoxin may be more efficacious than the human form in treatment, possibly because it can be given intravenously and in larger amounts than the human type. Higher initial cerebrospinal or nervous tissue concentrations therefore can be attained rapidly. Human tetanus immune globulin is used in smaller doses (3,000 to 6,000 units) than equine antitoxin (10,000 to 500,000 units) because it has a longer biologic half-life (25 days) than the equine form (7 to 14 days).

Human antitoxin is obtained from people who have been immunized with tetanus toxoid. It is concentrated and contains 165 mg. of immunoglobulin (mainly IgG) per milliliter and is available in 250 unit ampules. The optimal dose in treatment of tetanus has not been established. A dose of 3,000 to 6,000 units has been suggested, but 1,500 units yield an average serum concentration of 0.08 to 0.16 units per milliliter, and a level of 0.01 unit per milliliter is considered protective. We recommend a total of 3,000 to 6,000 units (24 to 48 ml.) be given intramuscularly at several sites to patients with tetanus, with 500 to 1,000 units given in the region of the wound. Human tetanus immune globulin should not be given intravenously. There is no rationale for additional or subsequent doses. Injection sites should be massaged, and heat may be applied to facilitate absorption. It should be given one or two hours prior to wound debridement so that protective levels of antitoxin will be present in the serum during surgery when toxin may be released into the circulation.

The use of intrathecal antitoxin is highly debatable. Although tetanus toxoid and tetanospasmin penetrate the cerebrospinal fluid, antitoxic antibodies fail to enter this compartment in significant amounts. Intrathecal injection of antitoxin has been avoided for fear of inducing allergic meningitis and cerebral edema, even though there is experimental evidence in support of this procedure. Mice with tetanus benefit from intrathecal equine tetanus antitoxin, and dogs with tetanus treated with intrathecal equine antitoxin and prednisolone have a higher survival rate than do those treated only with intravenous or intramuscular equine antitoxin. Ildirim has given equine antitoxin and prednisolone intrathecally to 28 neonates and three children with tetanus, along with intramuscular and intravenous equine antitoxin and large doses of prednisolone. Only three neonates died, which was less than half of the expected mortality rate.[7] These results are encouraging, but controlled studies are needed.

Active Immunization. The tetanus toxin is so potent that amounts sufficient to produce the disease do not produce immunity. Patients with tetanus should be immunized with tetanus toxoid in order to prevent future attacks, as recommended in the section concerning prevention.

Recent experiments have shown that large doses of tetanus toxoid given to unimmunized animals protected them against lethal doses of tetanus toxin, possibly by competing with tetanospasmin for binding sites. The clinical applicability of these experiments is still speculative, and the administration of large amounts of toxoid to patients is not recommended. It has been recommended that a booster dose of 0.5 ml. of toxoid should be given every three days to patients with tetanus, primarily because protective levels of antibody may be attained more rapidly. This is also of dubious value.

Aspects of Management Varying With the Severity of Tetanus. Criteria for categorizing patients with tetanus according to severity were described earlier. These are helpful in planning and standardizing therapy. Serious complications such as pneumonia or asphyxia are much more frequent in severe tetanus. The need for specialized treatment and close observation should be anticipated in severe cases, and may require transfer to larger centers.

Muscle relaxants and sedatives are the keystone in the treatment of *mild or moderate tetanus*. The therapeutic goal is to eliminate spasms and reduce rigidity for about a week until the bound toxin is eliminated. Dosage must be determined empirically and individualized according to physical signs. The patient can be titrated until trismus, opisthotonos, and rigidity of extremity and abdominal muscles disappear. Palpation of the rectus abdominis muscles is a helpful guide to dosage and interval.

Mild cases of tetanus can be managed with sedatives such as phenobarbital, secobarbital, or pentobarbital. Sodium thiopental has been used with success in moderately severe cases, and is usually administered as an intravenous drip at the rate of about 20 drops per minute (0.5 to 1.0 gm. per liter of solution) until the patient becomes sleepy but still obeys commands. This can be supplemented with an intravenous 10-ml. bolus of thiopental (2.5% solution, 250 mg.) if a convulsion occurs. This will produce relaxation in less than a minute. Paraldehyde is another popular and useful sedative. Eight to 12 ml. is administered every four hours orally or by nasogastric tube (usually diluted 1:10 in milk or juice). Its intramuscular use is limited because it may result in necrotic abscesses.

Many physicians prefer to use tranquilizers that have proven muscle relaxant and antispasmodic effects instead of sedatives. Since these drugs do not reliably prevent serious convulsions, which may have a fatal outcome, the patient must be observed at all times. Diazepam (Valium) is most frequently used because it produces few side effects and reduces hypertonicity and spasms without inducing cortical depression. It is administered parenterally in 10-mg. doses every four hours in mild cases. Moderate and severe cases usually require larger and more frequent doses (10 to 40 mg. every two hours intravenously). A continuous intravenous infusion is useful in titrating the patient to a sleepy state (at least 100 mg. per liter of solution per 24 hours). Large doses of diazepam can cause a syndrome of alert wakefulness and mute tetraplegia (the "locked-in syndrome").

Meprobamate may be used instead of diazepam in a 400-mg. intramuscular dose every two to four hours in adults. The usual dose in infants is 50 to 100 mg. and in children 100 to 200 mg. The effects of meprobamate and diazepam can be prolonged or accentuated with small doses of phenobarbital, such as 1 mg. per kilogram of body weight every four to six hours.

Most physicians use two different kinds of drugs, one given in maximal dosage as a baseline, and the other given intermittently as needed. A combination of diazepam and intravenous thiopental has been very useful.

Patients with *moderate tetanus* have dysphagia, but their episodic spasms do not embarrass respiration or cause cyanosis or dyspnea. Mild tetanus involving the head and neck is placed in the moderate category. Tracheostomy is performed routinely and electively, usually under general anesthesia and with insertion of a cuffed tube in moderate tetanus. This is to prevent aspiration of food, liquids, or oropharyngeal secretions, which may result in suffocation, atelectasis, or pneumonia. Important measures in tracheostomy care include humidification, daily change of tubing and reservoir solutions, aseptic techniques for tracheal suctioning, and chest physiotherapy.

Tranquilizers or sedatives are given as in mild tetanus, but larger doses are usually required. If the patient suffers severe spasm of respiratory muscles while receiving muscle relaxants, anoxia may be prevented by administering oxygen at high flow rates. Such patients should be advanced to the severe tetanus category. Serial determinations of arterial blood gases and measurements of the vital capacity (VC) and forced expiratory volume (FEV) should be used to decide whether patients are developing significant respiratory paralysis. If the vital capacity is less than 15 ml. per kilogram of body weight and the forced expiratory volume is less than 10 ml. per kilogram of body weight, mechanical ventilatory assistance should be provided.

Severe tetanus is characterized by an incubation period of less than 10 days and a symptom onset period of less than three days. Inadequate ventilation/perfusion and recurrent, severe tetanic contractions of the muscles of respiration advance a patient to the category of severe tetanus. The main complication and cause of death in tetanus is hypoventilation and anoxia due to respiratory arrest, which occurs during severe and prolonged rigidity and spasms. Tracheostomy with a cuffed tube is indicated in all these patients. Total paralysis with curariform drugs is usually required to treat severe tetanus when muscle relaxants or sedatives fail to arrest the tetanic convulsions. Total paralysis is much more popular in treatment of severe tetanus in Europe than in the United States.

Succinylcholine and d-tubocurarine are the curariform agents usually used. Their margins of safety are narrow, and they should be reserved for severe cases.

We prefer d-tubocurarine to succinylcholine in adult patients. Fifteen to 20 mg. is given either intravenously or intramuscularly every 30 to 60 minutes. Rectus muscle rigidity is a useful guide to dosage interval. A longer duration of paralysis can be achieved with larger doses, but abdominal distention occurs and is a limiting factor. In addition, d-tubocurarine can be given as an intravenous drip (1 mg. per milliliter of 5% dextrose and water). The interval between doses of d-tubocurarine usually increases as symptoms subside. After three to seven days of treatment, the frequency of administration of the curariform drugs can be decreased, and the patient can be observed closely for return of spasms and rigidity. The usual initial dose of succinylcholine is 20 to 80 mg. intravenously or intramuscularly. The dose must be individualized and repeated whenever muscular activity returns, usually within one to two hours. A convenient method is to deliver 0.5 to 2.5 mg. per minute (1 gm. per 500 ml. of 5% dextrose and water) in a carefully controlled intravenous drip. Morphine, triethylcholine, and mephenesin are usually inadequate in severe tetanus because these agents induce only brief or partial paralysis.

The induction of paralysis is expensive as well as dangerous, and complications are frequent. A patient deprived of spontaneous muscular activity is a difficult management problem. Close supervision by physicians is essential 24 hours per day. The assistance of an anesthesiologist is desirable. Mechanical ventilation must be continuous, and the patient should *never* be left unattended. Either a pressure or a volume-cycled ventilator can be used. Supplemental oxygen is usually unnecessary unless the patient has an underlying pneumonia or perfusion/ventilation defect. Arterial blood gases and electrolytes must be determined regularly. Tracheal suctioning should be rapid and brief (less than 30 seconds). Alarm systems to indicate ventilator failure should be checked daily. Nursing attendants should know how to deflate the tracheostomy cuff, disconnect the respirator, and ventilate the paralyzed patient manually whenever cyanosis or respiratory distress occurs. Anoxic encephalopathy has occurred in patients with tetanus following ventilator or tracheostomy cuff failure.

Management of Sympathetic Hyperactivity. This complication has been noted in severe tetanus, and may cause death, even in patients who have been paralyzed and adequately ventilated. Such patients develop episodes of severe hypertension, with diastolic pressures exceeding 150 mm. Hg, sweating, tachycardia, and serious arrhythmias very similar to the sympathetic discharge syndromes seen in pheochromocytoma and thyrotoxic crises. Myocardial necrosis, lesions in the conduction system, and toxic myocarditis have been noted in tetanus patients at post mortem and may be related to this syndrome.[9]

This syndrome has been treated successfully with beta-blocking agents such as propanolol and bethanidine. Our experience with these drugs has been favorable. Vital signs must be monitored closely, preferably with electronic monitors. The decision to institute beta blockade is made if the patient develops a serious arrhythmia or sinus tachycardia that is prolonged and greater than 130 beats per minute. Other causes of sympathetic hyperactivity should also be excluded by determination of arterial blood gases, hematocrit, temperature, and thyroid hormone levels.

Treatment can be begun intravenously with 0.2 mg. of propanolol. Continuous monitoring with subsequent increments of 0.2 mg. of propanolol will control the arrhythmia if it is due to vasomotor hyperactivity. A more rapid administration is dangerous. Propanolol may be given in 10- to 20-mg. doses every six hours by nasogastric tube for further control. These doses only induce a partial beta adrenergic blockade and antihypertensive effect. Other measures may be employed to control vasomotor hyperactivity, such as general anesthesia with halothane and nitrous oxide, an infusion of plasma or fluids, and administration of chlorpromazine. A combination of alpha and beta blockade is hazardous because the patient with vasomotor hyperactivity may need pressor amines for paradoxical hypotensive episodes. Antihypertensive drugs such as hydralazine (10 mg. intravenously) are effective. It is interesting that Cole and Youngman did not note sympathetic hyperactivity in 59 patients with tetanus who were treated with paraldehyde.[2] Further controlled studies of paraldehyde in patients with sympathetic hyperactivity are clearly indicated.

This syndrome should be anticipated and treated aggressively, because it is a preventable cause of death in severe tetanus.

Controversial Ancillary Measures. A number of other measures should be mentioned because they occasionally have been used in attempts to reduce the high fatality rate characteristic of severe tetanus.

Adrenal corticosteroids do not appear to influence the clinical course of tetanus, although some physicians give them for "adrenal exhaustion" in severe or prolonged cases. Sanders reported an improved survival rate with betamethasone; however, these data were uncontrolled and need further confirmation.[20]

Pascale described nine patients with tetanus who improved when given hyperbaric oxygen. Subsequent studies of barotherapy in mice and humans failed to document favorable effects, and we do not recommend it.[18]

Hypothermia has been employed in severe tetanus. We do not believe it has a place, except possibly in patients who develop hyperpyrexia due to vasomotor hyperactivity that cannot be controlled with antipyretic drugs. This is extremely uncommon. Fever is notably absent in tetanus, and a temperature exceeding 101° F should be viewed as an indication of superinfection.

Enhancement of cholinesterase production or activity is an attractive theoretical approach to treating tetanus. Leonardi has proposed that the biochemical block induced by tetanospasmin can be circumvented with pralidoxine, a cholinesterase-producing drug.[12] He believes that the toxin partially inhibits cholinesterase activity. The incubation period of tetanus in guinea pigs was prolonged and increased survival rates were obtained when antitoxin was given with pralidoxine methanesulfonate. Only a few patients have been treated with pralidoxine, and although these results are encouraging, further studies are needed.

Supportive Care. Providing optimal general supportive measures is one of the most important aspects of treating tetanus.[6] This may be needed for as short a time as five days or as long as six weeks. The patient should be followed closely, with a great deal of personal attention from physicians. The coordinated efforts of a variety of specialties are usually required. The team should include a general surgeon, an anesthesiologist and a pulmonary physician, a neurologist, and the primary physician. Physicians should be readily available for emergencies. A carefully planned regimen should be developed prospectively. Specialized units for treating tetanus are common in Europe but unusual in the United States.

The patient should be in a darkened, quiet private room to avoid noises and other external stimuli that might precipitate spasms. Personnel should know that patients with tetanus are often alert, aware of sounds, anxious, and sensitive to idle comments. Family members should restrict their visits. Vital signs, body weight, and fluid intake and output should be assessed frequently and recorded meticulously.[6]

Continuous, meticulous, and gentle nursing care is especially important. The nursing staff should be instructed *never* to leave the patient unattended or unobserved. The heavily sedated or paralyzed patient must be turned frequently to prevent pressure sores and ulcers. Once

7

spasms are no longer occurring, physiotherapists can administer chest therapy and passive exercises. Footboards and splints are useful in preventing contractures. Eyeshields and artificial tears should be used. Mouth care is important, and a padded tongue blade should be used to protect against biting and lacerations.

The patient is usually unable to control urination and may develop overflow incontinence and urinary tract infection. Patients with mild tetanus need to be catheterized intermittently. If indwelling catheters are needed, a continuous bladder rinse with a neomycin/polymyxin solution using a triple lumen catheter will delay the onset of catheter-induced infections. A closed drainage system should be used. Fecal impaction is frequent, especially if curariform drugs are used. Enemas, laxatives, and stool softeners are used routinely. Rectal examination with release of fecal impactions should be performed regularly.

Patients with tetanus are susceptible to dehydration, electrolyte imbalance, malnutrition and starvation. They are frequently deprived of nourishment because of trismus, dysphagia, inability to communicate hunger, and prolonged immobilization. Studies indicate that they retain salt and water in compensation for an inadequate circulating blood volume. Administered fluids may not remain within the vascular bed. Large volumes of blood or plasma may be needed to restore circulating volume, and serum proteins should be measured repeatedly.[6]

Nasogastric feeding may suffice in the mild case for prevention of negative nitrogen balance. Although patients with mild tetanus can obtain sufficient fluid and calories via nasogastric feedings, patients with moderate and severe tetanus may have marked paralytic ileus that is refractory to anticholinergic drugs, and nasogastric feeding may be impossible. Total parenteral nutrition has been employed in severe tetanus and is delivered through a polyethylene catheter that has been placed in a central vein by aseptic technique. Nutritional needs can be met with 5% protein hydrolysates and 20% dextrose and electrolytes. Blood glucose should be kept between 150 to 200 mg. per 100 ml. with the aid of small doses of insulin (50 to 100 units of regular insulin per 1,000 ml. of hypertonic fluid). The urine glucose should be kept between 1 and 2+ because these patients are often unable to respond physiologically or vocally to hypoglycemic episodes. Infections due to the intravenous catheter can be avoided by not withdrawing blood samples from the catheters, by changing dressings daily, and by applying antibacterial and antifungal ointments.

Pulmonary emboli are a frequent and important cause of death in tetanus. They seem to be more common in paralyzed tetanus patients than in patients paralyzed with other conditions. Most authorities therefore believe that patients with moderate or severe tetanus should receive anticoagulation therapy with heparin or coumadin, beginning about 24 hours after surgery or tracheostomy.

Neonatal Tetanus. Tetanus in the neonate is frequently associated with mortality rates exceeding 80%. The management of a small patient with tetanus presents many technical problems. Symptomatology may be meager and diagnosis delayed. Neonatal tetanus should always be placed in the severe category. Several studies indicate that heterologous or homologous antitoxins are effective in neonatal tetanus.[19] McCracken *et al.* found no differences between the results in infants in whom 10,000 units of equine antitoxin and those in whom 500 units of human antitoxin were used.[16] Dosages of antispasmodic and curariform drugs must be appropriate for neonates, and total parenteral nutrition is an important aspect of their care. The prognosis is not entirely bleak, because Smythe was able to decrease the mortality rate in neonatal tetanus from 100 to 20% during a 13-year period using the therapeutic measures discussed herein for adults with severe tetanus.[22]

References

1. Adams, E. B., Laurence, D. R., and Smith, J. W. G. 1969. *Tetanus.* Oxford, England, Blackwell Scientific Publications.
2. Cole, L., and Youngman, H. 1969. Treatment of tetanus. *Lancet,* 1:1017–1019.
3. Eckman, L. 1967. *Principles on Tetanus.* Bern, Switzerland, Hans Huber.
4. Edsall, G., et al. 1967. Excessive use of tetanus toxoid boosters. *JAMA,* 202:17–19.
5. Hardegree, M. C., Palmer, A. E., and Duffin, N. 1971. Tetanolysin: in vivo effects in animals. *J. Infect. Dis.,* 123:51–60.
6. Holloway, R. 1970. Fluid and electrolyte status in tetanus. *Lancet,* 2:1278–1280.
7. Ildirim, I. 1967. A new treatment of neonatal tetanus. Antitetanic serum and prednisolone given together intrathecally. *Turkish J. Pediat.,* 9:89–96.
8. Illis, L. S., and Taylor, F. M. 1971. Neurological and electroencephalographic sequelae of tetanus. *Lancet,* 1:826–830.
9. Kerr, J. H., et al. 1968. Involvement of the sympathetic nervous system in tetanus. Studies on eighty-two cases. *Lancet,* 2:236–241.
10. Kloetzel, L. 1963. Clinical patterns in severe tetanus. *JAMA,* 185:559–567.
11. LaForce, F. M., Young, L. S., and Bennett, J. V. 1969. Tetanus in the United States (1965–1966): Epidemiologic and clinical features. *New Eng. J. Med.,* 280:569–574.
12. Leonardi, G. 1971. Oxime treatment in tetanus. *Lancet,* 2:658–659.
13. Levine, L., et al. 1966. Active-passive tetanus immunization. Choice of toxoid, dose of tetanus immune globulin and timing of injections. *New Eng. J. Med.,* 275:186–190.
14. McCarroll, J. R., Abrahams, I., and Skudder, P. A. 1962. Antibody response to tetanus toxoid fifteen years after initial immunization. *Amer. J. Pub. Health,* 52:1669–1675.
15. McComb, J. A., and Dwyer, R. C. 1963. Passive-active immunization with tetanus immune globulin (human). *New Eng. J. Med.,* 268:857–862.

16. McCracken, G. H., Dowell, D. L., and Marshall, F. N. 1971. Double-blind trial of equine antitoxin and human immune globulin in tetanus neonatorum. *Lancet,* 1:1146–1149.
17. Nation, N. S., et al. 1963. Tetanus. The use of human hyperimmune globulin in treatment. *Calif. Med.,* 98:305–307.
18. Pascale, L. R., et al. 1964. Treatment of tetanus by hyperbaric oxygenation. *JAMA,* 189:408–410.
19. Patel, J. C., and Goodluck, R. 1967. Serum therapy in neonatal tetanus. *Amer. J. Dis. Child.,* 114:131–136.
20. Sanders, R. K. M. 1970. Tetanus: new treatment and prophylaxis. *Lancet,* 2:526–527.
21. Smith, J. W. G. 1964. Penicillin in prevention of tetanus. *Brit. Med. J.,* 2: 1293–1296.
22. Smythe, P. M. 1963. Studies on neonatal tetanus, and on pulmonary compliance of the totally relaxed infant. *Brit. Med. J.,* 1:565–571.
23. Vaishnava, H., et al. 1966. Controlled trial of antiserum in the treatment of tetanus. *Lancet,* 8:1371–1374.
24. Wright, G. P. 1955. The neurotoxins of *Clostridium botulinum* and *Clostridium tetani. Pharm. Rev.,* 7:413–465.

12

Wounds of the Soft Tissues

R. W. Dow

Soft tissue trauma is part of the injury complex in nearly all patients who require emergency treatment for trauma. In many situations, such as a simple cutaneous laceration or abrasion, the soft tissue injury is the only emergency problem. At other times the soft tissue trauma is only a small part of a complex of injuries requiring emergency management. In either event, soft tissue injuries are a common problem for the emergency physician.

The emergency physician's responsibility to the traumatized patient is complex. The scope of the injury must be defined, appropriate emergency procedures must be instituted in correct sequence, and the patient's subsequent course must be anticipated in order to organize effective after-care. Furthermore, these obligations must be met within a limited period of time and in circumstances that are usually not conducive to orderly planning or thought. Consequently, it is imperative that the approach to the injured patient be systematic.

The priorities of trauma management are well known. First, airway and ventilation problems are recognized and controlled. Second, major bleeding (either overt from a complex open wound, or occult from a ruptured spleen) is treated by volume expansion and control of the blood loss. Other circulatory problems (*e.g.,* tamponade or myocardial contusion) are considered and remedied. Third, cerebral, spinal, and peripheral nerve injuries are identified and stabilized. Fourth, other major visceral injuries are treated. Fifth, open bone and joint injuries are controlled. Sixth, closed fractures and dislocations are reduced and immobilized. Finally, the soft tissues are treated. When multiple injuries are involved, considerable judgment is required to place the appropriate staging of treatment.

Although soft tissue injuries occupy a low position in the priorities of trauma management, it is distressing to see the soft tissues totally ignored while other problems are fully investigated. During the initial evaluation of the trauma victim, there are frequent short periods of time during which one must wait for equipment or results of tests. This time can be utilized by the well organized physician to evaluate the soft tissue injuries and to protect these tissues from further contamination and damage. If the overall priority of injuries dictates that the soft tissues not be treated or evaluated promptly, they should be protected by simple dressings until they are definitely treated.

Assessment of Injury

When, within the overall priority, the physician's attention is directed to the soft tissue injury, assessment of the wound to define the extent of each soft tissue injury completely and accurately is the first step in appropriate management. Underlying injuries to bones, joints, major body cavities, tendons, or major vessels or muscles must be excluded or identified by physical examination and application of appropriate diagnostic aids. The potential for retained foreign body should be estimated by evaluation of the mechanisms of injury and by examination of the wound.

If major underlying injuries are detected during this initial phase of evaluation, the physician should carefully consider the ramification of these findings before proceeding with further treatment of the soft tissue problems. In general, such complex wounds require treatment techniques and follow-up care that are not readily available in the emergency department. (Care of these wounds is considered elsewhere in this book.) Occasionally, although injuries are confined to the soft tissue, the magnitude of the wound may dictate that care be administered in the operating room. The need for general anesthesia, surgical assistance, or specialized equipment usually dictates that the operating room facilities be used. Additionally, the emergency department physician is frequently unable to spend the time required for appropriate treatment of extensive though simple wounds, and this is a consideration in his decision to seek consultation for further care.

The soft tissue wounds that are appropriately treated in the emergency department consist mainly of simple abrasions, lacerations, and avulsions. The elements of initial treatment are the same regardless of the type of wound.

Decontamination of Wound

The first effort is to clean the wound. Except for the eyebrow, enough body hair should be removed by shaving to allow cleaning and access to the injured area. The skin around the wound is then cleansed with surgical soap and sterile gauze. Simple soaking of the injured area in soapy water does not provide adequate mechanical cleansing.

After the preliminary cleansing, adequate local anesthesia is obtained. In general, lidocaine without vasoconstrictors is an appropriate agent for use in the out-patient setting of the emergency department. Field block with these agents is easily accomplished and provides effective anesthesia. Sometimes the use of finger or wrist blocks facilitates this element of the patient's care.

When pain has been controlled, the wound is further inspected and cleaned. This aspect of wound decontamination includes further mechanical cleaning with soap, irrigation, and special attention to the identification and removal of foreign bodies. The excision of devitalized tissue is a part of the decontamination process and does not involve only those tissues with impaired blood supply. Badly crushed, fragmented, or contaminated tissue should also be removed with due consideration for the consequences in terms of cosmesis and closure. The depths of the wound should be carefully inspected for any previously unrecognized injury to specialized structures.

Closure of Wound

It is false economy to attempt to close a wound with inadequate debridement or excessive tension. If adequate cleansing and decontamination of the wound result in a defect that cannot be closed with facility, more complex techniques, such as split-thickness skin grafting or pedicle reconstruction, should be considered. If decontamination is inadequate because of the nature of the injury, the wound should be treated open.

The mechanical process of closure is dictated by the anatomic characteristics of the wound. Although coaptation of superficial tissues should be accomplished, excessive numbers of sutures should not be placed in the skin or deep tissues. These sutures are foreign bodies, and additional tissue trauma and devitalization invariably are produced during their placement. A conscious attempt should be made to keep the additional foreign bodies to a reasonable minimum. Absorbable fine sutures (plain catgut) are appropriate for deep tissue closures, but monofilament nylon is advisable for closure of the skin. Simple suture techniques are usually adequate.

Regardless of whether wounds are sutured or treated open, dressings should be made bulky enough to absorb the small amounts of blood and serum produced by the wound. The bulky dressing also aids in immobilizing the wounded part and protects the site from further inadvertent contamination. When wounds are in areas of motion, immobilization with plaster splints is advisable. Topical antibiotics or ointments should not be relied upon to promote healing of inadequately decontaminated wounds.

Prophylactic Agents

The addition of antibiotics to the treatment regimen is usually not appropriate when dealing with simple soft tissue wounds. When specialized structures (*e.g.,* tendons or joints) are involved, antibiotic therapy is advisable. These topics are covered in other chapters of this book.

Tetanus prophylaxis is an important aspect in the treatment of every soft tissue wound. Guidelines for use of active and passive tetanus immunization are presented elsewhere. It is to be emphasized that tetanus prophylaxis includes the decontamination process and is not merely the administration of a shot.

After Care

The final aspect of emergency care of soft tissue wounds involves instructing the patient and organizing follow-up care. The patient should be fully informed about all aspects of care for which he is responsible. He should be instructed about limitation of activity of the injured part. Generally it is prudent to elevate the injured part for 24 to 36 hours and to curtail motion in the area of injury for seven to ten days. The patient should be alerted to the possibility of complications, such as bleeding or infection, and he should be told what signs to watch for and who to contact if they appear. Conspicuous swelling, severe pain, fever, erythema around the injured area, blood-soaking of the dressing, or substantial wound drainage should prompt the patient to seek further attention.

Before the patient leaves the emergency department, specific instructions should be given for care of the dressing. Except in the most favorable circumstances with minor wounds, the patient is advised to leave the dressing in place and to keep it clean and dry until it is redressed under medical supervision 48 to 72 hours after injury. Sutures in areas of cosmetic importance may be removed and the wound supported with Steri-Strips at this time. Usually, however, sutures are left in place for five to seven days. When injuries involve poorly vascularized tissues, such as the leg, or areas with a considerable amount of tension across the wound, it is prudent to leave the sutures in place 10 to 12 days if well tolerated. Arrangements for such follow-up care should be completed prior to releasing the patient from the emergency department. If the wound is being treated open, more frequent medical supervision must be planned. In general, elevation of and limitation of activity of the injured area should be emphasized.

References

1. Baxter, C. R. 1972. Surgical management of soft tissue infections. *Surg. Clin. N. Amer.*, 52:1483–1499.
2. Meade, J. W. and Mueller, B. 1968. Necrotizing infections of subcutaneous tissue and fascia. *Amer. Surg.*, 168:274–280.
3. Rea, W. J. and Wyrick, W. J., Jr. 1970. Necrotizing fascitis. *Amer. Surg.*, 172:957.
4. Stone, H. H. and Martin, J. D., Jr. 1972. Synergistic necrotizing cellulitis. *Amer. Surg.*, 175:702.
5. North Atlantic Treaty Organization. 1958. Wounds and injuries of the soft tissues, Chapter 14 in *Emergency War Surgery, NATO Handbook*. Washington, D.C., U.S. Government Printing Office, pp. 207–218.
6. Committee on Trauma of the American College of Surgeons. 1972. *Early Care of the Injured Patient*. Philadelphia, W. B. Saunders Co.

13

Emergency Care of Severely Burned Patients

Irving Feller and Kathryn E. Richards

The burn injury is the third most common cause of accidental death in the United States. Each year, two million people are burned in this country. More than 200,00 burn victims seek medical attention, and approximately 75,000 are hospitalized with severe burns. Burn severity varies considerably depending upon the size (area), depth (partial- or full-thickness destruction of skin), age, part of the body burned, and the patient's medical history.

The minor burn is a painful nuisance that requires several days to several weeks to heal, but the serious burn is life-threatening, taxing the skills of the medical personnel, the hospital facility, and the economic resources of all concerned. Whether a person suffers a minor or a severe burn is often decided by chance as well as by circumstances of the accident.

Etiology and Prevention

The etiology of burn accidents usually interests a physician only when he undertakes the treatment of a patient. After prolonged involvement with the care of any of these unfortunate patients, however, he cannot help becoming concerned with the causes of the injury and the problems of prevention. Many things can and should be done to reduce the incidence of burn accidents, and these things can and should be based on authoritative information concerning etiology of burns.

Accurate collection and analysis of data are needed first to define the etiology of burns and then to establish necessary methods of prevention.

Prior to 1964, there was no way to obtain uniformly coded, nation-wide information on burn accidents. In 1964, the National Burn Information Exchange (NBIE) was organized to collect data on burn etiology. To date, more than 30 thousand cases have been submitted from 40 hospitals having specialized burn care facilities. Of these, 14,000 cases have pertinent data on etiology. Because the amount of data is extremely large, it is necessary to employ a system of analysis that presents the information in a meaningful way. Three basic questions must be asked to define the problems of etiology:

Who are the injured victims?
How did the accident occur?
Where did it occur?

The answers to these questions provide the clues to prevention.

Who are the victims? Age, sex, and race are the most common data used to answer these questions. When studying etiology, however, it is also important to identify the type of victim. Six types have been isolated using NBIE data:

1. the victim of personal acts
2. the innocent bystander
3. the intended victim
4. the victim of personal medical history
5. the fire-rescue victim
6. the victim of military action.

One who starts a fire using combustible fluids and burns himself is a victim of personal action, as is the child playing with matches who accidentally sets his clothing on fire.

Injuries to innocent bystanders occur when they are near a burning agent, but their own actions are not responsible for causing the accident. This type of victim is represented by the burn victim injured in a house fire resulting from a furnace explosion.

Intended victims are those deliberately injured by another, generally in civilian assaults. One fairly typical example is the husband who is burned when his wife pours scalding water on him during an argument.

The victim of one's personal medical history is best depicted by the patient who suffers an epileptic seizure and falls into a fire during the convulsion.

Injuries to professional rescue workers, such as fire fighters and policemen, are minimized by their training. These professionals and nonprofessionals do suffer a significant number of injuries, however, in attempts to save other victims, such as those trapped within burning buildings or vehicles.

Burns also result from enemy military action or military action during training. These are given a special classification because these accidents do not affect the average civilian in the United States. This country does have a large military force, however, and burns resulting from military weaponry do appear in NBIE data.

The advantages of studying etiology to determine methods of prevention may best be illustrated by following an analysis of burn accident data from preschool children between 3 and 6 years old.

Of the 10,000 cases in the NBIE used in this study, 1,350 victims were found to be between the ages of 3 and 6 years. Further examination of this group indicated that 45% were males and 55% were females. The next question is, what type of burns did they suffer? We find that 895 of these children were flame burn victims (Table 13-1) and that 618 of these were victims of their own actions (Table 13-2). Let us now look at the place of occurrence of these 618 accidents. Examination reveals that 412 victims were burned both at home and indoors (Table 13-3). Continuing with this selected group of patients,

Table 13-1.   Burns in Children 3 to 6 Years of Age

Type of Burn	Number of Cases	Percentage
Flame	895	66.30
Hot liquid	374	27.70
Electric	14	1.04
Chemical	10	0.74
Radiation	1	0.07
Hot surface	43	3.19
Not specified	13	0.96
	1,350	

Table 13-2.   Types of Victims in Flame Burns of Children 3 to 6 Years of Age

Type of Victim	Number of Cases	Percentage
Victim of own action	618	69.05
Innocent bystander	195	21.79
Intended victim	13	1.45
Victim of personal medical history	2	.22
Not specified	67	7.49
	895	

Table 13-3. Locations of Flame Burning in Children 3 to 6 Years of Age Who Were Victims of Their Own Actions

Location	Number of Cases	Percentage
Home, indoors	412	66.66
Home, outdoors	134	21.68
Away from home, indoors	7	1.13
Away from home, outdoors	12	1.94
Traveling in vehicle	1	.16
Not specified	52	8.41
	618	

we find that the common activity was playing (339), the burning agent was gasoline (61), and the igniter was open flame (267). Further analysis shows that fabric flammability was involved in 488, or 90% of cases. It has been established that fabric flammability makes the burn worse in 85% of cases.

This analysis suggests that the burn accident in this age group can be prevented at least in part by educating children in this age group, educating the parent to better supervise preschool children, and encouraging product safety, such as the use of flame-retardant cloth in children's clothing. The specific methods of carrying out these recommendations are not difficult once one has concrete data on the mechanisms of accidents. Educational brochures for parents could be given out in pediatricians' offices, distributed through the Public Health Department, and distributed to children in preschool and kindergarten classes. It is important to realize that the preschool child can be educated. When using flame-producing devices, the child is experimenting and trying to imitate what he sees his elders doing. The parent can be educated to instruct the child in the proper use of flame-producing agents, and to provide better supervision of the child. The need for laws to encourage manufacturers to provide flame-retardant clothing is apparent, and increased efforts must be made to accomplish this in the United States.

Emergency Care

Treatment of the severely burned patient is a complex task, devoid of operative glamour, but presenting more potential management problems than found in most surgical diseases. Despite the complexity of this injury, there may be a tendency to concentrate treatment on only one of the many problems at a given time. One comes to realize that this is not wholly effective, because other physiological derangements may become additive and ultimately destroy the patient. Thus, we see patients in whom the initial shock has been successfully combatted by a meticulous program of fluid therapy, but who die later of sepsis that might have been controlled if more vigorous measures had been directed early to its prevention. A highly coordinated therapeutic regimen is, therefore, necessary if optimal care is to be provided the extensively burned patient. To implement this concept of treatment, a burn team has been established at the University of Michigan Medical Center. The goals of the team are to provide continuous and vigorous treatment of the individual patient throughout his entire course, including final rehabilitation, and to observe and study the many complex surgical problems created by thermal injury.

Three basic derangements follow the loss of an appreciable area of full-thickness skin. The first is massive fluid shifts resulting from the flow of extracellular fluid from the blood into the damaged tissue. The second is the loss of normal skin function in the burned areas, which creates a predisposition to serious complications. The third is functional and cosmetic deficits caused by contractures and scar formation.

These derangements constitute the basis for a classification of burn therapy that emphasizes the changes that take place during the three phases of injury and recovery. The first phase can be called the *emergency period* and involves the accurate appraisal and correction of the massive fluid shifts that occur and produce shock. The duration of this period is two to four days. The second phase encompasses the time required to resurface all areas of full-thickness skin loss and is known as the *acute period*. It is during this interval that many of the complications occur that contribute most heavily to the high mortality and morbidity rates in severely burned patients. This is the most difficult area of treatment. We consider that the patient is acutely, not chronically, ill until all areas of full-thickness skin loss are resurfaced. This may require many weeks or months. The *reconstructive period* is the phase during which functional repair, cosmetic reconstruction, and social readjustment are accomplished, resulting in the best possible rehabilitation of the patient.

Ironically, the most satisfying phase of burn treatment today is often the emergency period. The advances in the knowledge of fluid therapy during the past two decades have made it possible to resuscitate most severely burned patients successfully; formerly many deaths occurred during this time. Other considerations pertaining to emergency care following trauma are equally important, however, in providing a complete and successful therapeutic program.

When the severely burned patient arrives at the emergency room, he presents many of the same problems encountered in patients with other types of injuries. The burn is obvious, but a quick and careful search must be made for other injuries as well and appropriate treatment of these instituted.

First Aid. When administering first aid to any seriously injured patient, *breathing, bleeding,* and *shock* are paramount considerations, usually in the order presented. Aseptic technique is employed in all phases of management. All clothing and dressings must be removed for a satisfactory appraisal of the extent of the burn as well as of possible associated injuries.

Breathing. The airway is more frequently a problem with the burned patient than is bleeding. The mouth and pharynx should be examined for foreign bodies and evidence of intraoral burn. The usual sequence of events is that burns of the head and neck that are seen early do not cause difficulty in breathing. Subsequently, however, edema increases insidiously, and within several hours the patient develops respiratory obstruction. We have found that endotracheal intubation is eventually required in many patients with head and neck involvement and is best done immediately in the emergency room when indicated. Positive pressure oxygen may be helpful in combatting pulmonary edema due to tracheobronchial injury. The use of oxygen should be considered in all patients. Initial blood gas levels are helpful to determine current oxygenation and to serve as a baseline value if the patient experiences respiratory insufficiencies.

Bleeding. Hemorrhage may occur internally as well as externally because of trauma at the time of injury and should be carefully evaluated and treated as indicated. As much as 10% of the red blood cell volume may be destroyed at the time of severe thermal injury, resulting in a relatively small blood loss initially due to the burn itself. The need for whole blood, therefore, is limited to approximately 500 ml. in a severely burned patient who does not have associated injuries.

Shock. This may be neurogenic at first but is due later to the extensive and rapid fluid shifts. Analgesics may be required if the patient is in pain and should always be given intravenously. Subcutaneous or intramuscular injections pool locally if the patient is hypotensive and then release suddenly when the systemic circulation returns to adequate function, resulting in dangerously high blood levels from accumulated doses. The secondary cause of shock is hypovolemia, resulting from the loss of serum to the extracellular spaces. The fluid therapy program to be discussed later is designed to control this problem.

After the immediate emergency matters have been handled and a preliminary evaluation has been made, time should be taken to reassure the patient and explain the problems to the family.

Differential Diagnosis of Depth of Burn. The percentage of the area of body surface involved, the patient's age and his past medical history are the three most important determinants of the severity of injury; emergently, they are the most serious considerations. The depth of burn is the most difficult to determine. There are signs and symptoms that indicate the level of tissue damage, but only with time, after spontaneous healing or appearance of granulation tissue, can the exact depth of injury and destruction be determined.

Depth of burn is best described in terms of partial thickness or full thickness. These are anatomically descriptive and therefore preferable to the popular references to first and second degree (partial-thickness) and third degree (full-thickness) burns, terms that were created from visual impressions. In a partial-thickness burn the tissue damage and destruction do not include the deeper dermal layers, which may regenerate new skin. In a full-thickness burn, the skin and its appendages have been destroyed and the subcutaneous tissues, muscle, and bone may also be involved. In these cases, skin grafting is necessary to replace the destroyed tissues.

In assessing the depth of burn immediately after the accident, the following signs and symptoms are helpful. Erythematous areas that blanch with fingertip pressure and then refill are shallow partial-thickness burns; the erythema indicates tissue damage where viability remains. Vesicles usually represent deeper partial-thickness injury, especially if they enlarge during the immediate postburn phase.

Full-thickness burns are characterized by a leathery surface that may be white, tan, brown, red, or black. There is no sensation of pain, because the pain fibers terminating in the dermis have been destroyed. Absence of pain in response to stimuli such as a pin prick or pulling out a hair indicates full-thickness skin loss. Deep partial-thickness burns may be anesthetic during the first few days, but sensation returns as the tissues recover. Small vesicles may be present, but they do not increase in size. These vesicles represent areas where the heat was intense enough to destroy all layers of the skin; the vesicles are caused by steam from tissue fluid. When severe scalds occur, there may be full-thickness skin loss with a red, discolored surface; however, this area does not blanch and refill when pressure is applied.

In general, the patient who has a painful erythematous surface with vesicles probably has a partial-thickness burn. If there is no complaint of pain and the surface is anesthetic, a full-thickness burn usually exists.

Fluid Therapy. Intravenous fluids should be started immediately in all patients with burns exceeding 15% of their body surface. Patients with smaller burns are observed initially and parenteral fluids given only as needed. Oral fluids suffice in patients with smaller burns.

Intravenous Catheters. Plastic intravenous catheters are used in all patients requiring immediate intravenous fluid therapy. Femoral or brachial cutdowns are employed into the deep venous system. When possible, percutaneous plastic catheters should be employed to lessen the hazards of infection. In addition, a second intravenous infusion is started in another extremity by the routine method, enabling the administration of colloid and crystalloid solutions simultaneously during the first few days. It is important to change the sites of the deep venous catheters after six days to avoid thrombophlebitis and sepsis.

Estimation of Percent of Body Burned. A chart is provided to facilitate estimation of the percent of body surface burned (Fig. 13-1). It is not necessary to distinguish full-thickness from partial-thickness skin loss at this time. In general, areas of full-thickness loss are anesthetized, dry, and perhaps charred. Areas of partial-thickness loss are painful and may have blisters. The chart takes into account the relative changes in surface area of parts of the body that accompany growth.

Calculation of Fluid Requirements. There are several formulas by which one can approximate the fluid requirements. *It must be emphasized that a formula provides only a working start for the administration of fluid; the patient's response to therapy is the most important factor in determining ultimate requirements.*

Colloid is considered to be whole blood, plasma, dextran, and 5% serum albumin. Electrolyte solutions used are Hartman's (lactated Ringer's) solution. Water is administered in the form of a 5% glucose solution.

Guides to Administration of Fluids. The question "What are the best guides to fluid requirements of burn patients?" is a loaded one, because it pits the formula users against each other and against those who do not use them.

The severe burn results in an outer layer of dead tissue and a deeper band, or zone, of damaged cell. The dead tissue is not important in the immediate fluid treatment, but the zone of damaged tissue below it is extremely important. It is here where plasma leaks from the injured blood vessel into the interstitial and intracellular spaces resulting in "burn edema."

The red blood cells stay within the vessel, resulting in a high hematocrit. The loss of fluid through the eschar into the dressings or the air is insignificant during the first few days compared with the volume that passes into the burn area. When the burn is greater than 20% of the body surface and a large injured tissue space is created, a large plasma loss occurs during the first day and continues at a slower rate for another day or two. When the fluid replacement has been adequate, the process reverses itself and much of the fluid returns to the vascular space

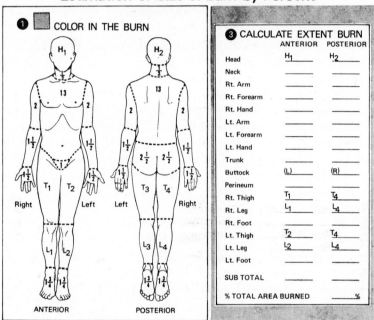

UNIVERSITY OF MICHIGAN BURN CENTER
ST. JOSEPH MERCY HOSPITAL BURN UNIT
I. FELLER, M.D., DIRECTOR

Name:
Hospital No.
Date:
Form completed by: _____

Estimation of Size of Burn by Percent

① ▧ COLOR IN THE BURN

H_1 H_2

13 13

2 2 2 2

$1\frac{1}{2}$ $1\frac{1}{2}$ $1\frac{1}{2}$ $1\frac{1}{2}$

$2\frac{1}{2}$ $2\frac{1}{2}$

$1\frac{1}{2}$ $1\frac{1}{2}$

T_1 T_2 T_3 T_4

Right Left   Left   Right

L_1 L_2 L_3 L_4

$1\frac{3}{4}$ $1\frac{3}{4}$ $1\frac{3}{4}$ $1\frac{3}{4}$

ANTERIOR   POSTERIOR

❸ CALCULATE EXTENT BURN

	ANTERIOR	POSTERIOR
Head	H_1	H_2
Neck	_____	_____
Rt. Arm	_____	_____
Rt. Forearm	_____	_____
Rt. Hand	_____	_____
Lt. Arm	_____	_____
Lt. Forearm	_____	_____
Lt. Hand	_____	_____
Trunk	_____	_____
Buttock	(L)	(R)
Perineum	_____	_____
Rt. Thigh	T_1	T_4
Rt. Leg	L_1	L_4
Rt. Foot	_____	_____
Lt. Thigh	T_2	T_4
Lt. Leg	L_2	L_4
Lt. Foot	_____	_____
SUB TOTAL	_____	_____
% TOTAL AREA BURNED	_____ %	

② CIRCLE AGE FACTOR

PERCENT OF AREAS AFFECTED BY GROWTH

AGE	0	1	5	10	15	Adult
H(1 or 2) = ½ of the Head	9½	8½	6½	5½	4½	3½
T(1,2,3 or 4) = ½ of a Thigh	2¾	3¼	4	4¼	4½	4¾
L(1,2,3 or 4) = ½ of a Leg	2½	2½	2¾	3	3¼	3½

Fig. 13-1. This chart provides for recording the distribution and accurately determining the percent of area burned. (Adapted from Lund, C. C., and Browder, N. C. 1944. *Surg. Gynec. Obstet.*, 79:358.)

during the following 7 to 12 days. If excessive fluids have been given and large amounts of fluid return to the vascular space suddenly during this period, hypervolemia, congestive heart failure, and pulmonary edema may result. The goal of fluid therapy for severely burned patients is to avoid hypovolemic shock during the first few days of therapy and to prevent hypervolemic complications later.

The successful treatment program requires that one know how much fluid to give and what fluids are needed. Each patient should be given the quantity and quality of fluid he requires to compensate for the losses he sustains during the first few days.

The rate of loss and the depth of burn cannot be predicted or measured, and herein lies the weakness of the formulas. The formulas attempt to predict a specific volume requirement for each patient.

Fluid therapy at the University of Michigan Medical Center is based on two principles, *i.e.,* that the fluid loss to the damaged tissue area is primarily plasma, and that the purpose of fluid therapy is to keep the patient out of hypovolemic shock. The fluid given is therefore plasma or a plasma substitute, and the quantity required is that which is sufficient to avoid hypotension.

In practice, the basic fluid administered to patients on admission to the hospital is a saline solution, preferably Hartman's in 5% glucose with 25 to 50 gm. of serum albumin added per 1,000 ml. of Hartman's solution. Plasma is also given during the first two days, with 250 to 500 ml. infused after every 100 gm. of albumin.

The patient's response to therapy serves as the guide for the volume of fluid required. The parameters followed are urine output (30 to 60 for children) and vital signs. The hematocrit is determined at six-hour intervals as a guide to but not as a primary indication of the quantities of fluid needed.

The patient is titrated so that his hourly intravenous intake will result in normal vital signs and a urine output of 20 to 60 ml. per hour. This requires careful observation of the patient's progress so that the therapy can be individualized. The nurses and physicians work very closely to accomplish this.

Central venous pressure measurements are used when indicated, such as in patients with heart disease. It is also important when the patient does not show an early satisfactory response to therapy.

Mannitol is used only when hematuria or hemoglobinuria is evident on the first catheterization. Usually 6 to 12 gm. are given intravenously, and it is rarely necessary to repeat the dose.

A urinary catheter is placed in all seriously burned patients on admission. An output of 20 to 60 ml. per hour is desirable depending upon the patient's age. The catheter can be clamped and drained either once an hour or once every two hours as indicated. The specific gravity should be determined with each measurement, and corrections must be made for high concentration of albumin when calculating the specific gravity.

Both the hemoglobin and hematocrit values are utilized to determine hemoconcentration. The determinations are repeated every 12 hours during the first day and as often as indicated thereafter, usually at 12 hour intervals. The hematocrit increases in most instances. The patient's response as measured by urine output, vital signs, and state of consciousness is more important than the hematocrit level. Although the

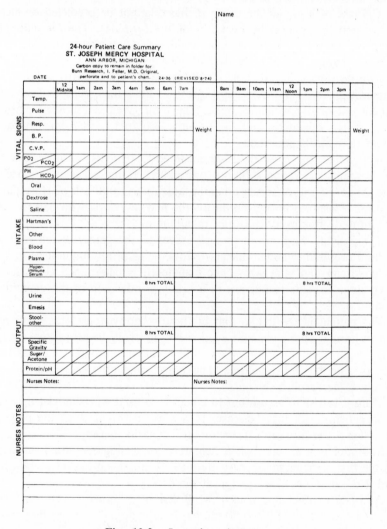

Fig. 13-2. *Legend on facing page*

latter does not serve as a specific parameter in prescribing fluid replacement, it does serve as a guide to the progress of therapy. With adequate fluid replacement, the high hematocrit level will remain constant and then return to normal.

Baseline chemical determinations are important in evaluating the patient's state of health on admission and in measuring changes due to therapy. Serum sodium, potassium, carbon dioxide concentration, blood urea nitrogen, protein levels, creatinine, blood sugar, blood gases, and

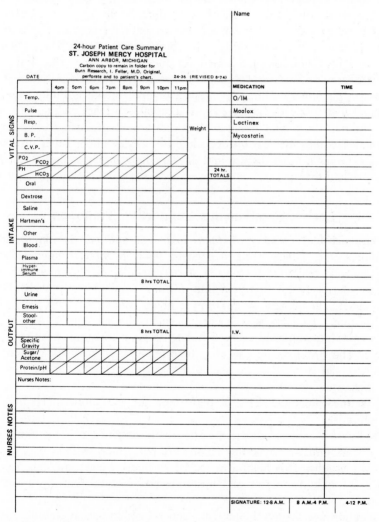

Fig. 13-2. A complete hourly summary of the patient's course is readily available on this chart at all times. The chart is placed in full view on the wall near the patient's bed. Later, it can be folded to fit on the standard hospital record.

coagulation profile are determined on admission and repeated each day for the first three days.

As mentioned previously, a predetermined formula serves only as a guide in fluid therapy. The patient's response, as judged by urinary output and vital signs, is the final determining factor in the administration of fluid during the emergency phase. It is therefore mandatory to evaluate the patient's progress at intervals no greater than every four hours, rewriting fluid orders as often as necessary. A special summary chart has been developed to aid in coordinating therapy (Fig. 13-2). This chart permits the accurate hourly recording of the many observations that have proved useful in evaluating the patient's course. Each chart has space for hourly recordings for a 24-hour period. The patient's course is advantageously followed for the first three or four days on these charts.

When pulmonary damage is suspected, fluid intake is limited to the volume that will provide the lowest acceptable urinary output (20 ml. per hour in the adult) because of the hazard of producing pulmonary edema. The past medical history should be reviewed for other diseases, such as organic heart disease and primary lung diseases, that might influence fluid therapy.

Early Miscellaneous Supportive Treatment

Antimicrobial Therapy. *Tetanus toxoid or antitoxin* is administered routinely, the choice being dependent upon previous immunizations. Prophylactic antibiotic therapy is started in all patients on admission. We are currently advising penicillin (5 million units intravenously every 6 hours). The patient is questioned about allergy to these or other medications. If there is a history of penicillin allergy, erythromycin (500 mg. intravenously every 6 hours) is good for gram positive coverage. The prophylactic use of antibiotics in burn patients remains a controversial issue. It is our belief that early infections can be limited by their use.

Electrocardiogram. This is performed for evaluation of injury or arrhythmias.

X-Rays. A chest radiograph is routinely obtained of all patients on admission. Other x-ray examinations are performed as indicated.

Photographs. It is helpful to record all injuries pictorially when possible. We obtain anterior and posterior views of the burned areas as soon as conditions permit.

Wound Care. When the patient's general condition has stabilized, the wound is gently washed with a surgical soap and water; only minimal debridement of dirt and loose tissue is attempted, leaving the intact blisters undisturbed. This can usually be accomplished in the patient's room. Analgesics may be given as indicated but are rarely required in severe burns. General anesthesia is seldom necessary and should be avoided if possible. The Foster or Stryker frame is employed if the burns are extensive. In general, burns of the hands and feet and trunk are covered by occlusive dressings whereas those of the face are managed by the open method. Sterile linen is used and isolation technique is required.

Clinical Management of Minor Burns

The difference between minor and severe burns is determined by the tissue damage and the patient's age and past medical history. A minor burn may be defined as one in which the full-thickness (third degree) loss is less than 5%, the partial-thickness (first or second degree) loss is less than 20% of the body surface, and the patient is over 2 but less than 60 years old. The very young and the old have higher mortality and morbidity rates for a given injury. Another factor to consider is the possible physiological abnormality that exists depending on the past medical history. For example, a 2% full-thickness burn would be serious for a diabetic patient, but only minor for a normal patient of the same age. The minor burn may be treated on an out-patient basis, but the seriously burned patient should be hospitalized.

Wound management is the major consideration for minor burns. There is no need for intravenous fluid therapy and prophylactic antibiotics. Tetanus immunization should be up to date in all injuries. The basic principles of wound management for minor burns are cleanliness and comfort. A partial-thickness burn is usually painful, because the pain fibers in the area of tissue damage are irritated. Analgesics may be necessary before the involved surface is cleaned, but care should be taken to avoid oversedation, because pain during cleansing helps to prevent excessively rough handling of the tissues. The partial-thickness wound can become a full-thickness wound when the added mechanical trauma during cleansing further damages the weakened tissues. This often happens with infants in whom the skin is thin.

Cool sterile saline containing a small amount of surgical detergent is used to cleanse the burned area. Loose skin is excised and debris removed. Intact vesicles represent partial-thickness injury and should not be disturbed; they make an ideal sterile, painless dressing. When the vesicle breaks the loose tissue should be excised.

One layer of a saline-moistened roll bandage, directly applied to the burned area and then covered with dry Kerlix gauze, provides a comfortable occlusive dressing. This dressing should be changed daily by soaking it off with warm water; a new one is then applied. The dressing changes remove the exudate and products of infection, allowing the wound to heal spontaneously. The partial-thickness burn requires approximately two weeks to heal. The appearance of granulation tissue after the necrotic surface is cleared indicates that the burn is full thickness and may require skin grafting.

During the daily dressing changes the normal skin surrounding the burn site is observed for evidence of spreading infection. If cellulitis appears, the proper antibiotics should be used; in most cases, gram-positive organisms are responsible. Oral antibiotics are usually satisfactory, and, of course, more frequent dressing changes with longer soaking periods hastens the control of infection. Oral analgesics should be used to minimize the patient's discomfort at any time during the treatment.

Ointments, other topical medications, and expensive dressings are not indicated. There are no chemicals that can restore viability to dead tissue, nor can they speed the healing process over what the body can accomplish. Many of the substances used to coat burns have actually increased the injury by their own chemical action on the already weakened tissues. It is not so much what is put on the wound but how the wound is cared for that is important.

Physical Examination

As complete a physical examination as is possible should be done on admission. A thorough knowledge of the patient's past medical history is necessary before extensive fluid therapy is undertaken. The history is obtained from the relatives in the emergency room and again from the patient when he is able to respond to questioning. Usually, the patient can give a history within the first few hours but not later, because the increasing edema incapacitates him.

Careful management of the patient during this phase will be rewarded by the onset of diuresis during the third or fourth day, signifying the successful termination of the emergency period. If the full-thickness loss is not great, the diuresis will begin earlier. Homeostasis has been restored temporarily. The removal of the burn eschar and resurfacing of the area with split-thickness skin are the next steps. The prevention and treatment of complications during the ensuing acute period become matters of extreme importance for survival.

References

1. Feller, I. 1969–1975. *International Bibliography on Burns and Supplements.* Ann Arbor, National Institute for Burn Medicine.
2. Feller, I., and Archambeault, C. 1973. *Nursing the Burned Patient.* Ann Arbor, Institute for Burn Medicine.
3. Feller, I., and Crane, K. 1972. *Planning and Designing a Burn Care Facility.* Ann Arbor, Institute for Burn Medicine.

14

Radiation Contamination and Acute Radiation Injury

Eugene L. Saenger

Radioactive contamination and acute radiation injury are comparatively rare events when compared to others discussed in this text. Apprehension in regard to this kind of physical trauma is great in the minds of both the public and the medical profession. Much of this concern stems from a lack of understanding of the physical properties and biological effects of ionizing radiation. Space restrictions preclude discussion of these aspects, but several references, both brief and extensive, are given.[1-3]

Definition

A radiation accident may be defined as an unforeseen occurrence, either actual or suspected, involving exposure of or contamination on or within humans and the environment to ionizing radiation. The accident will be considered as occurring over a short time period of seconds to as long as several days.[4] This definition, while perhaps lacking certain legal connotations, points out the problem of "actual" and "suspected" because it is often safer and less expensive to put an accident plan into operation when the occurrence is suspected than after it has been verified.

An installation with a well organized and well developed industrial medical program already has many if not most of the essential features needed for the care of possible radiation injuries. The ominous feature of radiation is, of course, that it is not readily detectable by human senses; thus it must be sought by special instruments or some malfunction of equipment recognizable in some other way. In many situations there are legal requirements for technical and professional personnel to aid in these matters. In general they are identified as health physicists or industrial hygienists in industry and as medical radiation physicists in hospitals and medical colleges. In most institutions, either one of these specialists is available or a responsible individual is designated as Radiological Safety Officer (RSO) with responsibility to activate emergency programs. Also, the Joint Commission on Accreditation of Hospitals[5] requires that each hospital have an approved plan for handling these emergencies.

There are two ways in which humans can be exposed to radiation. The source of radiation may be outside the body, in which case the radiation strikes the individual and is absorbed according to its physical characteristics. Radiation from x-ray generators, particle accelerators, sealed sources of radionuclides, and reactors are examples of this type. The radiation may be beta, gamma, or neutron. Particle accelerators may produce other particles, such as deuterons and mesons.

The second way in which humans can be involved is by surface or internal contamination with radioactive nuclides, which can be deposited on the skin, inhaled, ingested, or enter the body through wounds. They may also be formed within the body following exposure to an external source of neutrons; those most commonly detected are ^{24}Na and ^{32}P. Both external radiation exposure and radionuclide contamination may occur simultaneously.

In a suspected radiation accident the physician has the following responsibilities:

1. Evaluate the possibility of contamination.
2. Evaluate the possibility of neutron exposure.
3. Do simple decontamination.
4. Give emergency first aid.
5. Obtain the history and perform a physical examination.
6. Consider triage for massive accidents.
7. Consider hospitalization.

It is necessary to be ready to provide health physics and medical services for a situation that may arise only rarely or never. Many installations do not require full-time physicians. Reliance must therefore be placed on the help of physicians with appropriate levels of specialization who practice in the vicinity of the plant and who are interested in the problems peculiar to the installation. In addition, consultants from nearby or even distant centers may be retained for special considerations if needed.

The relationship between the physician and other plant personnel must be carefully defined. Often the physician is available only part time. He may be utilized only in emergencies as in the case of a surgeon. It therefore becomes necessary to provide him with sufficient information concerning the work of the installation and the particular kinds of accidents that might be anticipated so that he can function effectively. It is particularly important that a good working relationship be developed with the health physicists. These specialists often have far more detailed information than the physician about physical and chemical characteristics of radiation as either sources or contaminants, about metabolic pathways and dosimetry of radionuclides, and about methods of decontamination. Yet, legally, the physician is the only one who can diagnose and treat the patient, and the health physicist therefore must work, in a sense, under the direction of the physician with very close interpersonal relationships. The health physicist is often responsible for proper indoctrination of physicians. It is important that management give proper attention to these relationships.

The Accident

Two sets of rules are given here for use in the immediate accident period, representing levels of complexity of action and illustrating roles of plant personnel.

Simple Emergency Procedures

1. Survey and then evacuate potentially exposed personnel from accident area and give necessary first aid.
2. Notify medical officers, health physics (industrial hygiene) personnel, and management.
3. Close off radiation area. Turn off air supply. Seal area if contamination is likely.
4. Confine and survey all contaminated people. Then give first aid for injuries and burns.
5. Evaluate situation with regard to contamination by radionuclides, neutron exposure, and level of radiation exposure.
6. If contamination is present, perform simple decontamination and resurvey patients.
7. Put patients to bed. Conduct brief physical examination.
8. Save all samples of clothes, jewelry, blood, urine, feces, and vomitus. Label with name, time, and date.
9. Do routine blood counts.
10. Obtain careful history of accident.
11. Send patients to hospital if exposure of 100 R or more is suspected.

Rules Primarily, but not Exclusively, for Physicians

1. If radionuclide contamination is present, all exposed individuals should be surveyed and decontaminated before being examined and treated. If this step is neglected, personnel who must care for patients may become so contaminated themselves that they are rendered ineffective. Proper protective clothing should be available.
2. Do simple decontamination of patients if radionuclides are present. The operator should wear coveralls or a scrub suit, shoe covers, gloves, cap, and respiratory mask as indicated by initial survey before working with patients. If patient is ambulatory, confine him to a small area. Spread a sheet or paper for him to stand on. Patient then disrobes, putting clothing in a container suitable for later survey (such as a bag or wastebasket). Nose, mouth, and ear wipes are done. Then the patient washes and is resurveyed until clean. If patient is not ambulatory, he is placed on a sheet and his clothing is cut off but saved as already described for later surveying. The patient is washed by the operator with repeated surveys.
3. If there is evidence of massive exposure to external radiation or radionuclides, and if large numbers of individuals are involved, triage is needed. It may be necessary to limit drastically any extensive medical care to the moribund individual in order to utilize available facilities for the care of those potentially salvageable. Dose estimates of over 1,000 R for external radiation, or over 2,000 rads per hour (rem, R) for radionuclide contamination, indicate that little can be offered to such patients. In the latter case, contamination of treatment personnel may become a major problem.
4. Put patients at bed rest. Obtain careful history. Do brief physical examination.
5. Obtain routine blood count.
6. Hospitalize patients with severe nausea and vomiting.
7. No specific therapy is indicated for acute radiation injury within the first few days after exposure.
8. If a dose estimate of less than 100 rads can be estimated for certain individuals, they do not require emergency care of a major degree.
9. Individuals receiving only external exposure from alpha, beta, gamma, and x-radiation are not radioactive.
10. Individuals receiving neutron radiation are slightly radioactive but present no hazard to personnel caring for them.
11. Individuals contaminated with radionuclides present a hazard to personnel caring for them. The degree of hazard depends upon the level and type of contamination.

Guidelines for Protection of Workers Aiding in a Radiation Accident. Table 14-1 gives dose-limiting recommendations for normal peacetime operations. If these values are exceeded, the volunteer should be certain

Table 14-1. Dose-Limiting Recommendations*

Maximum permissible dose equivalent for occupational exposure	
Combined whole body occupational exposure	
Prospective annual limit	5 rems in any one year
Retrospective annual limit	10–15 rems in any one year
Long term accumulation to age *N* years	$(N - 18) \times 5$ rems
Skin	15 rems in any one year
Hands	75 rems in any one year (25/qtr.)
Forearms	30 rems in any one year (10/qtr.)
Other organs, tissues, and organ systems	15 rems in any one year (5/qtr.)
Fertile women (with respect to fetus)	0.5 rem in gestation period
Dose limits for the public, or occasionally exposed individuals	
Individual or occasional	0.5 rem in any one year
Students	0.1 rem in any one year
Population dose limits	
Genetic	0.17 rem average per year
Somatic	0.17 rem average per year
Emergency dose limits—life saving	
Individual (older than 45 years if possible)	100 rems
Hands and forearms	200 rems, additional (300 rems, total)
Emergency dose limits—less urgent	
Individual	25 rems
Hands and forearms	100 rems, total
Family of radioactive patients	
Individual (under age 45)	0.5 rem in any one year
Individual (over age 45)	5 rems in any one year

* From National Council on Radiation Protection and Measurements. 1971. *Basic Radiation Protection Criteria,* NCRP Report No. 39. Washington, D.C.

that the gain is considered in relation to the risk. An individual is permitted a single emergency exposure of 25 rads in a lifetime.[6]

Preexposure Data. All individuals who are involved in work with radiation should have a baseline medical and radiation history, physical examination, blood counts, and urinalysis recorded and available in the medical department of the institution so that in the event of accident, this information can serve as a baseline for future studies. Ideally the initial blood counts should be obtained at weekly intervals for three weeks to be certain that the average value is accurate for the individual in good health. The laboratory work forming this baseline should be repeated at intervals of six months to one year, depending on the routine hazards, so that the information is up to date. The name of the family physician and the closest responsible relative should be available on this record so that any emergency medical information can be obtained rapidly.

Role of the Physician. Within 30 to 60 minutes after notification that an accident has been suspected, the physician should have been advised as to whether the radiation exposure has occurred and whether there is likely to be internal deposition of radiation as well as external irradiation. This information will aid him in his planning. In any institution in which a health physicist is available, it is his duty to provide this information. In small installations, it may be the job of the Radiological Safety Officer who may well be the physician, his nurse, or someone trained in engineering and with a knowledge of the operation of survey instruments.

Triage. In situations in which the radiation injury is complicated by other injuries, the usual concept of triage, as employed in military medicine or in large-scale catastrophes, must be employed. It is necessary to reserve definitive treatment for patients whose likelihood of recovery is greatest, especially if facilities, equipment, and supporting medical personnel are limited. Within the first few hours of an accident it is possible that an estimate of the radiation dose received by the individual cannot be obtained. It is important in the history to learn from this worker his location at the time of the accident and some estimate of his scram time. At this point the nonradiation injury should be treated in a suitable manner and the patient transported to a hospital if necessary.

Dose Estimates. Estimating the dose in the various types of accidents is the greatest single problem for the physician responsible for patient care. Depending upon the dose received by various individuals, decisions will be made such as whether to hospitalize patients, take them off work, or utilize their skills in helping cope with the accident. It is relatively simple to estimate possible dosage from sealed sources of radioactive nuclides and from x-ray units, teletherapy units, and various types of accelerators. Such dose estimates can usually be made by calculation, given a rough estimate of the time and location of the individual injured.

The dose determination in accidents involving contamination with radioactive materials is more difficult because the nature of the contaminating radionuclide may not at first be known and the metabolic pathways of the substance may not be well understood.

Estimating the dose in mixed external and internal accidents is difficult because combined exposure to neutrons and beta and gamma rays is possible. This problem is greatest in a reactor exposure, particularly if there has been some disruption to the reactor or its container. Such dose estimates require the cooperation of skilled reactor physicists and health physicists. In general, the more complicated the accident, the more difficult it is to obtain highly accurate dose estimates.

In addition to the routine use of film badges and ion chamber dosimeters, the use of thermoluminescent dosimeters is recommended for personnel monitoring. These dosimeters are very small and can be combined with the usual film badges. Advantages include a wide dose range (about 100 mrads to 100,000 rads) and very little energy dependence. They have a long shelf life and are reusable.

The Acute Radiation Syndrome

Basic to the understanding of this syndrome are four considerations: the volume of the body irradiated and distribution of radiation, the dose, the dose rate, and the presence or absence of neutrons.

It is rare to find a patient who has received uniform whole body radiation except when given for treatment. In most circumstances the radiation is irregularly distributed and has an important effect on the clinical course. Irrespective of the different radiosensitivities of the various body tissues, the greater the volume of tissue irradiated for any given dose, the more severe will be the effect. Shielding of a relatively small portion of the body (the spleen or an extremity) gives significant protection, usually by protecting bone marrow. In addition, the individual tissue sensitivity must be considered. Bone marrow is the most sensitive followed by the mucosa of the gastroenteric tract and the cardiovascular and central nervous systems.

The clinical manifestations are directly related to the total dose; the higher the dose, the greater the effect and the more rapid the onset.

Another estimate of radiation effect in man is the LD_{50}. For high intensity radiation, the air dose is estimated at 400 to 450 R and the absorbed midline tissue dose at 250-300 rads.[7] It is assumed that treatment is minimal or nonexistent. Certainly, intensive therapeutic efforts would probably increase the LD_{50}. Our experience is too limited for precise values; these numbers at best provide guides for planning purposes and permit comparisons with animals and plants.

The changes are also proportional to the dose rate. The concept of dose rate is complicated in that the dose may be instantaneous, *i.e.,* at a very high rate or protracted, or it may be intermittent and in this sense is comparable to the type of exposure given in radiation therapy. With either protracted or intermittent dose rates, recovery is greatly enhanced; therefore the same dose that causes severe effects at a high rate is far less effective at lower rates. One must also realize that from the time a photon or particle interacts with and is absorbed within any part of the body, the initial physical and chemical events occur so rapidly that no evasive or protective action can be carried out. Any amelioration of radiation effects or salutary end result is in great part the result of a combination of factors, *i.e.,* volume of irradiated tissue, radiosensitivity, total dose, and dose rate.

Neutron exposure remains a special case for several reasons. Physicians have little experience in their detection and measurement. They occur in reactors, about critical and subcritical assemblies, in uranium and transuranic elements, and about certain particle accelerators. If their presence is suspected, detection is relatively easy because they induce radioactivity in the body. If exposure to neutrons is not suspected, one might conclude that the patient is grossly contaminated externally when there is only induced activity within the body. Levels of ^{24}Na so induced in a human being do not constitute a hazard to personnel giving aid. By determining the level of activity of ^{24}Na in blood, it is possible to estimate the level of neutron exposure and calculate an absorbed dose in rads. For practical purposes at this time the relative biological effects (RBE) of all neutrons of any energy for morbidity and lethality is assumed to be 1. There is no useful human evidence on this point; data on animals suggest that this value be utilized for these end points in spite of the use of higher values for genetic effects and cataract formation.

Techniques for estimation of ^{24}Na in blood should be available whereever neutron exposure may occur. One should be able to measure activation of other elements in various metallic objects carried on one's person, in similar objects in the area, and in body excreta, blood, and hair. The skills and facilities of the modern nuclear medicine laboratory are most helpful.

Diagnosis. Although it is difficult to make proper dose estimates by physical means it is desirable to attempt to classify the degree of injury, method of treatment, and prognosis based on history, physical examination, and simple, readily available laboratory tests. The approach presented here, developed by Thoma and Wald,[8] has been carefully tested and can be relied upon for clinical care.

The acute radiation syndrome is conveniently divided into four stages as shown in Table 14-2 where it is compared to a viral disease to emphasize its similarity to well known patterns of illness.

Patients are classified into five injury groups as shown in Table 14-3. This classification is of particular value in diagnosis and therapy because it separates patients in Group I, who require no therapy, and those in Group V, in whom definitive therapy is not needed, from all

Table 14-2. Comparison Between the Clinical Patterns of Viral Disease and Acute Radiation Syndrome

Viral Infection	*Acute Radiation Syndrome*	*Approximate Duration*

Inoculation or exposure
   Delay
   ↓
	Exposure
	   Delay (minutes
	   to hours)
	   ↓
		Minutes/hours

Prodromal stage (nonspecific system reaction)	Prodromal stage (of motion sickness) ↓	1–4 days

Incubation period	Latent stage (hours
	   to days)
	   ↓
		2–3 weeks

Manifest illness (typical clinical picture) ↓	Manifest illness (specific; weeks to months) ↓	second or third to sixth week
Convalescence	Recovery or death	8–15 weeks

Table 14-3. Clinical Radiation Injury Groups

Group No.	*Clinical Manifestations*	*Dose Estimate (rad)*	
I	Mostly asymptomatic; occasional minimal prodromal symptoms	<150	
II	Mild form of acute radiation syndrome; transient prodromal nausea and vomiting; mild laboratory and clinical evidence of hematopoietic derangement	<400	Hematopoietic
III	A serious course; hematopoietic complications severe, and evidence of gastroenteric damage in upper portion of group	400–600	Hematopoietic
IV	An accelerated version of acute radiation syndrome; gastroenteric complications dominate clinical picture; severity of hematopoietic complications is related to survival time after exposure	600–1500	Gastrointestinal
V	A fulminating course with marked cardiovascular and/or central nervous system impairment	>5000	Cardiovascular-cerebral

8

other patients. Those in Group II may require treatment and those in Groups III and IV require intensive care.

In regard to Group V patients, following further study of the deaths of two individuals, one at Los Alamos, New Mexico, and another at Wood River, Rhode Island,[9,10] the concept has been advanced that the patients did not die from injury to the central nervous system but rather from damage to the cardiovascular system. Both patients showed irreversible shock and cardiac failure in spite of intensive therapy; they also showed severe myocardial changes at autopsy. This concept has not influenced treatment or survival. It does point up a distinction between the acute changes of convulsive seizures and death noted within a few hours after doses of several hundred thousand rads have been given to the head or whole body of animals.

In planning the care of a patient, one should be guided by the time of change in the various manifestations of the acute radiation syndrome. In Group V patients, the prodromal and manifest illness stages are not distinguishable, and although supportive therapy is desirable, in our present state of knowledge no cure is possible. In all other groups the prodromal symptoms rarely last more than two days, and a latent period of at least 1 week follows. It is therefore possible to plan for appropriate treatment within the first few days after the event. Since radiation accidents seem to elicit concern and interest far exceeding those in similar kinds of injuries from other sources, the pressures and tensions surrounding the patient and physician seem often to be disproportionately increased. Hence the need for the establishment of orderly procedures should be recognized. Also, since it is highly likely that adequate estimates of dosimetry will not be immediately forthcoming, it is necessary

Table 14-4. Symptoms and Signs in Prodromal Stage of Acute Radiation Syndrome

Anorexia	Prostration
Nausea	Diarrhea
Vomiting	Abdominal pain
Weakness and fatigue	
Conjunctivitis	Sweating
Erythema	Oliguria
Fever	
Hyperesthesia	Paresthesia
Ataxia	Coma
Disorientation	Death
Shock	

Table 14-5. Symptoms and Signs in Manifest Illness Stage of Acute Radiation Syndrome

Anorexia	Sweating
Nausea	Oliguria
Vomiting	Weakness and fatigue
Diarrhea	Prostration
Abdominal pain	Weight loss
Abdominal distention	Hyperesthesia
Conjunctivitis	Paresthesia
Erythema	Ataxia
Jaundice	Disorientation
Fever	Shock
Infection	Epilation
Purpura	Coma
Hemorrhage	Death
Scalp pain	

to pool clinical observations and results of laboratory tests in a systematic approach.

Tables 14-4 and 14-5 list the important symptoms in the prodromal and manifest illness stages. If the frequency of occurrence of these changes is tabulated daily, one can estimate the severity of exposure. Details of the clinical manifestations are discussed in other published works.[4,7-13]

The only clinically useful laboratory procedures are routine hematologic tests. Peripheral chromosome cultures of circulating lymphocytes with scoring of dicentric and ring forms is of considerable investigative interest and is useful in estimating a whole body dose. Bone marrow studies are helpful, particularly in estimating dose distribution in severely exposed patients. By comparing the cellularity of marrow from the sternum, both iliac crests, and various spinous processes, for example, the distribution of radiation and the presence of viable marrow can be appraised.

The many examinations and tests can be confusing in the given patient; an orderly procedure is suggested in Table 14-6. The Type A procedures are recommended for routine use. Type B procedures are indicated only when the severity of the patient's illness suggests their usefulness.

Assuming a situation in which there is a total lack of dosimetric data, it is possible to assess the probable injury classification for a given patient by following the scheme presented in Figure 14-1, utilizing only clinical examination and routine blood counts over a period of one to ten days.

Table 14-6. Recommended Diagnostic Procedures for Clinical Management of Radiation Injury

	Group									
	I-II-III-IV			I	II		III		IV	V
Time (d)	1	2	3	STT	18–48	STT	4–48	STT	4	1
Type A Procedures										
History										
Symptoms	x	x	x	x	D	x	D	x	D	D
Signs	x	x	x	x	D	x	D	x	D	D
Past medical	x									
Physical examination					21d	3mo+	15–30d	6mo+	6d	D
Body weight	x		x	x	D	x	D	x	D	D
Urinary output	x	x		x	D		D		D	6hr
Laboratory tests										
Hematology										
Hematocrit	x	x	x	x	D	x	STT	x	D	6hr
Leukocytes	x	x	x	x	D	x	D	x	D	6hr
Differential count	x	x	x	x	D	x	D	x	D	6hr
Total neutrophils and lymphocytes	x	x	x	x	D	x	D	x	D	6hr
Platelets	x	x	x	x	D	x	STT	x	D	6hr
Bone marrow aspiration			30d	14d	14d	6mo	14d	6mo	7d	1d
Chromosomes			60d		30d	6mo	30d	6mo	7d	
Radioassay										
Blood ^{24}Na	x	x								
Whole body counting	x	x								

Type B Procedures

Laboratory tests									
Hematology									
Sedimentation rate	x	x	x	x	x	D	x	D	D	6hr
Reticulocytes	x	x	x	x	x	STT	x	D	D	6hr
Bleeding and clotting times	x					STT	STT	STT	3d	6hr
Biochemistry									
Blood									
Nonprotein nitrogen	x	prn	prn			prn		STT	STT	6hr
Sodium	x	prn	prn			prn		prn	prn	1d
Chloride	x	prn	prn			prn		prn	prn	1d
Potassium	x	prn	prn			prn		prn	prn	1d
pH or CO_2	x	prn	prn			prn		prn	prn	1d
Serum bilirubin	x	x		STT	x	STT	STT	D	6hr
Routine urinalysis	x	x	x	D	x	D	x	D	6hr
Occult blood in feces	x		D	12d+		D	D	All
Slit lamp ophthalmologic examination	x	6mo+		6mo+		6mo+	

Recommended frequency of time of performance:

STT = Standard testing times: 6, 9, 12, 15, 18, 21, 24, 27, 30, 33, 36, 40, 44, 48, 60, 90, 105, and 120 days; 6 months, 1 year, and annually.

x = at times indicated in column heading.

d = day(s).

D = daily during time indicated in column heading.

prn = as indicated by clinical course.

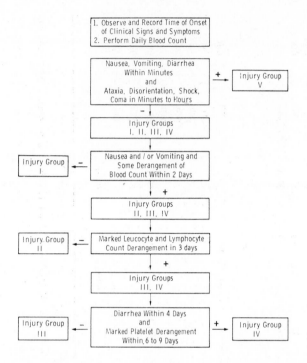

Fig. 14-1. Preliminary evaluation of clinical radiation injury following over-exposure. (From Saenger, E. L. 1963. *Medical Aspects of Radiation Accidents.* Washington, D.C., United States Government Printing Office, U.S. Atomic Energy Commission.)

The hematologic changes are well described in other published works.[4,7–13] Particular attention is directed to changes in the absolute lymphocyte count in the first 48 hours (Fig. 14-2). This test may be of great value in the very early period after exposure because of the rapid decrease to low levels after large radiation doses. The second especially useful method is profile scoring.[1,2] In this method, profile values are assayed for deviations of normality for common hematologic indices and are then scored. The method is of particular help in the evaluation of patients in whom radiation exposure is suspected but the time of exposure and dose are uncertain. It also permits one to follow the effects of treatment easily.

For patients with exposures exceeding 200 rads (and certainly in injury Groups III and IV) in whom rigorous therapy is contemplated, cultures of blood, nasopharynx, gingiva, teeth, skin, vagina, and excreta are indicated together with appropriate sensitivity tests for antibiotics. Serial erythrocyte sedimentation rates are helpful in the detection of

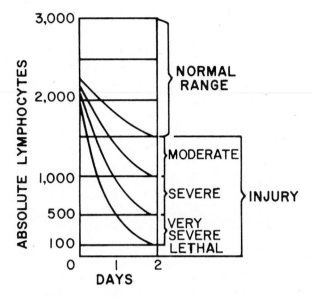

Fig. 14-2. Schematic relationships between lymphocyte levels and dose. (From Andrews, G. A., Auxier, J. A., and Lushbaugh, C. C. 1965. *Personnel Dosimetry for Radiation Accidents.* Vienna, International Atomic Energy Agency.)

latent infection. If homologous bone marrow therapy is contemplated, the most current tests of tissue compatibility are required.

Therapy. The extent of the therapeutic efforts is obviously determined by the apparent extent of the injury. Since these changes unfold gradually, one should provide hospital facilities and solicitous care for possible victims until the nature and extent of the injury are clarified. Nothing creates so much havoc as the neglect of an individual exposed to radiation who develops lesions much to the surprise of the attending physician.

Therapy is essentially nonspecific and supportive; *i.e.*, there is no specific antidote for radiation. Depending on the degree of exposure, there may be serious impairment of the hematopoietic, gastroenteric, cardiovascular, and cerebral systems. It is probable that only the hematopoietic and to a lesser degree the gastroenteric system can be helped by therapeutic efforts.

In Groups II and III, in which the injury involves chiefly the hematopoietic system, therapy is directed chiefly to the prevention of infection because of destruction of white cells and diminution or loss of immune competence. The measures can be very simple or extremely complex and expensive. The careful employment of diagnostic procedures described earlier greatly simplifies these management problems.

Group I and some Group II patients require little in the way of specific therapy except for being kept quiet and in a relatively clean environment, possibly at home. In Group II patients, one should search for infections and treat them appropriately and vigorously. When the white blood cell count is less than 1,000 per cubic millimeter, and until it increases to 2,000 per cubic millimeter, the use of bowel sterilization is indicated. Neomycin (4 gm. daily), oxacillin (2 gm. daily), and nystatin (1,500,000 units daily) is suggested. Nasal ointments containing neomycin, bacitracin and oxacillin should be instilled two or three times daily.

Whole blood or plasma should be given only for blood loss. Fresh platelets are indicated with low platelet counts (10,000 per cubic millimeter) or with bleeding if platelets are less than 60,000 per cubic millimeter. The use of white cells from leukemia donors and of cross circulation are experimental and should be considered only after consultation.

The use of bone marrow should also be regarded as an experimental procedure. It has been shown conclusively that a marrow autograft given immediately after irradiation will abort the hematologic depression.[14] The use of bone marrow from an identical twin before the tenth day after exposure to massive irradiation has continued to be effective without eliciting rejection phenomena in a patient followed for more than two years. The use of homografts has been effective, but the patient almost surely encounters severe rejection phenomena. It is possible that the homograft will provide temporary support during the time that bone marrow function and immune competence are lacking. In order for the graft to be successful, one must give in excess of 10^9 viable marrow cells. They should be given within 10 to 14 days postexposure, because the new cells require about two weeks to begin effective growth. Increased availability of this mode of treatment awaits additional refinement of tissue typing. Until then one should use expert consultation freely.

The other new therapeutic innovation involves the use of various levels of sterile environment. It is possible to set up a relatively clean ("sterile") room with the use of several portable laminar air flow units and strict adherence to sterile techniques for the patient. This approach, while relatively inexpensive in terms of major equipment, is enormously costly in terms of personnel, because sterile scrub nurses and circulating nurses or aids are required. The cost of small laminar flow units is about $1,500 each. The older life islands, such as those used on burn services, are more economical for nursing but are unsatisfactory for the adult, especially if he is not clinically ill. These units cost about $10,000. The large life island provides one of the best methods for patient care. It can be erected in a temporary space, the patient does not feel confined, and he has his own toilet facilities. A rigorous isolation technique can be maintained with simplified nursing procedures. The cost of such a unit in the United States is approximately $15,000 to $20,000.

The efficacy of these units in treating radiation injury has not been evaluated critically. Preliminary results with patients receiving prolonged intensive chemotherapy or immunosuppressive therapy suggest that this type of environment improves the course of treatment.[15]

Radioactive Contamination

In comparison with the injuries from external radiation sources, the injuries that might be expected from contamination have been at the worst minimal or essentially nonexistent in terms of overt damage due to radiation. There have been wounds, foreign bodies, and chemical burns but no evidence of the acute radiation syndrome, cancer, or other abnormalities attributable to contamination accidents in the modern nuclear energy industry. Those who have been exposed have received about 1 to 20 body burdens of various radionuclides. One may reasonably ask the reason for the concern. The urgency, the desire for prompt diagnosis, decontamination, and other forms of treatment in these situations result from the fear of late effects of the radionuclides, particularly if they become fixed in tissues so that they cannot be removed easily. Deleterious late effects have been demonstrated in radium dial painters, underground uranium miners, the Marshall Island natives, and many laboratory animals. All the efforts devoted to these patients are in the general province of preventive medicine rather than immediate cure. One must be reasonably certain that the treatment methods do not create more problems than the contamination.

The problem associated with adequate care for this type of exposure varies greatly depending on the nature and level of work in a given installation. The following outline describes the major considerations that must be evaluated in the care of these patients. The general principles of emergency care were presented earlier in this discussion. The most important point is that the nuclide is metabolized in the body according to its chemical form and not its radioactivity or isotopic form. Similarly, the choice of a decontaminating agent depends on the physical and chemical forms of the compound. Metabolic schemes for the many nuclides and their chemical forms are not always readily available. Help for less understood elements and compounds can be found in other publications.[16] The current literature often provides clues for specific compounds. Many compounds encountered industrially are relatively insoluble because they occur as oxides and metallic fragments.

Considerations in Radioactive Contamination

A. Type of contamination
   1. One specific nuclide
   2. A mixture of nuclides
   3. Are elements known or unidentified
B. Forms of contaminant
   1. Physical state—dry or liquid, nature of solvent
   2. Chemical form of contaminant—ionic state, valence, solubility, pH
C. Elapsed time since contamination
D. Number of persons contaminated
   1. Male
   2. Female
E. Extent of body area involved
   1. General
   2. Local
   3. Hands
   4. Head—face, eyes, nose, mouth, hair, etc.
   5. Other body orifices
F. Contamination in presence of other conditions
   1. Wounds—location, depth, area, vasculatory, amount of tissue destruction
   2. Ambulatory or nonambulatory status
   3. Burns—thermal, chemical
   4. Shock
   5. Extent of wound—major or minor, single or multiple
G. Entrance routes of radionuclides
   1. Inhalation
   2. Ingestion
   3. Injection
   4. Percutaneous absorption
   5. Contamination of wound

Factors Determining Effects of Radionuclides

A. Quantity entering body
B. Metabolic pattern
C. Radiation characteristics
   1. Radiations produced—alpha, beta, gamma
   2. Decay scheme and half life
   3. Tissue and organ susceptibility—the critical organs

Radiation Syndromes to be Anticipated

A. Acute radiation syndrome—could result from relatively massive internal doses; extremely rare; no known human example
B. Chronic low dose effects usually after many years—fractures, bone necrosis, anemia, and cancer (*e.g.,* radium dial painters)

Personnel Available to Aid in Decontamination

A. Level of previous training
B. Protective covering for personnel performing decontamination
   1. Hands—rubber gloves (surgical, obstetric, industrial)

    2. Plastic aprons, coats (may be disposable)
    3. Shoe covers
    4. Dust masks
C. Instrumentation
    1. Alpha, beta, gamma
    2. Mobile or fixed

Physical Facilities and Equipment

A. Location
    1. Within installation where accident occurred
    2. At plant or community hospital
B. Is layout designed for decontamination?
C. Water supply—quantity available
D. Effluent water—is storage necessary?
E. Airborne contamination—will it affect other areas in the building?
F. Chemicals for decontamination
    1. Previously stockpiled and familiar to operators
    2. Procured after event
G. Floor covering
    1. Kraft paper
    2. Plastic
    3. Masking or adhesive tape
H. Medical supplies
    1. Drugs
    2. Dressings, swabs, envelopes, test tubes, labels, marking pens
    3. Instruments
I. Protective coverings
    1. Plastic sheets
    2. Plastic pillow covers
    3. Paper
    4. Shoe covers
    5. Large paper or plastic bags
    6. Crayons, pencils, labels, tags

In order to assay properly for radioactive contamination, the necessary instruments must be available. Alpha activity cannot be found readily with a beta-gamma meter, and the converse is equally true. With high levels of activity, a relatively less sensitive detector is particularly useful. All sponges and solutions used at various levels of decontamination should be monitored. All exposed body surfaces and orifices should be wiped. Urine, feces, sputum, hair, and blood should be assayed.

A suggested plan of decontamination is as follows:

A. Gross decontamination
    1. Removal of contaminated clothing
    2. Washing and removal of contaminated hair
    3. Removal of gross wound contamination

B. Intermediate stage—at clean location if necessary
  1. Removal of contaminated clothing
  2. Further local decontamination, swabs of body orifices
  3. Supportive measures, first aid
C. Final stage
  1. Patient discharged with fresh clothing
  2. More definitive decontamination (surgical) and other therapy at dispensary or hospital

Therapy is first directed toward surface decontamination. One should be careful not to spread radioactivity to uncontaminated parts of the body. The use of disposable waterproof drapes may facilitate cleansing. The use of scrub sinks, eye irrigators, douche cans, and foot baths may be more efficient than showering. In serial order, the following agents may be used to try to remove dry particulates: dry wipes, sticky tape, water, detergents (such as Tide, Alconox, and Hemasol), soaps, hair clippers, and shavers, and sweating abrasives. Common household bleach (5% sodium hypochlorite) can be used full strength on intact skin and diluted 1:5 for use on the face and in wounds. Another solution[17] that has been useful is as follows:

Tartaric acid	3.0 gm./liter (0.2 M)
Citric Acid	4.2 gm./liter (0.2 M)
Disodium DTPA* or calcium disodium edetate	8.0 gm./liter (0.2 M)
Calcium chloride	2.2 gm./liter (0.3 M)
Adjust to pH 6 with concentrated NaOH	

* The calcium salt of diethylenetriamine penta-acetic acid. It requires an IND from the Food and Drug Administration. It is available to qualified physicians through the Division of Biology and Medicine, Atomic Energy Commission, Washington, D.C.

The Contaminated Wound. In contamination accidents it is not unusual for small radioactive particles to become embedded in a wound. Wounds may also need debridement or other surgical procedures. The particles may be so small that they cannot be seen and may be sufficiently radioactive as eventually to be a hazard to the physician and his assistants as well as to the patient. In these cases the help of the health physicist and nuclear medicine physician and their technicians will be most valuable because they can use the appropriate instruments to localize the offending contaminants.[17]

In preparing the operative site, shaving and washing are done in the usual manner except that all instruments are segregated until they can be surveyed for radioactivity. Similarly, solutions, gauze wipes, and other cleaning materials must be properly disposed of under the direction of the Radiological Safety Officer. Whenever possible the use of disposable equipment and drapes is recommended. During the debridement, the surgeon must scan each piece of tissue with radiation detectors to be certain that the offending particles are removed. All tissue should be saved and carefully labeled for radioactive assay and autoradiography. Only in this way can the incident be reconstructed so that the body burden of the patient can be determined.

The procedure is completed by excision and sampling until the contaminated area is excised or until essential structures are reached. When all the particles cannot be removed, fibrosis frequently develops and a small nodule can be palpated, making excision easier.

As with surgery of infected or cancerous tissue, it may be necessary to change instruments, drapes, and sponges frequently to avoid transferring contaminated particles. It is necessary to train the health physicist and technicians about sterile technique so that they can function effectively.

The use of eliminants is important. Inhalation and ingestion of particles almost always occur together. Also, within the next day or two larger particles are brought up from the tracheobronchial tree and are swallowed. Simple catharsis for two or three days using magnesium sulfate or other suitable agent therefore is most valuable. Other eliminants may be used also. Sometimes nonradioactive carriers, such as iodide for ^{131}I contaminations, may be useful.

Chelating agents are of practical value when used soon after exposure. The agent DTPA has been of particular usefulness for elimination of rare earths, especially plutonium and americium, when given intravenously in doses of 0.2 to 1.0 gm. daily for 1 to 5 doses. Ideally, one would like daily total urine collection and immediate assay for the duration of therapy, but this goal is rarely achieved. The DTPA is of greatest value when begun immediately after exposure. Its effect lessens markedly within weeks or months. It is mildly nephrotoxic, and monitoring hematuria and albuminuria is necessary.

The benefit of DTPA solution for inhalation therapy is at present unproved, and further work to demonstrate its value is indicated.

After the patient has undergone decontamination and is free of easily removed radioactivity, he should be followed by studies using the whole body counter. This method is, of course, valuable for gamma-emitting substances. With sufficiently large doses, powerful beta emitters, such as ^{32}P, ^{90}Sr, and ^{90}Y, can be found if special detectors and standards are available. At this time even the 13, 17, and 21 keV. x-rays can be measured under very special circumstances. These devices are widely available throughout the world and their use will help the patient both medically and psychologically.

Hospital Plans. A disturbing feature of certain incidents in the past has been the reluctance or refusal of hospitals to admit patients with actual or suspected contamination. Occasionally the induced radioactivity of ^{24}Na from neutron exposure has been interpreted as serious contamination. The degree, type, and consequences of contamination are difficult to assess. Contaminated patients should not be brought directly into hospital emergency areas. Special arrangements are required for hospitals to be prepared adequately for the care of such patients.[18] The development of a plan for radiation emergencies by each hospital is required for approval by the Joint Commission on Accreditation of Hospitals.

Long-Term Follow-Up. In most recorded radiation accidents, the actual physical damage has certainly been no greater and, in most cases, less than in many nonradiation industrial accidents. Yet, frequently the accident victim complains of persistent vague symptoms, particularly fatigue and weakness which, in our present state of knowledge, seem out of proportion to the physical changes observed.

Because of the apparent lack of knowledge about radiation accidents, particularly about adequate therapy for the radiation syndrome, and also because of the widespread interest that has developed as a result of possible somatic and genetic changes induced in living tissue by radiation, a definite long-term program of follow-up therapy is advisable for persons who have been injured by radiation. Certainly the patient should be seen every three to six months for a period of one to two years and then at least once yearly for an indefinite period of time. Follow-up studies should include attempts to determine radiation levels if there has been internal contamination, and complete history and physical examination and slit lamp examination of the lenses if there has been external beta, gamma, or neutron exposure. Serial observations of fluctuations in blood count, chromosome karyotyping, and occasional bone marrow biopsy may also be of value.

Frequently persons involved in radiation accidents have chronic complaints of fatigue, malaise, and other vague symptoms that may, in part, be of psychogenic origin. The remarks of friends, co-workers, and family contribute to the patient's confusion. A patient can be rehabilitated far more quickly when an intelligent and warm relationship with the responsible physician exists, especially if the patient is encouraged to report to him at regular intervals. An intelligent medical approach to such problems can obviously minimize the possibility of lengthy legal actions.

Each patient should be encouraged to report for reevaluation at least yearly. At these visits, the physician should obtain a detailed history and perform a complete physical examination. A complete hemogram and urinalysis should be done. New complaints should be thoroughly studied in cooperation with the patient's personal physician, who also should be furnished with complete medical reports.

The patient will continually be concerned about the long-term effects of radiation, such as sterility, genetic abnormalities in his children, and the likelihood of increased susceptibility to neoplasia and anemia. These problems should be discussed with the patient and his personal physician. Consultation with radiation experts should be encouraged and obtained freely. An open and frank attitude with the patient is of great importance.

Job rehabilitation should begin as soon as the patient can be encouraged to return to work. New techniques of rehabilitation for physical injuries should be employed. Group I patients can certainly return to preaccident jobs as can many patients in Group II. If the damage is great or if there is a persistent high body burden of long lived, retained radionuclides, the patient should be reassigned to work away from a radiation environment. In most cases a change of job should not be necessary.

The proper long-term medical care program is obviously best carried out in institutions that have excellent industrial medical departments. A strong, well organized department is of the greatest economy and value in all locations employing radioactivity. If such facilities are not justified because of the small size of the operation employing radiation, suitable arrangements for patient care and consultation should be made with qualified and interested physicians in neighboring communities.

Dose Estimates for Direct Contact With Sealed Sources

Direct contact of sealed sources with human tissues has caused very severe local injuries with loss of extremities or parts thereof. Usually such injuries have occurred with industrial sources of 10 to 150 curies. It is also possible for such injuries to occur with newer brachytherapy sources.

The usual injury is to the hand. Superficial erythema, edema, and bulla develop rapidly. There is relatively little change at depths of 2 to 4 cm. below the exposed part. The doses calculated from the usually available brachytherapy data do not provide sufficiently accurate estimates of dose distribution.

Table 14-7. Approximate Gamma Dose Rates to the Hand for 1 Curie in a Sealed Source*†

Nuclide	β max (principal) MeV	γ (principal) MeV	Γ R/hr.mCi at 1 cm.	surface‡	Dose Rate (R/min.) at 1 cm. tissue depth	3 cm. tissue depth
^{137}Cs	0.51, 1.2	0.662	3.26	513	28	3.7
^{60}Co	0.31	1.17, 1.33	13.00	2,075	114	16.0
^{192}Ir	0.67	0.468	5.10	813	43	5.5
^{226}Ra	0.4–3.2	0.047–2.4	8.25	1,310	72	9.7

* From National Council on Radiation Protection and Measurements. 1972. *Protection Against Radiation from Brachytherapy Sources,* NCRP Report No. 40. Washington, D.C.
† The industrial source housings are usually of stainless steel, and for the purpose of these calculations the activity is considered to be a point source. In considering these dose estimates a capsule with 1/4-inch wall (outside diameter), 1/32-inch thick stainless steel (type 304) is assumed.
‡ The total surface dose rate for the ^{226}Ra source is 1,900 R per minute based on a 45% increase due to electron production in the stainless steel wall.[20] For the other nuclides given in the table, the increase in surface dose rate due to electron production in the stainless steel wall is estimated to be between 25 and 45%.

Table 14-8. Surface Dose Rate Calculations for Radium Needles and Tubes*†

Activity (mg.)	Active length (cm.)	Outside diameter (mm.)	Wall thickness (mm. Pt.)	Surface Gamma Dose Rate (R/hr.)	Total Surface Dose Rates‡ (R/hr.)
Needles					
1	1	1.7	0.5	393	656
2	2	1.7	0.5	393	656
3	3	1.7	0.5	393	656
Tubes					
5	1.15	2.7	1.0	700	1,170
10	1.30	2.8	1.0	1,240	2,070
15	1.45	2.9	1.0	1,665	2,780
25	1.10	3.5	1.0	3,660	6,110

* From National Council on Radiation Protection and Measurements. 1972. *Protection Against Radiation from Brachytherapy Sources,* NCRP Report No. 40. Washington, D.C.
† Numerically integrated to correct for oblique filtration.
‡ Includes 67% increase in surface dose rate because of electron production in platinum wall.[20]

The following factors are to be considered as contributing to the radiation injury:

1. Beta particle effect is negligible.
2. Electron production in the capsule wall from the incident gamma photons increases the surface dose by 30 to 70% depending on the gamma energy and wall material.
3. There is a smaller dose for an extended source as compared to a point source with equal activity.
4. Gamma absorption in tissue is about 5 to 10% per centimeter.
5. The inverse square effect is the principal factor accounting for the relative lack of effect at depths below 2 cm.

Table 14-7 provides estimates of gamma dose rates for certain sealed sources of very high activity, such as those encountered commonly in industry. For comparison, Table 14-8 presents surface dose rate calculations for several typical radium needles and tubes commonly utilized in brachytherapy.

References

1. Casarett, A. P. 1968. *Radiation Biology*. Englewood Cliffs, N.J., Prentice-Hall.
2. Fabrikant, J. I. 1972. *Radiobiology*. Chicago, Yearbook Medical Publishers.
3. United Nations Scientific Committee on the Effects of Atomic Radiation. 1958, 1962, 1964, 1969, and 1972. *Ionizing Radiation: Levels and Effects.* UNSCEAR Report of the Official Records and Vol. I and II with appendices. New York, United Nations.
4. Saenger, E. L. 1963. *Medical Aspects of Radiation Accidents; A Handbook for Physicians, Health Physicists and Industrial Hygienists.* Prepared under AEC Contract AT(30-1)-2106, Washington, D.C., U.S. Government Printing Office.
5. Joint Commission on Accreditation of Hospitals. 1970. *Accreditation Manual for Hospitals.* Chicago, Joint Committee on Accreditation of Hospitals.
6. National Council on Radiation Protection and Measurements. 1971. *Basic Radiation Protection Criteria,* NCRP Report No. 39. Washington, D.C., National Council on Radiation Protection and Measurements.
7. Langham, W. H. (ed.). 1967. *Radiobiological Factors in Manned Space Flight.* Washington, D.C., National Academy of Sciences.
8. Thoma, G. E., and Wald, N. 1959. Diagnosis and management of accidental radiation injury. *J. Occup. Med.,* 1:421–447.
9. Karas, J. S., and Stanbury, J. B. 1965. Fatal radiation syndrome from an accidental nuclear excursion. *New Eng. J. Med.,* 272:755–761.
10. Fanger, H., and Lushbaugh, C. C. 1967. Radiation death from cardiovascular shock following a criticality accident. *Arch. Path.,* 83:446–460.
11. *Diagnosis and Treatment of Acute Radiation Injury.* 1961. New York, Columbia University Press.
12. Andrews, G. A., Auxier, J. A., and Lushbaugh, C. C. 1965. The importance of dosimetry to the medical management of persons accidentally exposed to high levels of radiation. In *Personnel Dosimetry for Radiation Accidents.* Vienna, International Atomic Energy Agency, pp. 3–14.

13. *Handling of Radiation Accidents.* 1969. Vienna, International Atomic Energy Agency.
14. Saenger, E. L., et al. 1973. Whole body and partial body radiotherapy of advanced cancer. *Amer. J. Roentgenol.,* 117:670–685.
15. Penland, W. Z. and Seymour, P. 1970. Portable laminar-air-flow-isolator. *Lancet,* 1:174–176.
16. International Commission on Radiological Protection. 1959. *Report of Committee II on Permissible Dose for Internal Radiation,* Publication No. 2. London, Pergamon Press.
17. Wald, N., et al. 1968. Problems in independent medical management of plutonium-americium contaminated patients. In *Diagnosis and Treatment of Deposited Radionuclides,* H. A. Kornberg and W. D. Norwood (eds.). New York, Excerpta Medica Foundation, pp. 575–585.
18. Saenger, E. L. 1963. Hospital planning to combat radioactive contamination. *J.A.M.A.,* 185:578–581.
19. National Council on Radiation Protection and Measurements. 1972. *Protection Against Radiation from Brachytherapy Sources,* NCRP Report No. 40. Washington, D.C., National Council on Radiation Protection and Measurements.
20. Shalek, R. J., and Stovall, M. 1969. Dosimetry in implant therapy. In *Radiation Dosimetry. Sources, Fields, Measurements and Applications,* Vol. III, F. Attix and E. Tochilin (eds.). New York, Academic Press, p. 749.

15

Acute Renal Failure*

Jeremiah G. Turcotte

Acute renal failure is a major cause of morbidity and mortality following severe injury. Despite the widespread availability of peritoneal and hemodialysis, mortality associated with the combination of oliguric renal failure and trauma approximates 50%.[1] Renal failure can result either from direct trauma to the kidney or indirectly as a consequence of circulatory shock, sepsis, and failure of other organ systems. This chapter reviews some principles of prevention and management of acute renal insufficiency resulting from causes other than direct trauma to the kidney and urinary tract. Emphasis is given to newer concepts, such as the role of the diuretics mannitol and furosemide in the management of these patients.

Differential Diagnosis

Renal failure has a multiplicity of etiologies. Patients may be oliguric when first admitted to the emergency department, or the apparent onset of renal insufficiency may be delayed several days. Dividing the differential diagnosis into two categories dependent upon the time of onset is useful in the management of these patients (Tables 15-1 and 15-2). For instance, if the onset of oliguria is immediate, lower urinary tract obstruction, injury to the kidneys or renal vasculature, and shock should be ruled out as etiologies before the patient leaves the emergency department. Understanding that the onset of renal failure is often delayed implies that baseline renal function studies should be obtained promptly and repeated serially when etiologies such as those listed in Table 15-1 are potentially present.

* This work was supported in part by the James Lynd Fellowship and the U.S. Public Health Service Grant No. SM01 RR-42.

Table 15-1.   Etiologies of Acute Onset Oliguria

Obstruction of lower part of urinary tract

Thrombosis, dissection, or stenosis of aorta or renal arteries

Severe contusions or fractures of both kidneys

Circulatory shock

Compensated hypovolemia (blood pressure and pulse may be normal, especially when patient is recumbent)

Acute drug or transfusion reactions

Severe sepsis or pyelonephritis

Disseminated intravascular coagulation

Progression of chronic renal disease

Table 15-2.   Etiologies of Delayed Onset Renal Insufficiency

Delayed or progressive effects of all etiologies listed in Table 15-1

Nonoliguric (high output) renal failure

Drug toxicity, especially from nephrotoxic antibiotics

Cryptogenic hypovolemia

Cardiac failure

Hepatorenal syndrome

Myoglobin nephrotoxicity secondary to necrotic or ischemic failure

Classifying the etiologies of oliguria into prerenal, renal, and post-renal causes also organizes our approach to diagnosis and management and focuses attention on pertinent pathophysiology (Table 15-3).

Some simple urine and plasma tests that are readily available in most hospitals are useful in differentiating prerenal from true acute renal failure and some other common causes of oliguria (Table 15-4). Specific gravity determinations can at times be misleading if the urine contains sufficient albumin or glucose to increase the urine density significantly. Osmolality is a more accurate test, but it is not routinely available. If the kidney is concentrating urine, the osmolality should be at least 50 milliosmols higher than the plasma osmolality.

If any doubt remains about the status of kidney function, a one or two hour creatinine clearance test may be performed; a clearance of less than 20 ml. per minute indicates severe impairment of renal function, but this test alone does not differentiate between the causes of renal insufficiency. In prerenal oliguria, the blood urea level increases faster

Table 15-3. Classification of Causes of Oliguria

Prenal causes of oliguria

  Hypotension

  Hypovolemia

  Cardiac failure

Postrenal causes

  Ureteral obstruction or transection

  Urethral obstruction or transection

  Ruptured bladder

  Compression of bladder or urethra from hematoma

Intrarenal causes (partial list)

  Fixed acute renal failure

    Acute toxic renal failure (drugs)

    Acute circulatory renal failure (shock, sepsis)

  Severe acute pyelonephritis

  Advanced chronic renal disease

Table 15-4. Comparison of Urine and Plasma Tests in Common Forms of Acute Renal Insufficiency*

	Prerenal Oliguria (decreased GFR)	*Acute Renal Failure (diffuse nephron damage)*	*Hepatorenal Syndrome*
Specific gravity	Concentrated >1.020	Fixed 1.010	Variable
Urine/plasma creatinine	>15–20	<15–20	<15–20
Urine/plasma urea	> 7–10	< 7–10	< 7–10
Creatinine clearance	>40 ml./minute	<40 ml./minute	Low, <10 ml. minute
Urine sodium	Low, <10 mEq./liter	>40 mEq./liter	Low, <10 mEq/ liter

* The pattern of urine and plasma tests is usually sufficient to determine the cause of oliguria. Any single test, especially specific gravity or urine sodium concentration, may deviate from these guidelines.

than the serum creatinine, probably because of back diffusion of urea in the tubule and the increased catabolism associated with common causes of prerenal oliguria, such as trauma, shock, and sepsis. The hepatorenal syndrome is characterized by very low urine sodium concentration and evidence of associated hepatic insufficiency. Other tests such as intravenous pyelograms and renal arteriograms are also pertinent when dealing with a patient who has multiple injuries.

Pathophysiology

Acute renal failure is a common cause of temporary renal impairment on most surgical and emergency services. The terminology used to describe this entity has been confusing and our knowledge of its pathogenesis incomplete.

Acute renal failure is the condition characterized by the fairly abrupt onset of diffuse nephron dysfunction, which may follow shock, sepsis, trauma, or the administration of nephrotoxic drugs. Prerenal and postrenal causes of oliguria should be ruled out before making a diagnosis of acute renal failure. Recently the term "acute vasomotor nephropathy" has been used to describe this entity by authors who emphasize shifts in the intrarenal distribution of blood flow as being important in the pathogenesis. Other synonyms include acute tubular necrosis, shock kidney, crush syndrome, and lower nephron nephrosis. Acute renal failure may be subdivided into toxic or circulatory types depending on whether the etiology is related to nephrotoxic drugs or to other causes such as hypovolemia, shock, and sepsis (Table 15-3).

Acute renal failure usually persists for a few days to six weeks. The condition is almost always reversible, but renal function may not return to previous levels. Patients with the fully developed syndrome usually excrete 100 to 200 ml. of urine daily. Some patients excrete considerably larger amounts, and when the output approaches 1,000 ml. daily the entity is referred to as high output or nonoliguric renal failure. Complete anuria usually indicates lower urinary tract obstruction or compromise of renal vasculature. Only rarely and in the presence of severe damage are patients with acute renal failure truly anuric. In busy emergency departments and in large transplant programs, the complete spectrum of acute renal failure can be observed; patients with severe renal damage may be nearly anuric, while others may continue to excrete 1,000 to 2,000 ml. of urine daily despite diminishing renal function. Renal biopsies demonstrate ischemic cortical glomeruli and interstitial edema. Only in severe cases is actual necrosis of tubules observed histologically.

The three most discussed theories of pathogenesis are (1) obstruction of tubules due to intraluminal casts and debris or to compression from interstitial edema, (2) back diffusion of glomerular filtrate through damaged tubules, and (3) alterations in renal hemodynamics.[2,3] Micropuncture studies have disproved to the satisfaction of most investigators that neither the first nor the second hypothesis is the primary mechanism involved. Both clinical and laboratory studies have conclusively demonstrated that a marked shift in blood flow away from the renal cortex with a concomitant decrease in the glomerular filtration rate correlates best with the observed reduction in renal function. An increase in intrarenal angiotensin may be the chemical mediator that leads to vasoconstriction of the afferent arteriole, decreased glomerular filtration, and a general diminution in blood flow to the cortex. This theory, although far from proved, has become more tenable since it has been learned that renin from the juxtaglomerular apparatus can be converted to angiotensin within the kidney. In our own experience with an active renal transplant program, as well as in other surgical patients, magnification arteriograms obtained in many patients in various phases of acute renal failure have confirmed that this condition is associated with a general decrease in renal blood flow and marked ischemia of the cortex.[4]

These hypotheses provide the rationale for much of the therapy advocated for acute renal failure. For instance, mannitol, a drug used in prophylaxis of acute renal failure, may in part exert its effect by clearing the tubular lumen of debris and preventing interstitial edema. Long-term salt loading, another effective prophylactic measure, may exert its beneficial effect by suppressing the renin-angiotensin system.

Prevention

It is easier to prevent acute renal failure than to reverse the syndrome after its onset (Table 15-5). In fact, no drug or treatment has been proved conclusively to alter the course of acute renal failure after it is clinically apparent and prerenal causes have been eliminated. For this reason, it is prudent to concentrate one's efforts on prevention whenever possible. When confronted with the injured patient, often shock or sepsis is already present; nevertheless, attention to preventive measures often can be helpful. A common problem is the patient with multiple injuries who is continuing to hemorrhage and requires many transfusions and often a major operation. Adequate blood replacement, administration of generous amounts of a balanced electrolyte solution, and perhaps use of an osmotic diuretic such as mannitol will protect the kidneys during this period of cardiovascular instability.

Table 15-5. Prevention of Acute Renal Failure

Prompt reversal of shock, hypovolemia, or cardiac failure
Treatment of sepsis
Generous hydration
Salt loading
Mannitol
Furosemide
Careful monitoring of nephrotoxic drugs

Adequate hydration is the keystone to prevention of acute renal failure. In virtually every experimental model of renal failure and every clinical circumstance that has been studied critically, hydration ameliorates and dehydration augments the induced renal failure. Adequate hydration can be assured only by carefully monitoring patients who are critically ill. Urine output should be maintained at 50 ml. per hour as a minimum. The first physical sign of dehydration is not clinically apparent until a deficit equivalent to 6% of body weight has occurred. For this reason, one cannot depend upon physical examination to guide fluid replacement. Blood pressure, pulse, central venous pressure, and hourly urine output can be monitored readily in all patients. Many trauma centers are finding that more sophisticated physiologic monitoring is necessary to assess accurately the clinical status of the patient. Serial determinations of mean arterial pressure, cardiac output, and pulmonary artery pressures, together with calculation of peripheral resistance and other indicators of cardiac status, can be obtained readily with the help of a trained technician and approximately $5,000 to $10,000 worth of equipment.

Long-term salt loading has been demonstrated to prevent renal failure in experimental animals. McDonald and co-workers prevented renal failure in rats by feeding a 1% saline solution for three weeks prior to inducing renal failure with 50% glycerol.[5] This model of renal failure has features that are analogous to "circulatory" renal failure in humans. Silber preserved renal function in kidneys transplanted into rats by salt loading the donor and recipient.[6] Because of these experimental observations we prefer to hydrate patients with balanced electrolyte solutions, such as lactated Ringer's solution, unless otherwise contraindicated, rather than use more hypotonic solutions. Salt loading, however, has been shown to be effective only when used for several days prior to renal injury.

Mannitol is a popular diuretic that has been used as a prophylactic agent for renal failure since the early 1960s.[7,8] Mannitol, a synthetic sugar, exerts its osmotic effect by acting as a nonresorbable solute in the tubular lumen. Recent studies have demonstrated that the major site of action is the ascending loop of Henle.[9] There is no doubt that mannitol exerts a protective effect in a number of experimental models, including methemoglobin, glycerol-induced myohemoglobin, and other pigment models of renal failure. For this reason, it is especially recommended for management of transfusion reactions and after prolonged ischemia of muscle leading to release of toxic myoglobin degradation products. Mannitol should be administered prophylactically rather than after renal failure is established if possible. The usual intravenous loading dose for adults is 25 gm., *i.e.,* 100 ml. of a 25% solution. Repeat doses of 12.5 gm. are given every four to six hours. One should be aware that each 12.5 gm. temporarily expands vascular volume by 225 ml. A disadvantage of using this or other diuretics is that urine volume can no longer be used as a guide to adequate hydration. Mannitol should be discontinued after the acute episode is passed or if oliguric renal failure persists. With very high circulating levels of mannitol, central nervous system damage has been observed in our clinic and at other institutions.

In recent years furosemide and ethacrynic acid have been utilized for both prevention and treatment of renal failure.[10,11] In a few cases ethacrynic acid has been reported to increase urine output after furosemide has failed to do so. Despite these reports we have virtually abandoned the use of ethacrynic acid because of the greater incidence of ototoxicity and questionable therapeutic advantage as compared to furosemide.

Furosemide is a "loop blocking" diuretic; that is, both the concentration and the dilution of urine are inhibited, and the site of action is thought to be the loop of Henle.[9] Furosemide is a potent natriuretic agent and also causes excretion of increased amounts of potassium, calcium, and magnesium. Hypokalemic metabolic alkalosis can occur with repeated administration. Hyperuricemia and glucose intolerance are other side effects. Experimental studies suggest that when furosemide is given concurrently with certain antibiotics, such as cephaloridine, the nephrotoxic effect of the antibiotic may be potentiated. Ototoxicity, although occurring infrequently, is the most feared complication of large dose furosemide therapy. Both the total dose and the rapidity of administration seem to be related to the occurrence of middle ear dysfunction. Intravenous doses of more than 100 mg. should always be given slowly over at least 15 minutes.[10] Most cases of ototoxicity have occurred when the total dose exceeded 1000 mg. per eight hours, or when the drug was administered more rapidly than 2 mg. per minute.

Management

Proper management of acute renal failure includes accurate diagnosis; appropriate fluid, electrolyte, and nutritional support; preventive measures; and definitive therapy with drugs, peritoneal dialysis, and hemodialysis. Our approach to this problem may be outlined as follows:

1. Prerenal causes of renal failure, chronic renal disease, lower urinary tract obstruction, and injury to the kidney or renal vasculature are ruled out in the emergency department or soon after admission to the hospital.
2. Baseline plasma and urine renal function studies are obtained and repeated serially for several days.
3. If cardiac failure is not a serious consideration, 25 gm. of mannitol is administered intravenously soon after the patient arrives as a prophylactic measure.
4. Shock, volume deficits, and significant electrolyte imbalance, especially hyponatremia below 120 mEq. per liter, are reversed promptly. If the patient's cardiovascular status is unstable, a central venous pressure line and a Foley catheter are inserted to assist in monitoring fluid replacement. In critically ill patients, a Swan-Ganz pulmonary artery catheter is inserted and pulmonary artery pressures and cardiac function studies monitored serially. Serial cardiac studies can also be obtained through a radial artery catheter.
5. Mannitol, 12.5 gm. every four to six hours, is administered during the acute phase, that is, while the patient's cardiovascular status is unstable, when administering multiple blood transfusions, or during major operative procedures.
6. Intravenous furosemide therapy is begun when the patient is oliguric and unresponsive to mannitol administration, or when oliguria occurs after the acute phase and the patient's cardiovascular status is stable. Usually 80 mg. of furosemide is used initially. The dose is doubled every one to two hours if oliguria persists until a maximal single dose of 600 mg. is reached. If the patient does not respond to this dose, the renal failure is considered fixed, and furosemide is discontinued. In a few patients we have used a single dose of 1,500 mg. when smaller doses were ineffective and seen them respond with a diuresis. The risk of ototoxicity, however, is increased with these very large doses. If diuresis occurs, an appropriate dose of furosemide to a maximum of 600 mg. is administered every four to six hours with the goal of maintaining an average urine output of approximately 50 ml. per hour.
7. Hyperkalemia is avoided by restriction of potassium intake and use of the cation exchange resin sodium polystyrene sulfonate when serum potassium approaches high normal levels.[12] Twenty

grams of resin plus 20 ml. of sorbitol solution are administered orally every four to six hours. One gram of resin removes approximately 1 mEq. of potassium. When oral intake is not possible, the resin can be administered by high retention enema. One hundred grams of resin mixed with 100 ml. of 70% sorbitol solution are combined with an equal amount of tap water or glucose solution. The enema should be retained for at least 30 minutes if it is to be effective. When hyperkalemia is present, patients should be kept on a continuous cardiac monitor and serum potassium determinations obtained at least twice a day.

8. Acute hyperkalemia is controlled by administering sodium bicarbonate intravenously and starting an infusion of glucose and insulin. Usually two or three ampules, each containing 44.6 mEq. of sodium, are given slowly by intravenous drip, and then an infusion of 10% glucose containing 20 units of regular insulin is started. Simultaneously, cation exchange resin therapy is begun.

9. Plans for dialysis should be made when it is apparent that renal failure is fixed. Dialysis should be instituted early and repeated frequently with injured patients because of the acute nature of the insult and the severe catabolism associated with trauma or sepsis. Patients with acute renal failure do not tolerate the uremic state as well as those with chronic renal failure and seem more prone to cardiac arrhythmias and hyperkalemia. The usual indications for dialysis are the onset of uremic symptoms, hyperkalemia not readily controlled medically, a blood urea nitrogen level exceeding 100 mg. per 100 ml., or a creatinine level of more than 10 mg. per 100 ml. Usually it is preferable to dialyze patients when one of these indications is anticipated rather than to wait and risk a major complication such as hyperkalemic cardiac arrest. Our axiom has been that it is better to perform one too many dialyses rather than one too few.

Peritoneal dialysis is still an excellent method for management of oliguric renal failure. As compared to hemodialysis, it is more efficient in removing water and potassium. In addition, the risks of heparinization, always a consideration when hemodialysis is employed in the recently injured patient, are avoided and the patient's cardiovascular status does not have to be as stable. If blood pressure is low or fluctuating, adequate flows through the dialyzer are difficult to achieve, and frequently fluid must be added rather than removed simply to maintain blood pressure during the dialysis. Hemodialysis is the method of choice in the stable patient when renal failure persists for more than a few days.

10. During the diuretic or recovery phase of acute renal failure, strict attention to fluid and electrolyte balance is necessary. The ability of the kidney to concentrate glomerular filtrate is one of the last functions to return. Consequently, the kidney is not functioning satisfactorily as a regulatory organ during this phase, and patients may lose excess fluid and electrolytes. Instead of restricting water, sodium, and potassium, extra quantities may need to be administered. During this time the patient is questioned regularly about dizziness, weakness, and other symptoms of orthostatic hypotension and hypokalemia. Daily measurements of body weight, serum electrolytes, and blood pressures in the recumbent and standing positions are obtained until a stable condition is reached.

11. Acute renal failure usually reverses itself within six weeks from the time of onset. An occasional patient, especially the elderly patient, may recover after a period as long as three months. For this reason, we usually maintain dialysis and other supportive measures for three months before considering renal failure to be irreversible and planning for measures such as transplantation or long-term hemodialysis.

12. The patient in acute renal failure must be maintained on an appropriate diet.[13] Because of the associated catabolism and other metabolic changes, restriction needs to be severe during the early phases of acute renal failure, especially following trauma or operation. During this phase the usual restriction for adults is a maximal oral or parenteral intake of 20 gm. of protein, 20 mEq. of sodium, and 20 mEq. of potassium. Concomitantly, as much glucose or carbohydrate as feasible is administered to provide calories.

When the patient's condition is stabilized and a regular dialysis program has been instituted, dietary restrictions can be liberalized. Depending upon the individual patient's tolerance and response to dialysis, daily intake can usually be increased to 40 to 60 mEq. of sodium, 40 to 60 mEq. of potassium, and 60 to 100 gm. of protein. In the early phase, water should be limited to 600 ml. daily plus urine output, and later, when the patient is stable, it can be increased to 1,000 to 1,500 ml. per day plus urine output, providing the extra water can be readily removed by dialysis. Approximately 0.5 gm. of protein per kilogram of body weight is needed daily to maintain nitrogen balance, but after injury or operation this need is increased markedly.

The biologic value of the protein is also an important consideration; proteins that contain a high proportion of essential amino acids, such as egg whites, are more effective in their nitrogen sparing effect than are proteins consisting mainly of nonessential amino acids. Since magnesium is excreted primarily through the kidneys, the intake of this ion must also be restricted. Antacids, such as magnesium hydroxide, therefore should be avoided or limited. If the uremic course is prolonged, attention must also be given to calcium and phosphorus metabolism. Recently interest has turned to providing these patients with an appropriate balance of essential amino acids and glucose intravenously. Abel and co-workers have claimed to have improved survival using this program.[14]

Comment

Despite our increased understanding and improved therapy, the mortality rate from acute renal failure remains distressingly high. In patients who are elderly or have undergone major operations or severe trauma, only 10 to 20% of those whose courses are complicated by acute renal failure will survive. The explanation for this high mortality rate remains unknown and should be a high priority area for intensified research. At the present time our best hope for improved results depends upon prevention, early definitive therapy, careful monitoring of patients in intensive care units, and avoidance or treatment of complications before severe consequences ensue.

References

1. Editorial. 1973. Prognosis of acute renal failure. *Brit. Med. J.*, 2:435–436.
2. Flamenbaum, W. 1973. Pathophysiology of acute renal failure. *Arch. Intern. Med.*, 131:911–928.
3. Linton, A. L. 1974. Acute renal failure. *Canad. Med. Assn. J.*, 110:949–951.
4. Bookstein, J. J., et al. 1975. Angiography of renal transplants. *J. Radiol.*, 116:271–277.
5. McDonald, F. D., et al. 1969. The prevention of acute renal failure in the rat by long-term saline loading: A possible role of the renin angiotensin axis. *Proc. Soc. Exp. Biol. Med.*, 131:610.
6. Silber, S. J. 1975. Transplantation of rat kidneys with acute tubular necrosis into salt-loaded and normal recipients. *Surgery,* 77:487–491.
7. Powers, S. R., Jr., et al. 1964. Prevention of postoperative acute renal failure with mannitol in 100 cases. *Surgery,* 55:15–23.
8. Luke, R. G., et al. 1965. Mannitol therapy in acute renal failure. *Lancet,* 1:980–982.
9. Grossman, R. A., and Goldberg, M. 1974. The use of diuretics in renal disease. *Kidney,* 7:1–6.
10. Brown, C. B., Ogg, C. S., and Cameron, J. S. 1974. High dose furosemide in acute reversible intrinsic renal failure. A preliminary communication. *Scot. Med. J.,* 19:35–39.

11. Kjellstrand, C. M. 1972. Ethacrynic acid in acute tubular necrosis. Indications and effect on the natural course. *Nephron*, 9:337–348.
12. Levinsky, N. G. 1966. Management of emergencies. VI. Hyperkalemia. *New Eng. J. Med.*, 274:1075.
13. Gulyassy, P. F. 1972. Nondialytic management of chronic renal failure. *Kidney*, 5, No. 4, July.
14. Abel, R. M., et al. 1973. Improved survival from acute renal failure after treatment with intravenous essential L-amino acids and glucose. *New Eng. J. Med.*, 288:695–699.

16

Trauma to the Central Nervous System

G. W. Kindt and H. H. Gosch

An important segment of traumatology deals with injuries to the central nervous system. The nature of such injuries often requires rapid and sound judgement in order to prevent irreversible neurologic damage or death. This chapter is concerned with the usual mechanisms of injury, as well as the diagnosis and immediate treatment of patients with an acute central nervous system injury.

Epidemiology

In 1973 a total of 117,000 accidental deaths were recorded in the United States.[1] The motor vehicle accounted for 56,400 of these fatalities, while a total of 19,900 deaths were attributed to falls from heights. The number of fatalities has shown a steady increase over the previous years. These figures are from only two sources of accidental deaths and do not include fires, drownings, and certain industrial and sporting fatalities. For a comparison, the number of deaths in auto accidents in 1973 exceeded the number of battle deaths of the U.S. forces during the ten-year Viet Nam conflict.

The frequency of head injuries in motor vehicles accident victims can be seen in data collected by the automotive crash injury research program of the Cornell Aeronautical Laboratory, Inc.[2] In 57,597 reported cases of injuries to passenger car occupants, the percentage of body area injured was as follows:

```
Head ................................................................................. 70.8%
Neck ................................................................................. 10.8%
Thorax ............................................................................... 38.6%
Abdomen ............................................................................ 17.1%
Upper extremity ................................................................. 38.9%
Lower extremity ................................................................ 50.4%
```

The Cornell study demonstrates the extreme vulnerability of the head to injuries, either as the only part involved or more frequently as one of several areas injured. In an analysis of the causes of deaths in automobile accidents, Huelke and Gikas found fatal head injuries in 64% of victims.[3]

The spinal cord is also vulnerable to injury in vehicular accidents. Diving in shallow water was at one time the main cause of cervical spine injuries with resulting paraplegia or quadriplegia. Review of recent records at the University of Michigan Hospital, however, revealed the motor vehicle to be the current main cause of such trauma.

Central nervous system injuries are a prominent cause of morbidity. Since the brain and spinal cord are capable of little functional healing, injuries are often permanent, with the result that paraplegics and brain injured patients fill our rehabilitation and nursing home units.

What can be done about this dismal situation of central nervous system injuries? Ideally, accident prevention is the answer. Advances are being made, but the number of accidents continues to increase as the population and the number of vehicles increase. One way of reducing the mortality and morbidity rates in accidents is to further educate all personnel dealing with the accident victim about the mechanisms of injury and early care of the injured.

Mechanism of Injury

Over the past two centuries a succession of theories evolved to explain the mechanism of widespread brain damage. The lack of a suitable experimental model, however, hindered a clear definition of the nature of brain damage during concussion, contusion, and contrecoup. One of the first rational methods of correlating clinical observations with controlled experimental results was reported by Russell,[4] who described the motions of the brain within the cranial cavity following trauma. Our present understanding of the mechanisms of brain injury are based on his studies.

The brain and spinal cord consist of a semisolid mass, anchored to various areas of the skull and vertebral canal by nerves, blood vessels, and dentate ligaments in the spinal canal. A sudden accelerating force, such as a blow to the restrained or moving head, causes deformation and movement of the brain in relation to the surrounding skull. Brain tissue, with its high water content, is practically noncompressible, but it has a great tendency to change shape. With a frontal blow, the brain continues to move along the line of acceleration after the skull has stopped its forward progress. This phenomenon has been documented in many experimental animals in our laboratory.[5] The vertex of the skull and the dura were removed and replaced by a tight, clear polycarbonate calvarium without deficit to the monkey. Simulating a head injury in the anesthetized animal and observing the brain by high speed cinematography demonstrated the deformation and movement as the injury occurred. Correlating these observations with the human head subjected to similar forces in the decelerating vehicle provides a plausible explanation for some of the dynamics leading to diffuse or local brain damage. The main areas of injury are where tissue elasticity is exceeded and disruption of the delicate tissues is produced.

Concussions. A relatively minor injury in a critical location can lead to cerebral concussion. This term is usually defined as a period of unconsciousness due to a transient and reversible disruption of neuronal activity in the brain stem region or, more precisely, in the reticular activating system of the brain stem. The brain stem reticular formation has been shown experimentally to depress electrical activity following concussion to a greater extent and longer than do cortical and other subcortical structures.[6] This sensitivity to trauma of the reticular system explains the loss of consciousness following relatively minor blows to the head. Because anatomic disruption of nerve tissue apparently does not occur with concussion, the process is reversible. Physiological silence of neuronal activity during this period, however, prevents stimuli from reaching higher centers of brain function. Patients remain unconscious for variable periods until neuronal function is restored.

Contusions. Cerebral contusion denotes damage to or destruction of nervous tissue. In a patient with a head injury such damage is clinically most often observed beneath the area of trauma, at the basal portions of the brain, or at the pole opposite the side of the blow (contrecoup area). The temporal and frontal lobes are contused as the cerebral hemispheres slide over the sharp, bony protrusion of the sphenoid ridge between the temporal and frontal fossae. The contrecoup injury occurs at the frontal and temporal lobe tips in a person striking the back of his head. Perhaps the mechanism for brain contusion is simply the brain moving within the cranial vault and striking the rigid skull.

Another theory for the cause of coup and contrecoup injuries was advanced by Gross.[7] He stressed the importance of the inbending of the very rigid skull, which then snaps back into place. This sudden re-

9

turn of the skull to the normal position may produce cavitation within the tissue directly beneath the site of injury, as well as opposite to the site in the contrecoup region. Immense pressures are produced (30,000 atmospheres) when these cavities collapse within fluids. This theory may explain the pulp brain seen at the site of the coup and contrecoup injuries when the skull is intact. When the skull is fractured, the energy of the blow is absorbed by the skull, and severe brain injury may not occur. Clinically, we note that many accident patients rendered deeply unconscious may have severe brain damage but do not have skull fractures.

Lacerations. The most severe form of cerebral injury is cerebral laceration. Just as in the laceration of other tissues, this constitutes an open tear or break in the continuity of the tissue. If a vital area of the brain, such as the motor strip or visual pathway, is lacerated, the accompanying neurologic deficit or dysfunction is severe and permanent.

Intracranial Hematomas. Mass lesions, as a result of head injuries, include epidural, subdural, and intracerebral hematomas. The epidural

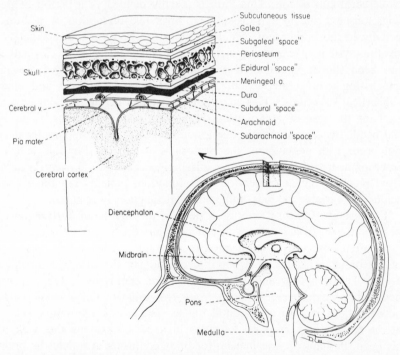

Fig. 16-1. A schematic diagram of the coverings of the brain, as well as deep brain structures often involved in head injuries. The layers and potential spaces commonly involved in hematoma development are shown in the magnified segment. The parts of the brain affected by concussion are labeled in the sagittal section.

hematoma usually results from damage to the meningeal arteries (Fig. 16-1) and is often associated with a skull fracture. Arterial bleeding leads to a rapidly expanding hemorrhagic mass between the dura and the skull. The mass produces pressure on the brain, as well as distortion, and may compromise vital brain stem functions.

Cerebral veins (Fig. 16-1), which cross the subdural space and enter the midline sagittal sinus, may rupture and lead to the formation of a subdural hematoma. These vessels are stretched beyond their elastic limits as the brain moves with respect to the skull after a blow to the head. In the elderly patient with generalized cerebral atrophy, movement of the cerebral hemispheres is enhanced. Such a patient also has a tendency to form a subdural hematoma even after an apparent minor injury.

The intracerebral hematoma results from rupture of small vascular channels within the brain substance. The mass lesion is produced by coalescence of hematoma, contused cerebral tissue, and edema fluid.

Skull Fractures. These injuries are related intimately with central nervous system trauma. The fracturing of the skull may be a protective mechanism by which the energy of a blow is dispersed away from the brain. At other times the fracture may tear a meningeal artery, resulting in a fatal epidural hemorrhage. Fractures can be classified as linear, depressed, or compound. Linear fractures are often associated with blunt trauma to the head, such as the head striking the pavement. Compound and depressed fractures are usually the result of a relatively sharp object striking a localized area of the head. Cerebral contusion and laceration, as well as intracerebral hematoma, may be associated with the fracture.

Spinal Cord Injuries. These injuries result from a variety of forces that produce alterations in the vertebral alignment. The necessity of the cervical spine in providing both support and mobility for the head renders it particularly susceptible to traumatic deformation. Flexion and hyperextension with a concomitant rotational movement, if of sufficient magnitude, can rupture the ligamentous supporting structures and dislocate the vertebral bodies. It is, however, not the bony destruction, but rather the extent and degree of spinal cord damage that dictates the patient's prognosis. The most common sites of spine fractures are at the low cervical and thoracolumbar regions. (See chapter on spinal injuries.) The cervical spinal cord is more susceptible to a compression fracture when the spine is flexed than when it is extended. The typical diving injury occurs with the neck flexed and results in a compression fracture of the fifth or sixth vertebral body with complete and permanent paraplegia. The thoracolumbar junction is the site at which the spine gives way when one falls in the sitting position.

Pathology

The central nervous system tissue is very soft and susceptible to injury, as well as incapable of regeneration. It is protected from injury to a degree by being suspended within cerebrospinal fluid and being covered by the very sturdy cranial vault and spinal column.

The importance of brain stem centers in the production of concussion has been demonstrated, but whether histologic changes occur is unclear. Transient chromatolysis and cell shrinkage in the area of the brain stem reticular formation have been found by some investigators and denied by others. Cerebral contusion, however, leaves it mark on the central nervous system with areas of tissue fragmentation and hemorrhage. The more severe cerebral laceration is seen at autopsy of victims with severe injuries.

The epidural hematoma results from the rapid accumulation of blood in the potential space between the inner table of the skull and dura

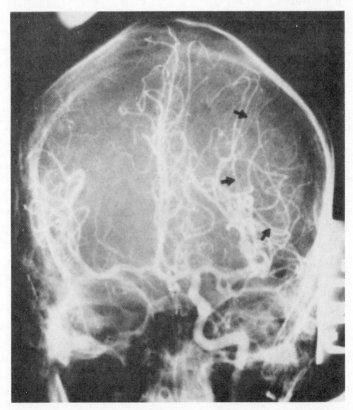

Fig. 16-2. Cerebral angiogram demonstrating epidural hematoma. The arrows along the depressed cortical arteries outline the epidural mass.

mater, as demonstrated in Figure 16-1. The most frequent location is the temporal area, but any portion of the cerebral hemispheres or cerebellum may be compromised by such a mass. The localized, expanding mass can accumulate rapidly to a significant size as a result of arterial bleeding from the middle meningeal vessels. Figure 16-2 shows the anteroposterior arteriogram of a patient with such a lesion. The vascular architecture is grossly altered as the epidural mass compresses and shifts the cortical arteries to the side opposite the lesion. When the hematoma compresses the cerebral hemisphere it causes the medial aspect of the temporal lobe to protrude through the tentorial notch and compress the third nerve and the brain stem. Protrusion of the temporal lobe in this manner is referred to as the tentorial pressure cone, which can be secondary to any type of supratentorial mass. Compromise of vital brain stem functions leads to rapid clinical deterioration unless normality is

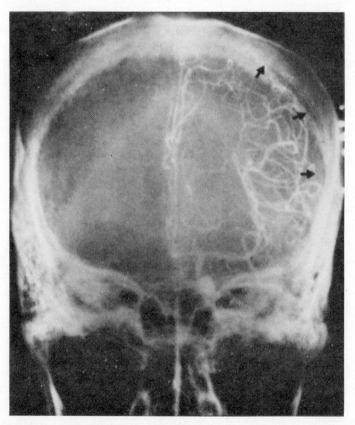

Fig. 16-3. Cerebral angiogram demonstrating an acute subdural hematoma. The hematoma outlined by the arrows in this case extends over the cerebral hemisphere.

quickly restored, making this one of the most acute emergencies of surgical practice.

The subdural hematoma expanding between the dura mater and pia of the cerebral cortex has a similar effect, as shown in Figure 16-3. This hematoma usually progresses more slowly than the epidural type because the bleeding is of venous origin, but the consequences, if treatment is neglected, are similarly tragic. This lesion can be classified as acute or chronic, depending on its discovery and production of symptoms after the initial injury. The acute subdural hematoma has a high mortality rate despite therapy because concomitant diffuse cerebral contusion is usually present in such injuries. The patient with a chronic subdural hematoma does not develop symptoms immediately but becomes symptomatic several weeks later and has a much better prognosis following removal of the clot, which becomes enveloped by a pseudomembrane of connective tissue and thin-walled vessels. The red cell membranes of the clot lyse and release molecules of the breakdown products of hemoglobin. The fluid becomes hypertonic and expands the subdural mass. Transudation of plasma and bleeding from the small vessels in the enveloping membrane continue the process, resulting in eventual pressure and decompensation of the brain unless treated.

A traumatic intracerebral hemorrhage is secondary to disruption of vessels within the cerebral substance. A roentgenogram of an intracerebral hemorrhage is shown in Figure 16-4. The hemorrhage may at times separate the fiber bundles within the cerebrum and cause little permanent deficit if removed. At other times the mass is a mixture of contused, edematous brain, as well as hemorrhage.

Skull fractures can be the direct cause of brain disease. The linear nondepressed fracture by nature of its location may cause damage to the meningeal vessels or dural sinuses, producing hemorrhage and brain compression. Fractures of the base of the skull occur most frequently in the frontal and middle fossae and tend to extend into one of the foramina or sinuses. A basilar fracture has the potential of presenting a special problem if associated with a dural tear and spinal fluid leak. The possibility of an ascending infection and meningitis can remain a threat months or years after the initial injury. Cranial nerves, particularly the olfactory, abducens, facial, and auditory nerves, are injured in 5 to 10% of basilar fractures.

Compound fractures are associated with scalp lacerations and the displacement of bone fragments and foreign material into the brain substance. Such material in the presence of localized contusion and hemorrhage results in infection unless properly debrided. Open fractures usually present more of an emergency than do depressed fractures with the scalp intact. Bone fragments in compound lesions may have lacerated

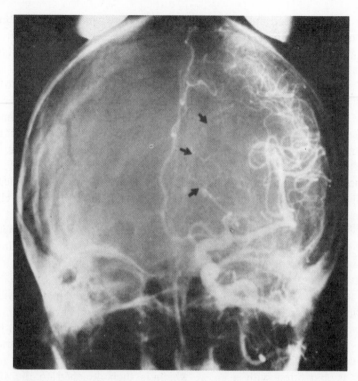

Fig. 16-4. Cerebral angiogram demonstrating an intracerebral hematoma. The mass lesion, as designated by the arrows in this case, separates the deep cerebral vessels.

the dura and penetrated the brain to variable depths. Associated hematomas and contused cerebral cortex are frequently associated with these lesions.

Trauma to the spinal cord is usually due to compression along the anteroposterior axis. The microscopic pathology reveals edema, diapedesis of red cells, petechial hemorrhage, and globular hematomas within the cord substance. These changes are seen first in the central gray matter of the cord and spread peripherally with increasing severity of trauma. The white matter of the posterior columns is often the last part of the cord to function in severe cord lesions that are incomplete. Continuous pressure from dislocated vertebrae or disc herniation may produce further damage because of spinal artery compression and ischemia.

Emergency Care

Scene of Accident. The dangers of moving an accident victim with a central nervous system injury have long been emphasized. Patients are often left untouched until the ambulance arrives, which may take hours. Perhaps some of these patients die from airway obstruction or external hemorrhage that could have been managed by a person with training in first aid and less fear of moving the patient.

A significant brain injury is likely if a patient is unconscious or lethargic at the scene of the accident, regardless of whether there is evidence of external trauma. Unconscious patients are prone to vomiting and aspiration; it is therefore imperative that they be provided with an adequate airway. A pressure dressing may be required to prevent exsanguination from a scalp laceration.

The patient rendered unconscious in an accident must be handled as a suspected vertebral fracture victim until proven otherwise. (See chapter on spinal injuries.) The reason for considering a spinal injury is that the forces necessary to produce the brain injury are also in the range of those that cause spinal injuries. The conscious patient who complains of pain in the spine or numbness and weakness of the extremities is likely to have a spinal cord injury.

A method used to extract from a vehicle the injured patient with a questionable spine injury has been well described by Farrington.[9] The equipment used consists of a collar, a short spine board, and a long spine board with appropriate straps. (See chapter on spinal injuries.) A patient who is sitting in a vehicle and is suspected of having a neck injury is first fitted with a collar which is then attached to the short spine board inserted behind him, and he is carefully extracted. A patient not fixed in the sitting position is rotated gently and slid onto a long spine board. The goal in the extraction process, with or without the equipment, is to keep the spine immobile, in line, and under slight traction at all times.

The patient with central nervous system injury should be transferred to the proper medical facility immediately. Although respiratory distress and shock are more urgent situations, the head injured patient may bleed intracranially, producing irreversible brain damage and death within minutes or a few hours. If a patient with a spinal cord injury is properly immobilized, his existing neurologic deficit rarely increases.

Emergency Department. All patients with a potential brain or spinal cord injury must receive the urgent initial care that other emergency patients receive. These procedures include securing an adequate airway, stopping external hemorrhage, and treating shock.

After one has attended to these emergencies, the remainder of the history and the physical and neurologic examinations can be completed. The pertinent details of the accident should be obtained so that the type of injury can be anticipated. Items of importance in vehicular accidents include finding out whether the patient was a pedestrian or an occupant of the vehicle, the speeds involved, the patient's position in the vehicle, and whether or not he was ejected from the vehicle. The item of greatest importance in the history of the head injury patient is his state of consciousness when first observed following the accident. If the patient was unconscious from the instant of the accident and has remained that way, it is unlikely that any immediate surgical procedure will be necessary. If the patient had a lucid interval and then became obtunded or unconscious, however, an expanding lesion is likely, and prompt measures may be necessary if a life is to be saved.

The history of the patient with a spinal cord injury from the time of the accident to arrival at the emergency department is of equal importance. The patient who was paralyzed from the time of the accident is unlikely to benefit from any surgical procedure. The patient who at first was walking and then became progressively weak, however, may have a lesion requiring an urgent decompressive laminectomy.

Careful attention should be paid to certain items during the routine neurologic examination. A dilated pupil, fixed to light stimulus, on a patient who also has bilateral Babinski signs and a deteriorating level of consciousness is the classic picture of an acute, expanding intracranial hematoma. Any deepening in the level of consciousness should be viewed with alarm. A slowing of the pulse and an increasing blood pressure in the unconscious patient is an ominous sign that may indicate brain stem ischemia. Urea administration or arteriography may be appropriate.

Disturbances in tone are common in patients with head injuries. Decerebration is often the result of a primary brain stem injury. The decerebrate posture can also occur following compression from an expanding clot because of brain stem compression. Again, it is important to know whether or not the decerebration is a delayed phenomenon or has been present since the accident.

The presence of a hemiplegia or hemiparesis may be due to conditions such as a cerebral contusion, cerebral laceration, contusion of the cerebral peduncle, or even traumatic occlusion of the carotid artery in the neck. A common lesion that causes hemiplegia and may require urgent therapy is an expanding intracerebral hematoma. Such a lesion usually produces a progressive paralysis with depression of consciousness.

The patient with a spinal cord injury may be expected to have spinal pain in the area of the injury. Pain is not always present, however, even in the conscious patient and cannot be verified in the unconscious patient. Spinal injuries commonly occur in the lower cervical area or at the thoracolumbar junction. Patients complaining of pain in these areas should be examined with care to prevent increasing a neurologic deficit.

Motor and sensory functions should be examined carefully to determine whether the neurologic deficit is increasing or decreasing. The sensory examination should include evaluation of the sensations of pain, touch, temperature, vibration, and position. A level of change in sensory modalities should be mapped carefully. The activity of deep tendon reflexes should be noted, because with an acute spinal cord lesion the deep tendon reflexes can be expected to be absent below the lesion. (See chapter on spinal injuries.)

Total dysfunction of the spinal cord below the level of a fracture is common after a spinal fracture, and unfortunately the injury is often permanent. A fracture with dysfunction of the spinal cord at the level of the third to fourth cervical vertebra or above is usually not compatible with life because of a loss of phrenic nerve function. (See chapter on spinal injuries.) A lesion between the fourth and fifth cervical vertebrae produces complete quadriplegia. A spared fifth cervical root preserves deltoid function for abduction of the shoulder. A lesion below the sixth cervical vertebra allows for use of the biceps and flexion of the elbows. If the seventh cervical vertebra is intact, the upper extremities are functional.

The common compression fracture at the thoracolumbar junction causes damage in the region of the conus medullaris of the spinal cord. (See chapter on spinal injuries.) Such a patient has impaired lower sacral segments, including loss of bladder function. The lumbar segments distal to the lesion may continue to function because the nerves of the cauda equina are more resistant to injury than is the conus tissue. More proximal thoracic spinal lesions cause complete dysfunction of the distal part of the spinal cord. These thoracic fractures are often associated with a mass or gibbus deformity over the thoracic spine, which is easily observed externally.

Since little can be done about a complete lesion of the spinal cord, it is important to determine whether any motor or sensory modalities are functioning below the lesion. An incomplete traumatic lesion of the cervical part of the spinal cord often affects the central gray matter first, which may produce motor and sensory loss of the upper extremities but leave the lower extremities intact. A more severe crush injury of the spinal cord produces loss of function below the lesion except for the senses of motion and position, which are carried in the posterior columns. When even slight function remains below the lesion, the prognosis is much better than when no function remains.

Triage of Patients. After evaluation in the emergency department, patients can be divided into three categories: those who can be released from the emergency department, those requiring operations, and those requiring observation in the hospital.

Patients Who Can Be Released From the Emergency Department. Patients whose neurologic examination and x-rays are negative can usually be released from the emergency department. This excludes patients who might have other conditions requiring hospitalization. The negative neurologic examination includes a normal mental status, because the patient who is confused or lethargic may need to be hospitalized. A patient released from the emergency department after a minor head injury should be closely checked by a reliable person for at least the first 24 hours. Changes in the neurologic condition of the patient should prompt immediate notification of the physician.

Patients Requiring Operations. Open fractures of the skull or spine require immediate operative debridement and wound closure to prevent infection. Debridement is ordinarily required for all missile wounds except for occasional cases in which missile fragments have traversed several centimeters of soft tissue before entering the central nervous system.

Another indication for an emergency operative procedure is an expanding hemorrhage within or compressing the central nervous system. There is no effective surgical therapy for the central nervous system damage that occurs at the instant of the accident. Surgery is of aid only to the patient who develops a hemorrhage secondary to the trauma. Such a patient is expected to deteriorate neurologically after the injury. The patient with an acute subdural or an epidural hematoma classically has a lucid interval after the trauma followed by progressive lethargy and coma. A definitive study, such as an arteriogram, is preferred prior to removal of the hematoma. A lumbar puncture is seldom helpful and may be dangerous to a patient with central nervous system trauma.

Emergency operative treatment for a spinal cord injury is also reserved for the patient with a progressing neurologic deficit. This deficit may be due to an expanding hemorrhage or mechanical compression of the spinal cord. Patients with cervical spinal fractures should be placed in skeletal traction promptly to realign broken fragments and dislocations. A spinal tap with manometrics helps to determine if the spinal canal is open.

Patients Requiring Observation. The remainder of the patients not requiring immediate operations and not released from the emergency department should be admitted for close observation. If these patients later show signs of deterioration, they may then require an operation. They should receive a close hourly check of vital signs, state of arousal, pupil size and reaction, and ability to move their extremities. They require supportive therapy with particular attention to proper airway maintenance. Dexamethasone is usually given if contusion of the central nervous system is present.

The patient with the spinal cord injury is immobilized in traction and placed on a frame that can be rotated to prevent decubitus ulcers. He is catheterized frequently under strict asepsis until his bladder begins functioning or until a urinary diversion can be performed. If the fracture is unstable, he is prepared for a later spinal fusion.

References

1. National Safety Council. 1970. Accident Facts. Chicago.
2. Kihlberg, J. K. 1968. Multiplicity of injury in automotive accidents, in *Impact Injury and Crash Protection*, E. S. Gurdjian (ed.). Springfield, Ill., Charles C Thomas.
3. Huelke, D. F., and Gikas, P. W. 1968. Causes of deaths in automobile accidents. *JAMA*, 203:98–105.
4. Russell, A. G. 1932. Cerebral involvement in head injury. A study based on the examination of two hundred cases. *Brain*, 55:549–603.
5. Gosch, H. H., Gooding, E., and Schneider, R. C. 1970. The Lexan calvarium for the study of cerebral responses to acute trauma. *J. Trauma*, 10:370–376.
6. Ward, A. A. 1958. Physiological basis of concussion. *J. Neurosurg.*, 15:129–134.
7. Gross, A. G. 1958. A new theory on the dynamics of brain concussion and brain injury. *J. Neurosurg.*, 15:548–561.
8. Kahn, E. A., et al. 1969. *Correlative Neurosurgery*, 2nd ed. Springfield Ill., Charles C Thomas.
9. Farrington, J. D. 1967. Death in a ditch. Bull. Amer. Coll. Surg., 52(3): 121–130.

17

Vascular Injuries

Calvin B. Ernst

A turning point in the management of vascular injuries was reached in the early 1950s. At that time the United States was involved in the Korean War, and some of the incurred injuries involved the vascular system. In contrast to previous conflicts, however, the combatants injured during the Korean War were greatly benefited by an innovation that ultimately saved many lives. This was rapid transfer from the scene of injury to a hospital by a medical evacuation helicopter.

This was also the period during which modern vascular surgery was developed. Diagnostic techniques were developed and therapeutic and technical advances followed to ameliorate symptomatic peripheral vascular disease. Of necessity, young surgeons were educated in the principles of vascular reconstructive procedures.

Since victims of battlefield injuries were promptly and efficiently evacuated from the site of injury to a definitive treatment facility, the lag time (the time from injury to definitive medical attention) was sometimes as short as two or three hours, and averaged 12 hours. Consequently, patients with injuries that in past wars would have been fatal were delivered to hospitals that were staffed with personnel knowledgeable in the management of vascular injuries and equipped with the facilities that enabled surgeons to treat the extensive wounds, preserving life and limb.

Among the varied injuries, those involving the vascular system were for the first time definitively treated on a large scale with results far superior to those obtained in the past. For example, during World War II, out of almost 2,500 vascular injuries, only 81 were treated definitively by direct operation. And of these 81 injuries, only three were resolved by end-to-end anastomosis of the severed vessel. The end results are reflected in the high amputation rate of almost 50% during the

Table 17-1. Amputation Rates (Percents) for Arterial Wounds During the Last Three Wars

Artery	World War II	Korea	Vietnam
Axillary	43%	7%	5.1%
Brachial	27%	0%	5.7%
Femoral	53%	12%	12.5%
Popliteal	73%	32%	29.5%
Overall	49%	13%	13.9%

Note: The rate for popliteal injuries has been persistently high. Since the 1940s, the overall amputation rate has progressively declined. The rates for the Republic of Vietnam reflect the increased severity of injuries over those in previous conflicts.

World War II experience. In contrast, with the improved methods of treatment, the amputation rate for the Korean War was a very satisfactory 13% (Table 17-1). The combination of aeromedical evacuation and skilled surgeons, therefore, was the genesis of modern management of vascular injuries. This experience was repeated in the Vietnam War in which vascular injuries were similarly expeditiously managed with an even lower mortality rate and a comparable morbidity rate.

From the military experience with vascular wounds have come principles for management of civilian vascular injuries. This is reflected in the decreasing mortality and morbidity rates for civilian vascular injuries, which are directly related to prompt evacuation and skilled definitive treatment (Table 17-2).

In the discussion of the etiology, diagnosis, and management of vascular injuries, the venous and arterial systems are considered together because of their contiguity. With few exceptions, the arterial injury receives the surgeon's attention because of the devastating consequences that occur if arterial flow is not promptly restored. Venous injuries assume a less important position on the scale of treatment of vascular injuries. This chapter, therefore, deals with the management of arterial injuries.

Table 17-2. Mortality and Amputation Rates (Percents) in Civilian Practice vs. the Vietnam Experience

	Civilian Practice				Military
	Ferguson[1] 1950–1959	Morris[2] 1950–1959	Patman[3] 1949–1961	Dillard[4] 1958–1966	Vietnam[5] 1965–1969
Mortality	15.5%	11.3%	8.4%	8.4%	1.7%
Amputation	9.8%	6.8%	3.8%	3.0%	13.9%

Etiology

The etiology of vascular injuries is varied and depends upon the community under consideration. In urban areas arterial injuries are the result of man's inhumanity to man as reflected in the high frequency of gun shot and stab wounds. Conversely, in rural areas, vascular injuries secondary to crush injuries and fractures are more prevalent.

There are three basic etiologies of vascular injuries: penetrating, blunt, and iatrogenic (Fig. 17-1).

Penetrating Injuries. These are injuries that pierce the skin, such as gun shot and stab wounds (Fig. 17-1). Stab wounds can be caused by fragments of glass, knives, or strips of metal. There is a distinct difference between the type of penetrating vascular injury seen in military and in civilian practice, and the two are compared in Table 17-3. High velocity weapons, such as the M16 rifle, cause extensive tissue damage resulting from the tremendous energy dissipated when the missile strikes the tissue. The greater the velocity of the missile the more devastating the injury. It is common for structures several inches from the path of the bullet to be damaged. In contrast, civilian gun shot wounds are usually of the low velocity type and, therefore, have less tendency to cause extensive contiguous injury. Penetrating wounds account for 80 to 90% of vascular injuries.

Etiology Of Arterial Injury

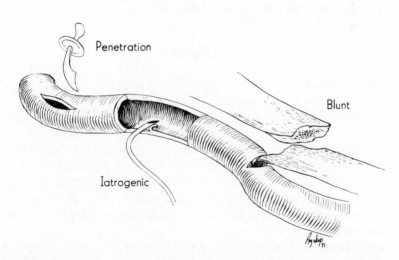

Fig. 17-1. Etiology of penetrating, blunt, and iatrogenic arterial injuries. A small intimal flap is elevated by the catheter tip in the iatrogenic segment.

Table 17-3. Comparison of Civilian and Military Vascular Wounds

Civilian	Military
Low velocity missiles	High velocity missiles
Minimal soft tissue damage	Major soft tissue damage
Frequent stab wounds	Few stab wounds
Short lag time	Variable lag time
Closed injuries	Open injuries

Blunt Injuries. The second etiology of vascular injuries is a blunt force, namely, crushing injuries to extremities or fractures of long bones (Fig. 17-1). These injuries cause laceration of vessels by loose bone spicules or entrapment of the vessel between unstable bone ends as a patient is being transported or extracted from the accident site. These vascular injuries are usually brought to the attention of a general or vascular surgeon by the orthopedic surgeon and make up a relatively small proportion of vascular injuries seen, approximately 10 to 20%.

Iatrogenic Injuries. The third etiology of vascular injuries is iatrogenic (Fig. 17-1). With the advent of more sophisticated diagnostic procedures, such as arteriography, during which vessels are punctured in order to introduce a catheter to outline the vascular tree with contrast material, a small number of vessels are inadvertently injured and require repair by a vascular surgeon or general surgeon. Figure 17-1 illustrates such an injury with a catheter piercing the vessel wall and turning back a small portion of the intima.

Classification

The classification of vascular injuries depends upon the time period in which the injury is recognized and the nature of the anatomic damage to the vessel wall. For example, if the injury is recognized late, one may find a chronic lesion, such as an aneurysm, or a totally occluded vessel. The same injury when recognized early would be an acute third degree contusion or an acute occlusion. It should be emphasized that the category "chronic" is actually an overlooked early or acute injury and ideally should not exist. If our diagnostic abilities were 100% correct in the emergency situation, no patient would have a chronic or overlooked acute injury.

Acute Injuries. Figure 17-2 is a classification of arterial injuries in which they are divided into acute and chronic forms. Table 17-4 shows the relative incidence of the four major classifications of acute vascular

Classification Of Arterial Injury

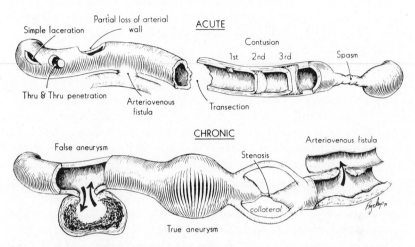

Fig. 17-2. Classification of arterial injuries. Upper vessel segment depicts acute injuries. Lower vessel segment depicts chronic (overlooked acute) injuries. Note the three degrees of contusion depicted by graded levels of vessel wall damage (see text).

injuries from two large series of civilian vascular trauma. Transection and laceration of vessels are the most common vascular injuries. Contusion and spasm, although definite entities, are distinctly unusual and account for less than 10% of vascular injuries.

Transection and laceration may be considered as a single category because one is often an extension of the other. In this combined category are simple laceration, partial loss of the arterial wall, through-and-through penetration, complete transection, and arteriovenous fistula (Fig. 17-2, upper portion).

Arterial contusions are divided into three categories as proposed by Sencert in 1918.[6] These are called first degree, second degree, and third

Table 17-4. Incidence of Civilian Arterial Injuries in Two Large Series

Type of Injury	Patman[3]	Morris[2]
Transection	42%	49%
Laceration	51%	44%
Contusion	5%	5%
Spasm*	2%	2%

*Note the rarity of this injury.

degree contusions (Fig. 17-2, upper portion). In a first degree contusion only a very small portion of the intima of the blood vessel is torn. This can lead to deposition of thrombotic material, occluding the vessel at the site of injury, or dissection of blood under the intima, causing an occluding intimal flap.

In a second degree contusion there is complete circumferential transection of the intima with its subsequent slight retraction. This leads to thrombosis at the site of injury or subintimal dissection as in a first degree contusion. Furthermore, in a second degree contusion the underlying muscle of the vessel wall is completely exposed, and it can cause focal spasm and thus decrease the blood flow or stop it completely.

A third degree contusion is characterized by a complete circumferential tear of both intima and the media leaving only the adventitia intact. Thrombosis and obstruction of the vessel may result. If thrombosis does not occur, the thin filmy adventitia may distend to cause a true fusiform aneurysm (Fig. 17-2, lower portion).

Spasm is a distinctly rare form of acute vascular injury but it is mentioned in reports of vascular trauma. It can occur with the three degrees of contusion or without intimal injury. It is important to realize that spasm accounts for only a small percentage of vascular injuries. When one is confronted with a patient with a vascular injury, it is therefore unwise to delay treatment in the hope that the injury is a spasm that will spontaneously resolve. If one follows this reasoning, he will be wrong 98% of the time and seriously jeopardize the viability of the patient's limb.

Chronic Injuries. If the vascular injury is not recognized when it occurs, it may come to the clinical horizon at a later date in the chronic forms of a false aneurysm, a true aneurysm, a stenosis, or an arteriovenous fistula (Fig. 17-2, lower portion). A false aneurysm has also been called a pulsating hematoma in the acute phase. Initially, there is a partial laceration of the arterial wall and as the blood spurts out it is contained in a large subcutaneous hematoma. With time this unrecognized acute hematoma develops into a fibrous tissue-lined cavity that communicates directly with the lumen of the vessel (Fig. 17-2, lower portion). Such a lesion is a false or pseudoaneurysm and has none of the constituents of a normal vessel wall. A true aneurysm may be the end result of a third degree contusion as noted previously. A third form of chronic arterial trauma is stenosis, which evolves from a scarred complete or partial occlusion. If the acute injury was partial and at a site circumvented by collateral channels, the extremity may survive but with a suboptimal level of blood flow. Finally, an acute arteriovenous fistula, if overlooked early, becomes chronic and often associated with hypervolemia and heart failure.

Sites Of Arterial Injury

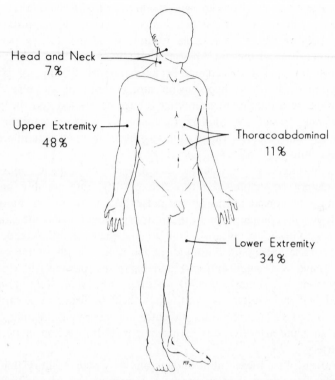

Fig. 17-3. Sites of civilian arterial injuries compiled from more than 1,100 vascular wounds. Note predominance of extremity locations (exceeding 80%).

Sites of Injury

Practically any artery in the body may be injured, but the most vulnerable are those of the extremities. Data from more than 1,100 civilian arterial injuries indicate that more than 80% involve either the upper or the lower extremities (Fig. 17-3). Head and neck vessel injuries almost equal those of the thoracoabdominal area; the two areas combined account for less than 20% of vascular injuries. Since extremity vascular injuries predominate, the obvious therapeutic implication is that hemorrhage can be easily controlled because the vessels are in an accessible portion of the body.

Diagnosis

The diagnosis of vascular trauma is usually clear, but occasionally it is challenging and difficult. Recognition of extremity vascular wounds is simplified by recalling the five P's of vascular trauma: pallor, pain, paresthesia, paralysis, and pulselessness. Another helpful finding is a temperature difference between two extremities or between different levels in the same extremity. It must be recalled, however, that approximately 50% of patients who have vascular wounds are in shock (hypoperfusion and hypotension) at the time they are initially examined by a physician. This must be taken into account because physical findings of generalized hypoperfusion and hypotension mimic those of vascular injury. After initial resuscitative measures have been completed and the patient is normotensive and has good perfusion, existing vascular injuries then become evident. Clearly, blood spurting from an open wound signifies a vascular injury.

In diagnosing vascular wounds, a high index of suspicion must exist and it cannot be emphasized too strongly that questionably palpable pulses must be considered as absent pulses. An associated hematoma in an anatomically contiguous area of an artery should signal the examiner to the possibility of a pulsating hematoma, which, if overlooked, could become a false aneurysm. Although penetrating wounds of the extremity may have very small entrance and exit sites, particularly when occurring in an anatomic region of an artery and vein, they should be palpated and auscultated. A continuous thrill or bruit, or a thrill and bruit with systolic accentuation, indicates an underlying vascular injury, such as an acute arteriovenous fistula or partial transection or occlusion of an artery.

There are other more subtle indications of vascular injury that must be sought. Sometimes the key person is the individual who initially sees the patient at the scene of the accident. If initial physical findings are remembered and passed on to the physician when the patient reaches the hospital, a great service may be done for the patient. The physician who examines the patient initially must speak with the persons responsible for initial resuscitation and transportation of the acutely injured patient. The history might include the comment that bright red blood had been spurting from the wound. Perhaps by the time the patient reaches the hospital he is in such a hypoperfusive and hypotensive state that it is not recognized that an arterial injury exists although it was quite evident initially. Furthermore, noting the condition of an injured extremity when the patient is initially seen and again when he arrives at the hospital emergency ward is important. For example, initially an injured extremity may be pink and warm, but en route to the hospital it becomes pale and cool from fracture fragments impinging on an artery. Similarly, a pale and cool extremity that becomes viable and pink after splinting at the scene is also an indication of an arterial injury. This latter sequence of events is vitally important because it indicates an underlying vascular injury that may be partially reversed but is still potentially dangerous and may progress to complete arterial occlusion. Progressive swelling in the region of a puncture wound, a stab wound, a gun shot wound, or an angulated fracture of an extremity indicates an enlarging hematoma whose source might be a complete or partial arterial injury.

Most vascular injuries are diagnosed readily by a thorough history and physical examination. Occasionally, however, special studies such as arteriography are useful in managing arterial injuries. Arteriograms can be most efficiently employed if one thinks about utilizing them to localize the *site* of the injury, rather than utilizing them to *make* the diagnosis. If the diagnosis is suspected on physical examination, and the patient's condition is satisfactory, exploring the artery is superior to delaying therapy by obtaining arteriograms. It must be remembered that many vascular injuries occur at night when the hospital is not staffed to supply the responsible physician or surgeon with all the diagnostic armamentarium that is available to him during the daytime.

Probably one of the most difficult situations in which to diagnose an arterial injury is that in which palpable peripheral pulses exist in an extremity with a vascular injury. As can be seen from Table 17-5, the incidence of a palpable pedal pulse with an associated significant vascular injury ranges from 18 to 61%. Saletta and Freeark[7] reported the highest incidence because they evaluated tangential vascular wounds, which are more likely to have associated palpable distal pulses. Nevertheless, a realistic figure for significant arterial injuries accompanied by palpable distal pulses is 20 to 25%. In this situation the history, a high degree of suspicion, and the utilization of arteriography in selected patients help minimize the overlooking of an acute arterial injury.

The diagnosis of arterial injuries in areas other than the extremities may be difficult. For this reason, penetrating wounds of the head and neck must be considered to have an associated component of vascular

Table 17-5. Incidence of Palpable Pedal Pulses Associated With Arterial Injury*

	Pedal Pulse Palpated	
	Patients Reported	*Percentage*
Saletta[7]†	28/46	61%
Patman[3]	69/256	27%
Dillard[4]	15/85	18%

* The overall incidence is 25%.
† This study reported partial arterial severance.

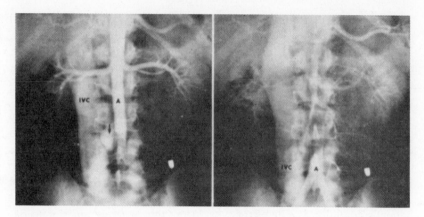

Fig. 17-4. Two frames from a serial retrograde axillary aortogram demonstrating an aortocaval fistula (arrow): IVC, inferior vena cava; A, aorta. Note the simultaneous opacification of the aorta and vena cava in frame 1 (left). Frame 2 (right) further demonstrates opacification of the vena cava, the aortic bifurcation, and the common iliac arteries. The 0.22 caliber bullet causing the fistula appears in the left lower quadrant.

trauma and, therefore, must be surgically explored. Penetrating wounds of the thorax and abdomen involving large arteries usually cause death before the patient reaches the hospital, There are occasions, however, when a patient with an intrathoracic or intraabdominal vascular injury presents himself for treatment. For the diagnosis in these situations, the responsible physician or surgeon must rely on the signs and symptoms of intrathoracic and intraabdominal trauma, which are discussed in other chapters. Here, arteriography may play a major role in management of the injury (Fig. 17-4).

Management

The management of vascular injuries, just as that of other acute injuries, is divided into two phases: the initial on-the-scene management and the subsequent definitive hospital management.

On the Scene. Treatment of the injured patient starts at the scene of the accident and continues en route to the hospital regardless of the type of injury. At the scene, be it on the highway, at home, in a cornfield, or in a local bar, common sense and general principles of good first aid should be employed.

First and foremost in managing vascular trauma is the cessation of hemorrhage. Since most vascular injuries result from penetrating trauma, external blood loss may be massive with the patient rapidly progressing into a low perfusion syndrome. It is imperative that the person assisting at the scene of the accident know how to stop arterial bleeding. Fortunately, most vascular injuries involve the extremities where the blood vessels are accessible and hemorrhage can be readily stopped by applying digital pressure over the site of bleeding. Ideally, a sterile gauze sponge is used, but a clean handkerchief or clean garment folded into a pad serves as well. A tourniquet is rarely required to alleviate hemorrhage, and digital pressure *must* be employed first. In the past, tourniquets have been overused and in many instances misused, resulting in further ischemic damage to an already compromised extremity.

Since vascular injuries sometimes accompany fractures, it is important that broken bones be splinted before the patient is moved. "Splinting them where they lie" minimizes blood vessel and nerve damage from entrapment or penetration by moving fracture fragments. Any rigid strut, board, tree branch, or similar object can serve as a splint, but ideally, a ready-formed splint or an aerosplint should be used.

At the scene of the injury, the condition of the patient's injured extremity should be observed and recorded. Several questions are of diagnostic significance. Was the extremity initially pale and cool, indicating a vascular injury? Was it initially pink and warm, and then in transit to the hospital did it become pale and cool, indicating a vascular injury? Was the extremity initially pale and cool and then after being splinted become pink and warm? This also indicates a vascular injury that must be investigated upon arrival at the hospital. Was the blood coming from the wound bright red, indicating arterial bleeding, or was it maroon, indicating venous bleeding? Did the extremity rapidly swell at the site of a penetrating wound or angulated fracture? Recognition of a rapidly progressing hematoma is particularly important in injuries of the neck. Unrelenting progressive bleeding into the neck results in airway occlusion, necessitating tracheostomy for relief.

Finally, about half the patients who have vascular injuries are in a state of hypotension and hypoperfusion. Appropriate procedures should therefore be employed at the accident scene to minimize the detrimental effects of these conditions. (See chapter on shock.)

Hospital Management. Upon the patient's arrival at a hospital, definitive diagnostic and therapeutic procedures are undertaken. Aggressive, prompt attention must be given to airway problems, life-threatening intrathoracic or intraabdominal injuries, and acute reversible head injuries. After hemorrhage from an injured vessel has been stopped, efforts are directed to lifesaving procedures if necessary. It must be realized, however, that limb survival is inversely proportional to the time interval from injury to restoration of arterial blood flow. If it appears that the patient will succumb because of another injury, the priority of treatment is directed to the potentially lethal injury, realizing full well that the patient might lose an extremity because there was not adequate time to treat the vascular wound. Certainly, for want of a limb, a life should not be lost.

The usual course of events permits prompt attention to the vascular injury. Therapy must be instituted in the emergency department at the time of the patient's arrival. (See chapter on intraabdominal injuries.) Placement of a large-bore intravenous catheter for rapid administration of blood and fluids and the measurement of central venous pressure is mandatory. If the patient is in a hypotension-hypoperfusion syndrome, urinary catheter drainage for evaluation of renal perfusion must also be instituted. If general anesthesia is to be employed in repairing the vascular injury, the stomach should be emptied by an appropriate tube to prevent aspiration of gastric contents.

During resuscitation and restoration of normal cardiovascular dynamics in the emergency department, the blood bank is requested to prepare sufficient blood and the operating room is readied in anticipation of immediate operation. The diagnostic maneuvers outlined previously will, in most instances, localize the vascular injury, and time should not be lost in obtaining extensive, sophisticated preoperative diagnostic studies. If one is suspicious of an arterial injury that cannot be definitively diagnosed preoperatively and the patient is otherwise able to tolerate an operative procedure, the suspected vascular injury should be explored, realizing that in a small percentage of cases a completely normal vessel will be found at the time of exploration. On the other hand, if prompt, efficient arteriograms can be obtained and the lag time is short, contrast studies are of great benefit in localizing the unclear vascular injury.

Operative Management. Since there is a relationship between the time elapsed and extremity salvage it is imperative that arterial flow be restored promptly. If delay is unavoidable, the safe ischemia time of the tissues distal to the injury can be prolonged by perfusing the distal limb vessels with heparinized, cooled, lactated Ringer's solution.

A very important principle in operative management of vascular wounds is debridement of all nonviable tissue. Dead tissue is an ideal culture medium for bacterial growth; therefore, copious irrigation of the damaged tissue must accompany excision. Sometimes it is difficult to distinguish viable from nonviable muscle. In this case, if debridement has been extensive, it is prudent to reexplore the wound 48 to 72 hours later and then excise any remaining nonviable tissue. In this way unnecessary mutilation and sacrifice of tissue is prevented.

The type of repair employed is dictated by the nature of the injury. Vascular injuries not associated with severe crushing, contusion, or fractures can usually be managed by simple arteriorrhaphy or a very short segmental arterial resection and primary end-to-end anastomosis of the vessel (Fig. 17-5). If the vessel is resected and primarily sutured, it is important to realize that excessive suture line tension will compromise the repair. The anastomosis therefore must be done without tension. Because arteries such as the superficial femoral and the brachial can be easily mobilized in young patients, approximately 3 to 5 cm. of vessel may be resected without compromising a primary tensionless anastomosis. If more extensive resection is required, however, or if the patient is elderly and has arteriosclerotic brittle vessels and the anastomosis cannot be performed primarily, reversed saphenous vein interposition must be employed (Fig. 17-5).

In civilian practice the incidence of severe, extensive arterial injuries from gun shot wounds is low because of the low velocity of the missiles.

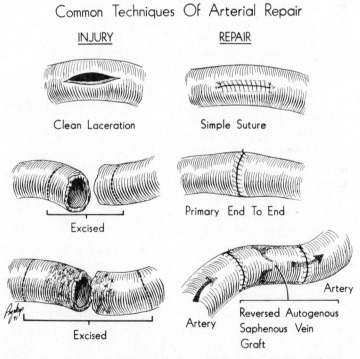

Common Techniques Of Arterial Repair

INJURY   REPAIR

Clean Laceration   Simple Suture

Excised   Primary End To End

Excised   Artery   Reversed Autogenous Saphenous Vein Graft   Artery

Fig. 17-5. Commonly employed techniques of arterial repair. The type of injury is indicated on the left and the repair on the right. Top: clean laceration without loss of vessel wall, and repair by simple closure. Center: transection with jagged edges requiring limited excision of vessel wall and repair by primary end-to-end tensionless anastomosis. Bottom: transection with extensive adjacent vessel damage requiring long-segment excision, and autogenous vein interposition to restore vascular continuity. Note vein segment is reversed so that valve is in the direction of blood flow.

Furthermore, stab wounds account for many of the penetrating injuries involving blood vessels. Penetrating injuries in civilian practice, therefore, can usually be managed by simple suture or segmental resection and primary anastomosis (Fig. 17-5). Occasionally, however, there is extensive damage to an artery either from the occasionally high velocity gun shot wound or from a shotgun blast. This requires extensive debridement of the blood vessel and utilization of a reversed saphenous vein graft for restoration of vascular continuity (Fig. 17-5). Extensive crush injuries also require excision of an inordinate length of artery, necessitating a reversed saphenous vein graft.

A sufficient length of greater saphenous vein is removed and cleaned of areolar tissue. The vein is reversed so that the valves are in the direction of the blood flow when interposed between the severed ends of artery. It is important to take the vein from the contralateral uninjured extremity because arterial injuries are frequently accompanied by venous injuries, and preservation of maximal venous return in the injured extremity is essential to a successful vascular repair. Similarly, to preserve maximal venous return, large veins, such as the common femoral or the popliteal, must be primarily repaired. If it is impossible to repair these vessels, an autogenous vein graft is utilized to bridge the venous defect. If major veins are not repaired, the ensuing acute venous hypertension may result in amputation because of progressive swelling, decreased capillary flow, and necrosis.

Autogenous venous grafts function very well and are the best replacements for extensive vascular injuries. Prosthetic materials such as Teflon and Dacron are rarely required in repairing vascular wounds. In open wounds particularly, their use should be avoided because a prosthetic material, being a foreign body, serves as a nidus for infection. Injuries to major vessels, such as the thoracic or abdominal aorta, however, may necessitate prosthetic materials for repair. Nevertheless, in young patients the thoracic and abdominal aorta may be mobilized for 2 or 3 cm. lengths, permitting limited resection and primary anastomosis.

The skin in clean, fresh wounds may be sutured primarily with little risk of subsequent infection. Open contaminated wounds should not be closed primarily, that is, sutured at the time of the original operation. Here the skin is left open, packed with gauze, and then closed three to five days later—a delayed primary closure. This technique decreases the incidence of wound infection and possible failure of the vascular repair. Finally, in open wounds the addition of broad-spectrum bactericidal antibiotics is recommended to help combat infection.

When possible associated fractures should be stabilized prior to vascular repair. If the order is reversed, that is, if vessel repair precedes fracture fixation, the added risk of vascular anastomotic disruption during fracture manipulation is introduced. If a fracture is open and grossly contaminated with debris, as in a thrashing machine injury, it is unwise to utilize a foreign body, such as internal metallic fixation of the fracture. Stabilization of the fractures in this setting must be performed with balanced skeletal traction or plaster cylinder immobilization. The vascular reconstruction can be done while the patient is in traction.

Other valuable adjuncts in managing the vascular wound in the operating room are the use of heparin solution, regional perfusion, and balloon tipped (Fogarty) catheters. Since approximately 30% of acute vascular injuries are associated with distal clotting, utilization of balloon-tipped catheters to extract distal thrombi is exceedingly important if a good result is to be obtained.

Fasciotomies. Although the most common form of vascular injury is that which directly involves the artery or vein, a more subtle form of arterial obstruction must be mentioned. Arterial insufficiency may result from extrinsic obstruction of the small arterioles and nutrient vessels supplying the muscle. Extrinsic obstruction results from constricting or restricting casts or dressings. Additionally, venous obstruction and subsequent venous hypertension result in subfascial edema, ultimately decreasing capillary perfusion.

The muscles of the extremities are enveloped by fascial sleeves (Fig. 17-6). Occasionally following the repair of vascular injuries, the sur-

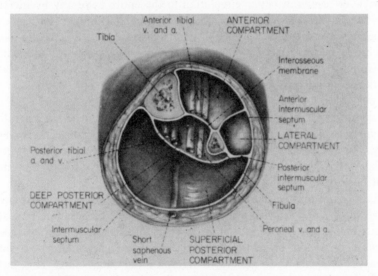

Fig. 17-6. Diagram of a midcalf cross section. The four osteofascial compartments are formed by attachments of intermuscular septae, crural fascia, interosseus membrane, and bones. The peroneal and posterior tibial vessels lie within the deep posterior compartment. The intermuscular septum attaches to the tibia deep to the superficial posterior compartment at this level.

geon must longitudinally incise these fascial barriers to allow the muscle to expand, thereby decreasing the devastating extrinsic compressive effects of subfascial edema and hemorrhage. Indications for the use of fasciotomies have been determined from extensive experience with severe vascular injuries. Absolute indications for fasciotomy are: (a) arterial injury and concomitant venous interruption, (b) arterial injury with severe distal soft tissue contusion; and (c) progressive postoperative intracompartmental edema producing vascular compromise. Arterial trauma with prolonged delay between injury and repair is a relative indication for four-compartment fasciotomy. The maximal permissible delay appears to be 10 to 12 hours. When faced with these four indications, fasciotomy should be performed in the operating room at the time of the original operative procedure.

Postoperative Care. During the postoperative period, strict attention to the overall physiologic balance of the patient is extremely important. Adequate cardiac output, renal perfusion, and cerebral perfusion must be maintained. Of utmost importance is maintenance of adequate hydration and normal renal function. Renal failure is a real threat following restoration of blood flow to ischemic muscle, particularly if the lag time has exceeded 12 hours.

The extremity in which a vascular repair has been accomplished must be elevated to a level of at least 45 degrees above the right atrium. This maneuver results in better circulation to the entire extremity by increasing venous return to the heart, thereby minimizing edema. Evidence of acute compartment compression with progressive edema in the postoperative period requires return to the operating room for immediate fasciotomy.

If the peripheral pulses in a young patient have not returned in six to eight hours, he should be returned to the operating room and the repaired vessel reexplored. Prompt return of the patient to the operating room is mandatory if a previously palpable pulse becomes imperceptible. At this time arteriography is exceedingly helpful because it may point out an overlooked associated injury or distal thrombi that may still be extracted easily.

Early anastomotic disruption, which usually occurs in the first seven days after the operative procedure, necessitates reoperation. Anastomotic disruption is invariably due to local infection secondary to inadequate debridement of damaged tissue. When managing a disrupted anastomosis, it is an error merely to reinforce the suture line. This inevitably fails. Instead, a new anastomosis is created, preferably in an area of viable uninfected tissue. In this regard an extra anatomic bypass must be frequently employed to preserve a limb; that is, the vein graft is routed around the normal anatomic path of the damaged vessel.

Broad-spectrum bactericidal antibiotics are continued for seven to ten days. If it was not possible to determine tissue viability with certainty during the original operation, the patient is returned to the operating room on the third postoperative day and a second procedure performed. By this time nonviable tissue is clearly demarcated and easily removed.

Patients with vascular injuries of the lower extremities without fractures begin gradual ambulation on the second or third postoperative day. Upper extremity injuries do not confine the patient to bed and he must ambulate freely. When the patient must be immobilized in a plaster cast or balanced skeletal traction, the cast or traction must be inspected daily. Close surveillance of orthopedic devices prevents motion of bone fragments in the postoperative period, which might possibly jeopardize the vascular repair.

Mortality, Morbidity, and Results

The mortality rate from vascular injuries has been progressively decreasing over the past several years (Table 17-2). The arterial injury itself rarely causes death unless exsanguinating hemorrhage occurs. Since about half the patients that have vascular injuries are in hypovolemic shock upon arrival at the hospital, this is a contributing factor. Nevertheless, death is usually the result of additional injuries that involve the head, chest, or abdomen. Of the patients who succumb from only a vascular wound, almost all have been in deep shock.

Results of management of vascular injuries depend on many factors, including the age of the patient, type of trauma, level of injury, type of repair, and associated fractures and venous injuries.

An older patient with occlusive vascular disease who sustains a severe crushing injury or fracture of the leg and vascular injury has a poorer prognosis than does a younger patient. Often elderly people have marginal blood flow to an extremity, and when a vascular injury occurs, the marginal situation becomes an irretrievable one.

The type of trauma also influences the outcome. As indicated previously, a sharp, clean stab wound is more easily repaired and with much less morbidity than a severe crushing injury in which a large segment of an artery is lost. The anatomic level of injury has profound prognostic implications. Table 17-1 indicates the high amputation rate with popliteal artery injuries. On the other hand, brachial artery injuries seldom result in limb loss.

The type of repair influences the final result to a lesser degree, but it is also important. For example, if a tangential wound results in partial loss of the arterial wall and a lateral arteriorrhaphy is attempted, a stenotic area in the vessel follows, resulting in arterial insufficiency with intermittent claudication. Evidence from the Korean conflict and from ballistic studies indicates that a severely contused blood vessel should be resected to a grossly normal vessel. In so doing, normal viable vessel is utilized for the repair, but it must be remembered that insufficient vessel may be available for a primary end-to-end tensionless anastomosis, and saphenous vein interposition may be required. Selection of improper types of repair frequently results in failure.

Associated injuries to bone and vein have a direct bearing on the eventual outcome of the vascular repair. If bone ends entrap or callous formation envelops the arterial repair, late failure ensues. Only recently have venous injuries been considered important enough to repair. During the Korean War venous repairs were infrequently performed. It is becoming more and more apparent, however, that large veins must be repaired, because if they are not, venous hypertension occurs with potential failure of the vascular anastomosis resulting in loss of the extremity. Furthermore, if large veins are simply ligated, the incidence of chronic venous insufficiency in the postoperative period increases, and this in itself may be disabling to a young patient.

In spite of the varied pitfalls in dealing with vascular wounds, the overall results are gradually improving with steadily declining mortality and amputation rates (Table 17-2).

The management of trauma consumes a greater proportion of our time today than it did one or two decades ago, and with increasing automobile accidents and man's increasing social inhumanity to man, the management of the injured patient will continue to be a formidable problem. Vascular injuries comprise a small but significant proportion of these patients. Aggressive early management of vascular injuries will maintain low mortality and morbidity rates and eliminate the necessity of caring for the sequelae of overlooked or inadequately treated vascular injuries.

References

1. Ferguson, I. A., Byrd, W. M., and McAfee, D. K. 1961. Experiences in the management of arterial injuries. *Ann. Surg.,* 153:980–986.
2. Morris, C. G., Jr., et al. 1960. Surgical experience with 220 acute arterial injuries in civilian practice. *Amer. J. Surg.,* 99:775–781.
3. Patman, R. D., Poulos, E., and Shires, G. T. 1964. The management of civilian arterial injuries. *Surg. Gynec. Obstet.,* 118:725–738.
4. Dillard, B. M., Nelson, D. L., and Norman, H. G., Jr. 1968. Review of 85 major traumatic arterial injuries. *Surgery,* 63:391–395.
5. Rich, N. M., Baugh, J. H., and Hughes, C. W. 1970. Acute arterial injuries in Viet Nam: 1000 cases. *J. Trauma,* 10:359–369.
6. Sencert, L. 1918. *Wounds of Blood Vessels.* London, University of London Press.

7. Saletta, J. D., and Freeark, R. J. 1968. The partially severed artery. *Arch. Surg.*, 97:198–205.
8. Patman, R. D., and Thompson, J. E. 1970. Fasciotomy in peripheral vascular surgery. *Arch. Surg.*, 101:663–672.

Bibliography

Cohen, A., Baldwin, J. M., and Grant, R. N. 1969. Problems in the management of battlefield vascular injuries. *Amer. J. Surg.*, 118:526–530.

DeBakey, M. E., and Simeone, F. A. 1946. Battle injuries of the arteries in WW II. *Ann. Surg.*, 123:534–579.

Drapanas, T., Hewitt, R. L,. Weichert, R. F., III, and Smith, A. D. 1970. Civilian vascular injuries: a critical appraisal of three decades of management. *Ann. Surg.*, 172:351–360.

Ernst, C. B., and Kaufer, H. 1971. Fibulectomy-fasciotomy: an important adjunct in the management of lower extremity arterial trauma. *J. Trauma*, 11:365–380.

Morton, J. A., Southgate, W. A., and DeWeese, J. A. 1966. Arterial injuries of the extremities. *Surg. Gynec. Obstet.*, 123:611–627.

Perry, M. O., Thal, E. R., and Shires, G. T. 1971. Management of arterial injuries. *Ann. Surg.*, 173:403–408.

Rich, N. M., Hughes, C. W., and Baugh, J. H. 1970. Management of venous injuries. *Ann. Surg.*, 171:724–730.

Smith, R. F., Szilagyi, D. C., and Pfeifer, J. R. 1963. Arterial trauma. *Arch. Surg.*, 86:825–835.

Smith, R. F., Szilagyi, D. E., and Elliott, J. P., Jr. 1969. Fracture of long bones with arterial injury due to blunt trauma. *Arch. Surg.*, 99:315–324.

Treiman, R. L., Doty, D., and Gaspar, M. R. 1966. Acute vascular trauma. A fifteen year study. *Amer. J. Surg.*, 111:469–473.

18

Injuries of the Face

William C. Grabb

Of the many types of facial trauma that the plastic surgeon is called upon to treat, those injuries caused by automobile accidents are by far the most common and usually the most severe.

This chapter is divided into the management of soft tissue injuries and facial bone fractures.

Soft Tissue Injuries

As a rule of thumb, patients who sustain severe facial lacerations in automobile accidents usually do not have accompanying facial bone fractures. The converse is also true, *i.e.,* that facial bone fractures are usually not accompanied by severe facial lacerations. The combination of facial injuries and knee lacerations is common in accident victims who were in the guest passenger seat.

Most patients with lacerations of the face are treated in the emergency department. Upon arrival at the hospital, the patient's blood pressure, pulse rate, and respiratory rate should be obtained and a complete physical examination carried out. Although the facial injuries are obvious, more serious conditions, such as respiratory obstruction, shock, ruptured internal organs, intracranial bleeding, and spinal cord injuries, are more life threatening and should be treated first. Though patients with extensive facial injuries are literally covered with blood from their wounds, we have never known of such a person dying from this cause.

In order to avoid the complication of infection, facial lacerations should be sutured ideally within eight hours of the accident, and this can usually be accomplished. They can be sutured up to 24 hours later if an antibiotic such as penicillin is administered.

Prior to repairing the lacerations the face is washed. Sterile drapes are placed about the injured area and anesthesia of the wound is ob-

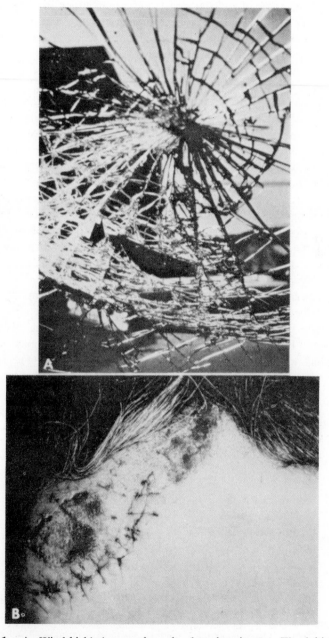

Fig. 18-1. A, Windshield damage from head-to-glass impact. The initial point of impact is the center of the spider web. Arrow points to tissue on the glass at the point where the laceration was sustained. B, Laceration and avulsion of skin of forehead sustained by impact with the windshield glass.

tained by injection of a local anesthetic agent either directly into the skin at the site of the wound or by a regional nerve block of the supraorbital, infraorbital, or mental nerve. This anesthetic agent should contain a small amount of adrenalin to reduce bleeding.

The technique for suturing facial lacerations involves closing the wound in layers.[1] Facial muscles involved in deep lacerations are reapproximated with fine absorbable catgut sutures, after which the subcutaneous tissue is similarly sutured and then the skin. Skin sutures are usually of fine nylon and are placed and tied carefully so that crosshatch scars do not occur on the facial skin.

The slicing trapdoor facial laceration is most commonly caused by impact of the passenger with the windshield in pre-1966 automobiles. The head strikes the windshield, breaking the windshield in a spider web pattern, and then continues downward in an arc with the slicing cut usually caused by an edge of broken glass about 4 to 6 inches below the center of the spider web (Fig. 18-1A and B).[2] Typically these lacerations occur on the forehead of women, the most frequent occupants of the passenger seat (Fig. 18-2).

More extensive parallel facial lacerations occur in a similar fashion, but typically lower on the face and in an oblique direction (Fig. 18-3).

Multiple short superficial lacerations are the product of modern technology. These less severe lacerations are caused by impact with the automobile windshield in cars built since 1966 (Fig. 18-4). This improved windshield with its thicker (30 mil), looser bonded plastic inter-

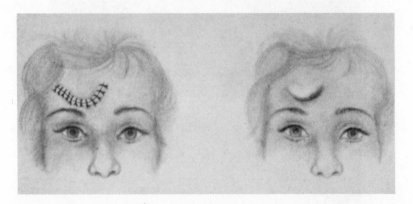

Fig. 18-2. A slicing trapdoor type of laceration sustained by impact with the windshield glass. These lacerations tend to heal in a U-shaped scar that contracts, causing the enclosed skin to become elevated. Secondary revisions of these scars are necessary to improve their appearance. (Courtesy of Frank Robinson and Ethicon, Inc.)

layer requires about twice the head-to-glass impact speed (25 to 30 m.p.h.) to penetrate the windshield, and it causes only multiple short superficial lacerations, usually on the forehead (Fig. 18-5).[3] Typically these lacerations require only a few or no sutures.

Accidental tattoo is caused by grease, dirt, paint, or asphalt being ground into the deeper layers of the skin (Fig. 18-6). It remains there permanently unless removed by deep scrubbing with a brush.

Avulsion of facial tissue occurs occasionally in vehicular accidents when a portion of the nose, forehead, cheek, lips, or ears is sliced away by impact with sharp glass or metal (Fig. 18-7). Although there are some successful replacements of this tissue, a skin graft or skin flap is usually required for late reconstruction.

Facial nerve lacerations occur when there is a deep cut in the cheek (Fig. 18-8). When the nerve is cut, the facial muscles are paralyzed unless the nerve is repaired.[4]

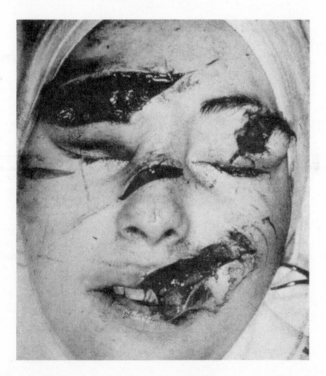

Fig. 18-3. Parallel facial lacerations following head-to-windshield impact. Persons with severe facial lacerations sustained in an automobile accdent only rarely have accompanying facial bone fractures.

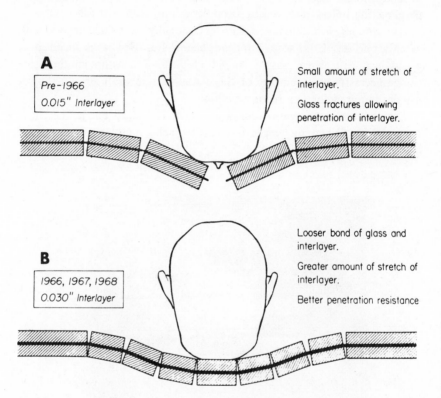

Fig. 18-4. A, Pre-1966 automobile windshield. Note the cutting of the plastic laminate by the broken glass. B, Post-1966 windshield, which requires more than twice the head-to-glass impact speed of the old windshield to perforate the laminate.

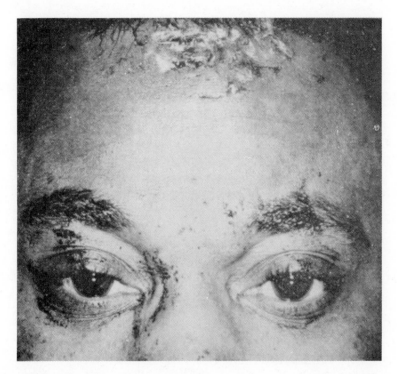

Fig. 18-5. Superficial short, multiple lacerations of the forehead that are typical of those caused by collision with the newer type of windshield glass.

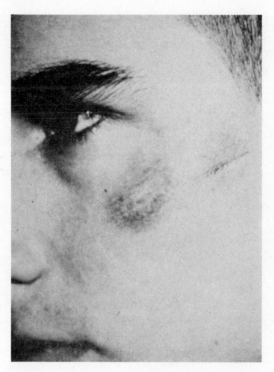

Fig. 18-6. Asphalt, dirt, and other materials can be ground into the facial skin, resulting in a permanent tattoo.

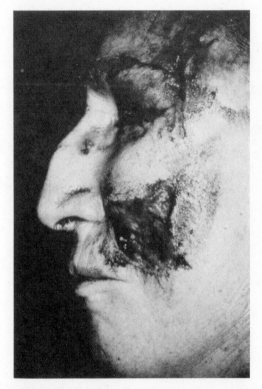

Fig. 18-7. Portions of the soft tissues of the face can actually be sliced away by impact with glass or sharp metal.

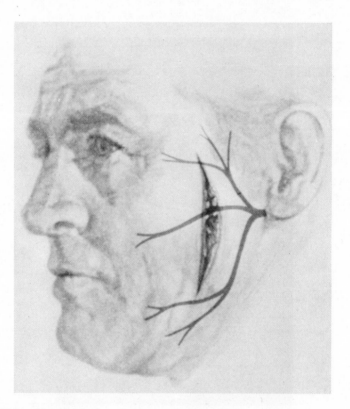

Fig. 18-8. The facial nerve innervates all the muscles of the face that provide the normal facial expression. Laceration of this nerve causes paralysis of the facial muscles involved. Early repair of this nerve following injury is important. (Courtesy Frank Robinson and Ethicon, Inc.)

Revision of Scars. Most scars at first are raised and red, but over a period of several months they mature and become flat and white. There is no way to remove a scar completely, but we can operate after six months or so to revise scars and make them narrower and therefore less noticeable. These scars can also be sandpapered.

Facial Bone Fractures

The bones of the face are most commonly fractured in automobile accidents by impact with the dashboard, steering wheel, or some other unyielding area of the vehicle. The bones involved are the mandible, maxilla, zygomas, and nasal bone (Fig. 18-9).

When we see patients with this type of injury in the emergency department we make the diagnosis of a fracture by examining the patient and obtaining x-rays of the facial bones.[5] Examples of these fractures are illustrated in Figures 18-10 to 18-13.

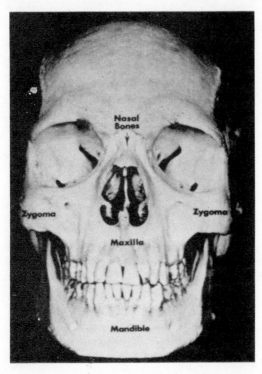

Fig. 18-9. The various facial bones are not of uniform strength. The thinner bones in the nasal and orbital areas are structurally more susceptible to fracture than are the heavier bones, such as the mandible and lower portion of the maxilla.

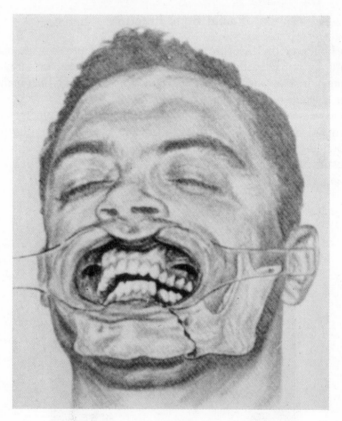

Fig. 18-10. Mandibular fractures commonly occur in the teeth-bearing portion of the bone. Fractures may occur, however, in any portion of the mandible. (Courtesy Frank Robinson and Ethicon, Inc.)

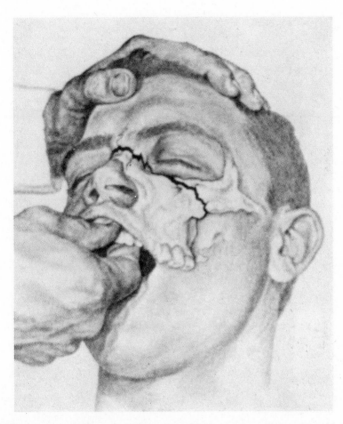

Fig. 18-11. A Le Fort type II fracture. The examiner is grasping the maxilla in his right hand to demonstrate the marked mobility of this fractured bone. (Courtesy Frank Robinson and Ethicon, Inc.)

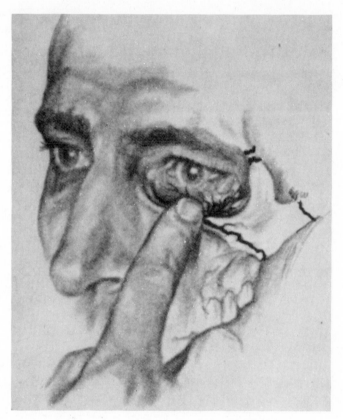

Fig. 18-12. The zygoma tends to fracture at its suture lines where it joins adjacent bones. The examiner's finger is on the zygomaticomaxillary suture line where separation of these two bones can be palpated. (Courtesy Frank Robinson and Ethicon, Inc.)

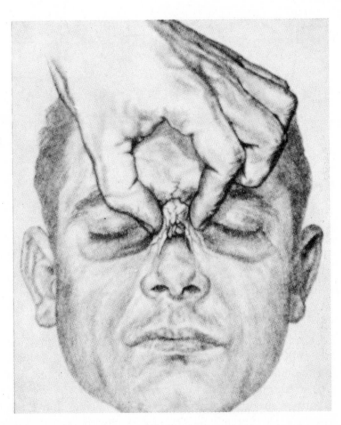

Fig. 18-13. The nasal bones have little strength and can easily be pushed to one side or broken into many small fragments. (Courtesy Frank Robinson and Ethicon, Inc.)

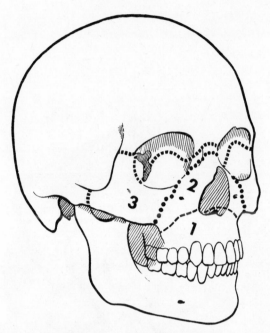

Fig. 18-14. Le Fort's classification of maxillary fractures. A Le Fort type I fracture (1) is a transverse fracture through the lower portion of the maxilla. A Le Fort type II fracture (2) involves complete separation of the maxilla from the adjacent bones. A Le Fort type III fracture (3) is a complete cranio-facial disjunction with separation of the facial bones from their cranial attachments.

The Le Fort classification of maxillary fractures was first described in the early 1900s (Fig. 18-14).[6] Le Fort demonstrated that the heavier portions of the maxilla give strength to the bone, and fractures are most likely to occur through the thinner parts. The Le Fort type I (transverse) fracture occurs transversely through the maxilla above the teeth. A Le Fort type II (pyramidal) fracture is caused by a force to the upper part of the maxilla with a fracture line through the upper part of the nasal bones, then downward and laterally through the floor of the orbit and zygomaticomaxillary suture, and continuing downward along the lateral wall of the maxilla. A Le Fort type III (craniofacial disjunction) fracture is a complete separation of the facial bones from their cranial attachments. Maxillary bone fractures are not always pure Le Fort types I, II, or III, but may be a combination of two of these types of fractures (*e.g.,* Le Fort type II on the right and type III on the left).

The blowout fracture of the orbital floor causes the contents of the orbit, including the globe of the eye, to be displaced downward.[5] The periorbital fat, bony floor of the orbit, and inferior rectus muscle actually herniate into the maxillary sinus (Fig. 18-15). With the eye on the injured side at a lower level, the patient has double vision (Fig. 18-16). Treatment consists of reconstructing the orbital floor with a graft of cartilage or bone, or a silicone implant.

Cerebrospinal fluid rhinorrhea can be associated with severe fractures of the nasal or frontal bones.[5] The leakage of the cerebrospinal fluid from around the brain into the nose is due to extension of the fractures

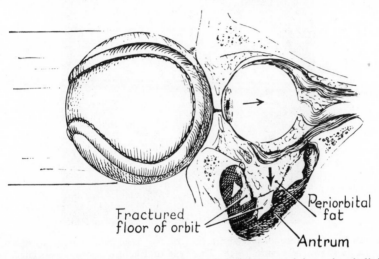

Fig. 18-15. A blowout fracture of the orbital floor caused by a baseball impact. The weakest portion of the orbit, the orbital floor, breaks away, allowing the orbital contents to drop into the maxillary antrum. Often the vision of the eye is unimpaired.

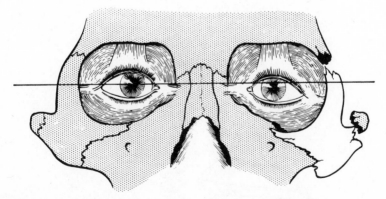

Fig. 18-16. A blowout fracture combined with a fracture of the left zygoma. The eye on the injured side has dropped down, causing double vision. In a true blowout fracture only the orbital floor is broken, the orbital rim remaining intact.

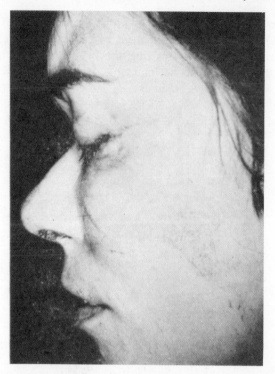

Fig. 18-17. Inwardly displaced fracture of the nasal bone caused by the type of trauma shown in Figure 18-18. This type of fracture is often associated with fracture of the cribriform plate and roof of the orbit. These latter fractures are usually the cause of cerebrospinal fluid leakage into the nose.

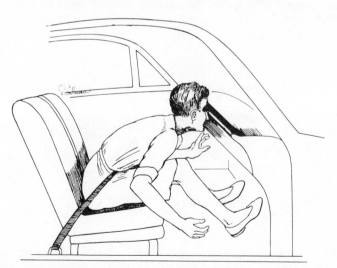

Fig. 18-18. Impact of the head against the dashboard. There is evidence that this type of injury is more common in persons wearing lap seat belts.[7]

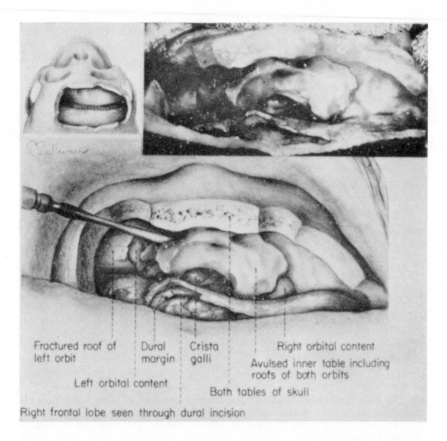

Fractured roof of   Dural   Crista   Right orbital content
left orbit   margin   galli
                                               Avulsed inner table including
       Left orbital content   roofs of both orbits
                                Both tables of skull

Right frontal lobe seen through dural incision

Fig. 18-19. Insert, top left: site of craniotomy exposure for patient shown in Figure 18-17. This patient required an intercranial operation to stop the flow of cerebrospinal fluid into the nose. Insert, top right: photograph of the inside of the skull at the time of operation, showing the fractures of the cribriform plate and roofs of both orbits. Lower diagram: the structures in the cranium shown in the photograph above.

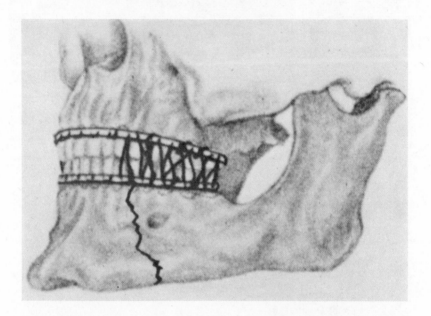

Fig. 18-20. Treatment of mandibular fractures consists of wiring the jaws together for four to six weeks, during which time the fractures heal. The patient can take food that has been ground in a food blender. (Courtesy Frank Robinson and Ethicon, Inc.)

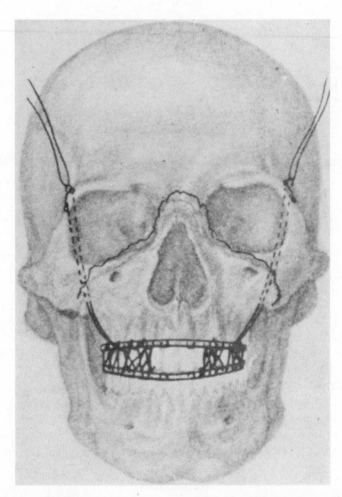

Fig. 18-21. Maxillary fractures are treated by wiring the teeth together and then suspending the maxilla with a heavy wire attached to the frontal bone. Fixation is maintained for four weeks. (Courtesy Frank Robinson and Ethicon, Inc.)

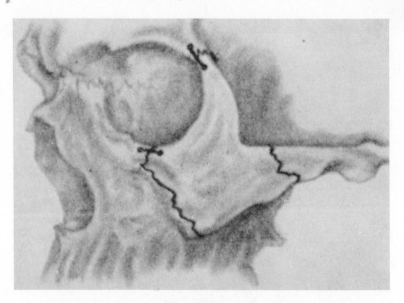

Fig. 18-22. For fractures of the zygoma, open reduction and interosseous wiring of the fractures at the zygomaticomaxillary and zygomaticofrontal sutures is required. These fine wires are left in place permanently. (Courtesy Frank Robinson and Ethicon, Inc.)

into the thin cribriform plate or the roof of the orbit (Figs. 18-17 to 18-19). A complication of this type of fracture is meningitis, with organisms from the nose gaining access through the fractures to the tissues around the brain.

Treatment of facial bone fractures is usually carried out in the operating room one or several days after the accident when the patient's condition permits. The methods of treatment are illustrated in Figures 18-20 to 18-22. In general they consist of reducing the fracture and then holding it in position for the four to six weeks required for healing.[5]

References

1. Grabb, W. C., and Smith, J. W. (eds.). 1968. *Plastic Surgery—A Concise Guide to Clinical Practice.* Boston, Little, Brown & Co.
2. Huelke, D. F., Grabb, W. C., and Dingman, R. O. 1966. Facial injuries due to windshield impacts in automobile accidents. *Plast. Reconstr. Surg.,* 37:324.
3. Huelke, D. F., et al. 1968. The new automobile windshield and its effectiveness in reducing facial lacerations. *Plast. Reconstr. Surg.,* 41:554.
4. Converse, J. M. (ed.). 1964. *Reconstructive Plastic Surgery.* Philadelphia, W. B. Saunders Co.
5. Dingman, R. O., Natvig. P. 1964. *Surgery of Facial Fractures.* Philadelphia, W. B. Saunders Co.
6. Le Fort, R. 1901. Étude Expérimentale sur les Fractures de la Mâchoire Superiéure. *Paris Rev. de Chir.,* 23:208, 360, 479.
7. Schneider, R. C., et al. 1968. Lap seat belt injuries; the treatment of the fortunate survivor. *Michigan Med.,* 67:171.

19

Ocular Trauma

Roger F. Meyer and John W. Henderson

It is important for all physicians, and especially those concerned with the management of injured patients, to be familiar with the nature and treatment of eye injuries. Even though the eye is protected by a bony orbital rim, cushioning of the orbital contents, and lids and lashes, it is still vulnerable. Protective devices, such as safety goggles and shatter-resistant spectacles, have prevented many eye injuries, but their incidence is still high.

Examination Techniques

An attempt should be made to determine, from a history provided by the patient or his relatives, how the eye was injured. The circumstances of the accident usually suggest the nature of the injury.

Whenever possible, an estimate of the patient's visual acuity should be made. A record of such an estimate may have medicolegal significance.

Pain and photophobia caused by the injury may produce blepharospasm so severe that the eye cannot be examined. This can usually be relieved by the instillation of sterile topical anesthetic drops, enabling the patient to cooperate. Topical anesthetics are toxic for the epithelium, however, and should never be prescribed for use at home.

When examining an injured eye, one should never exert direct pressure on the globe. If the injured patient is unable to open the eye, it may be necessary to separate the lids. The examiner can raise the upper lid safely by pushing up on the brow against the superior orbital rim, and he can retract the lower lid safely by pulling the cheek down with gentle pressure against the inferior orbital rim. With the thumb and forefinger pressing gently on the orbital rims, the lids can be safely opened without causing further damage to an injured eye.

The transparent ocular structures (cornea and lens) can be examined effectively if a penlight is focused on the eye at an oblique angle. Slow movement of the light at the proper angle will cast shadows on the iris from even very small corneal defects.

The adequate examination of uncooperative patients, such as frightened small children, may be difficult. If a lacerated globe is suspected, it may be necessary to examine the patient under briefly maintained general anesthesia. If a severe injury is not suspected, the lids may be separated manually under topical anesthesia by the described method.

When the injury is severe, it is important to bear in mind that further damage can be caused by unnecessary manipulation.

Chemical Burns

Chemical burns of the eye occur commonly in industry and in the home. When a patient with a chemical burn is first seen, regardless of the nature of the chemical, immediate, copious irrigation is of the utmost importance. Do not look for chemical antidotes or special solutions since time in these cases is of first importance. If no other means are available, the entire face can be submerged in tap water and the

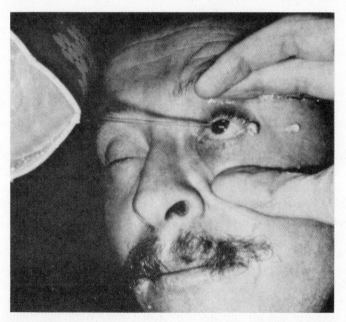

Fig. 19-1. Immediate irrigation with copious amounts of water is the most important initial treatment of any chemical burn. Note that lids must be held open for irrigation to be effective.

eyes opened and closed repeatedly, or the face and eyes can be held beneath a faucet. Sterility should be ignored temporarily. The important thing is to dilute the chemical and wash it away as quickly as possible. At least 2 liters of water should be used in the irrigation, and it should be continued for at least 30 minutes. If particles of material are still present, they must be removed with a cotton-tipped applicator.

Topical anesthesia may be necessary to alleviate lid spasm and permit adequate irrigation. The lids must be held open widely so that the water can irrigate the eye effectively; otherwise the patient will squeeze and only the lids will be irrigated (Fig. 19-1). In severe alkali burns, continuous irrigation by means of polyethylene tubing inserted through the lid may be necessary for 48 to 72 hours. This is necessary because alkalies continue to coagulate tissue as long as a trace remains.

The major difference in clinical behavior between acid and alkali burns is related to their penetration. The penetration of acids is limited by the buffering reaction of the coagulated protein. As a result, acid burns are usually sharply demarcated, essentially nonprogressive, less likely to have late relapses of inflammation than alkali burns, and more likely to heal rapidly and with less vascularization and scarring (Fig. 19-2).

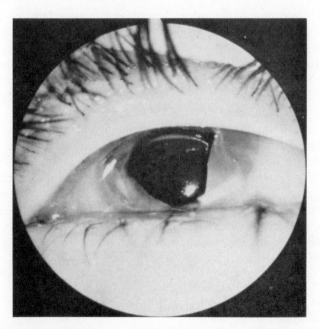

Fig. 19-2. Acute acid burn of cornea and conjunctiva. Corneal epithelium has sloughed centrally, and underlying stroma is only mildly edematous. Acid burns tend to be sharply demarcated and nonprogressive, and usually heal rapidly.

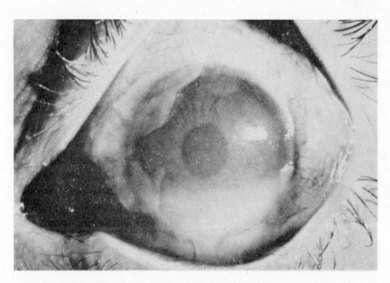

Fig. 19-3. Acute alkali burn of cornea and conjunctiva. Note damaged epithelium peeling off nasally, and severe clouding of inferior corneal stroma. Alkali burns tend to penetrate deeply, progress slowly, and heal with extensive scarring.

Alkalies are potentially more dangerous because they destroy the fatty acids essential for the integrity of the cellular membrane and dissolve the ground substance between cells. Their penetration is deep and their action prolonged. The alkali burn can therefore be very damaging (Fig. 19-3). Despite an initially benign appearance, it tends to be progressive; intense inflammation, corneal ulceration, and perforation of the globe may occur days or even weeks after the accident.

After the all-important immediate irrigation of any chemical ocular burn, a broad-spectrum antibiotic solution should be instilled. If the eye appears to be seriously injured, atropine drops should also be used.

Do not use steroids, either alone or in steroid-antibiotic combinations; although they may contribute to the patient's comfort by reducing posttraumatic inflammation, the potential hazards are great. Secondary infection, delayed wound healing, ulceration with perforation of the globe, and glaucoma are complications all too often associated with the use of topical corticosteroids.

Thermal Burns

Thermal burns from flames, hot grease, or steam usually involve the lids more than the globe and are treated like burns of the skin elsewhere on the body. Late contractures of the lids may cause trouble as a result of corneal exposure and desiccation. Treatment with a bland ophthalmic ointment, such as 5% boric acid, or tarsorrhaphy of the lids will protect the cornea from drying.

Ultraviolet Burns

Ultraviolet ocular burns may follow exposure to an electric arc-welding flash, a sunlamp, or the sun. Pain and tearing begin 6 to 12 hours after exposure and may be severe enough to awaken the patient. Ultraviolet radiation is absorbed mainly by the cornea and produces a superficial breakdown of its surface. The corneal reflex is dull when examined with a penlight, and the cornea shows diffuse, punctate staining with fluorescein. In severe cases, it may be necessary to instill a drop of sterile topical anesthetic in order to make an adequate examination.

Treatment should include cold compresses, occlusion, topical antibiotic drops, and oral analgesics. Steroid drops are strongly contraindicated. The patient must never be sent home with a bottle of topical anesthetic drops; if used in excess, they can disrupt the semipermeability of the corneal epithelium, allowing trivial trauma to progress. Unfortunately, this process can continue insidiously while the patient remains comfortable. With proper management, the cornea is rarely scarred permanently from an ultraviolet burn.

Lid Lacerations

The most important consideration in the evaluation of a lid laceration is whether or not the underlying globe has also been damaged. If the globe is intact, the lid laceration may be repaired by direct suturing as in other lacerations of the skin. The lids have an excellent blood supply, which minimizes the danger of infection, permits primary closure, and usually makes debridement unnecessary.

A laceration through the entire thickness of the lid that includes the lid margin requires closure by layers. The deep layer, consisting of the tarsal plate and conjunctiva, must be closed first by means of interrupted mild-chromic catgut sutures. When the sutures are tied, the knots should be buried in the substance of the lid so as not to abrade the corneal surface. A fine silk suture is placed through the gray line on each side of the laceration to insure accurate approximation of the lid border. If the deep layer is not closed by itself first, unsightly notching of the lid border will result. The next step is to close the orbicularis muscle

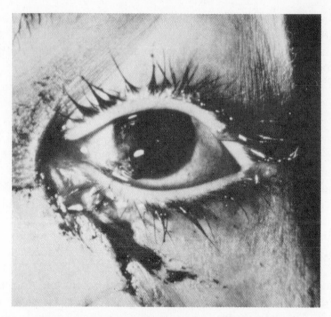

Fig. 19-4. Acute laceration of inner end of lower lid. Lower lacrimal canaliculus is severed and requires meticulous repair. Laceration of eyeball is indicated by protrusion of iris tissue, blood in anterior chamber, and displacement of pupil.

and skin with interrupted fine silk sutures. A pressure dressing is then gently applied.

If a laceration has passed through the inner corner of the eyelid, there is danger that the lacrimal canaliculi may have been severed (Fig. 19-4), and if these structures are not repaired, scar tissue may close them during the healing process and permanent epiphora result. To make this repair, a small polyethylene tube is passed through the punctum and both ends of the cut canaliculus. The tube is kept in this position while the tissues are rejoined and is left in place for several weeks. Careful observation is maintained to be sure that there is no erosion of the punctum.

Corneal Lacerations

Lacerating injuries of the eyeball that have penetrated the cornea, sclera, or both, produce characteristic signs, including shallowing or loss of the anterior chamber due to leakage of aqueous humor, and a distortion of the pupil in the direction of the laceration due to entrapment of the iris in the wound. There may be prolapse of the iris or ciliary body through the wound, which appears as dark brown or black pigment on the outside of the eyeball. Transparent jelly visible in the wound is likely to be the prolapsed lens or vitreous body. Blood may be present in the anterior chamber and always indicates a potentially serious eye problem.

When a laceration of the globe is detected, both eyes should be covered with sterile dressings and protective shields to immobilize the injured eye and prevent further damage (Fig. 19-5). No attempt should be made to remove blood clots or penetrating foreign bodies because manipulation can convert a simple laceration into one complicated by prolapsed ocular contents (Fig. 19-6).

The patient should be moved immediately by litter to appropriate surgical facilities where detailed examination and meticulous surgical repair can be performed under general anesthesia in an operating room. If there is an open wound, the application of ointments is to be avoided because they may become trapped in the interior of the eye. Tetanus prophylaxis is indicated whenever there is a penetrating ocular injury.

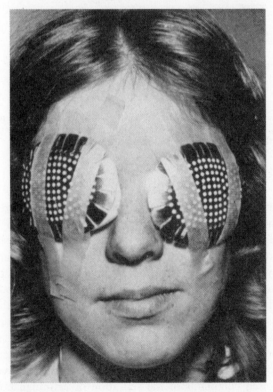

Fig. 19-5. When laceration of the globe is detected, cover both eyes with sterile dressings and protective shields to immobilize the injured eye and prevent further damage.

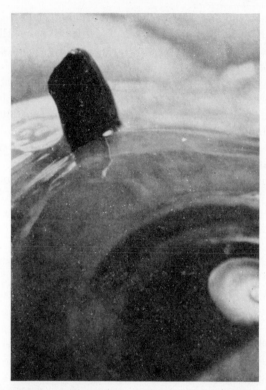

Fig. 19-6. Penetrating ocular foreign body. Do not attempt to remove blood clots or penetrating foreign bodies. Manipulation can convert a simple laceration into one complicated by prolapse of intraocular contents.

Foreign Bodies

The entrapment of foreign bodies beneath the upper lid or on the surface of the eye is one of the most frequent causes of eye injury. When a foreign body strikes the eye, it may take any of several courses, depending on the size of the particle and its speed on impact. If it strikes the eyeball, it may bounce off and become lodged beneath the upper or lower lid. Conjunctival foreign bodies are often lodged on the posterior surface of the upper tarsal plate, and eversion of the upper lid is then necessary to expose and remove them. They can be removed by a stream of sterile saline solution or can be wiped off with a moist cotton swab after the instillation of a sterile topical anesthetic.

Foreign bodies that become embedded in the cornea are very painful. The patient often complains of the sensation of a foreign body beneath the upper lid. This is due to movement of the lid over the foreign body, which causes pain with every blink. The instillation of a drop of sterile topical anesthetic is often necessary before an adequate examination can be made. Well focused, oblique, moving illumination is best for visualizing the corneal foreign body if a slit-lamp and corneal microscope are not available. Small corneal foreign bodies that are difficult to visualize may be outlined with sterile fluorescein; when the fluorescein is washed from the eye with saline solution, a green stain remains.

Corneal foreign bodies that cannot be removed by irrigation should be carefully lifted out with a fine hypodermic needle fitted on a syringe. For this purpose a slit-lamp affords the best magnification and illumination, but a bright light and magnifying loupe are usually satisfactory. If a foreign body containing iron has been present in the cornea for any length of time, a rust ring may penetrate the surrounding tissue. Since this devitalized tissue can be irritating and cause infection, it should be removed. A dental burr is useful for this purpose.

If the corneal foreign body is located in the central 5 mm. of the cornea, it is especially important to minimize trauma at the time of removal because at this location the patient's visual axis is involved. If the injury affects Bowman's membrane, scarring will result and even small corneal scars in the pupillary area can distort vision.

After the foreign body has been removed, a topical antibiotic solution instilled into the conjunctival sac is helpful in preventing secondary corneal ulceration. Topical corticosteroids must not be used; they are of no value after corneal foreign body removal, and they introduce significant unnecessary hazards, such as secondary infection and glaucoma. A dressing is usually not necessary unless the wound is extensive, in which case a gentle pressure dressing minimizes irritating movement of the lid over the injured cornea.

Intraocular Foreign Bodies

Small particles traveling at high speeds, such as those released by the hammering of stone or metal, produce small wounds that are easily overlooked. Such high-velocity, tiny fragments can cause serious eye injury and yet be almost painless. If a patient complains of blurred vision or persistent discomfort after having pounded metal on metal, an intraocular foreign body should be suspected. The cornea, sclera, iris, and lens should be inspected carefully with a slit-lamp in an effort to find an entrance wound. The corneal wound may be very small, but a hole in the underlying iris (Fig. 19-7), or an early traumatic cataract, may be noted. Direct ophthalmoscopic visualization of the foreign body through a well dilated pupil may be possible (Fig. 19-8). Any hemorrhage in the conjunctiva should be suspected as the point of entrance of

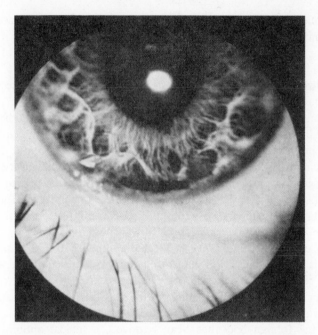

Fig. 19-7. Corneal and intraocular foreign bodies. Note metallic foreign body at 7 o'clock. Black hole in underlying iris at 6 o'clock indicates foreign body penetration.

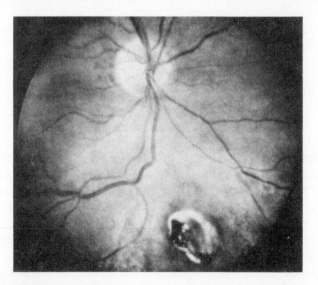

Fig. 19-8. Intraocular foreign body. Direct ophthalmoscopic visualization through well dilated pupil.

a foreign body, and the orbit must be x-rayed for the detection of a retained radiopaque intraocular foreign body.

Once an intraocular foreign body has been detected, or if one is suspected of being present, the patient should be referred to an ophthalmic surgeon. The eye should be covered with a protective shield to avoid further trauma until the foreign body can be removed at surgery. Since all foreign bodies must be assumed to be contaminated, broad-spectrum antibiotics should be used prophylactically. A tetanus booster should be given whenever a perforating eye injury occurs.

Contusions

Contusion injuries of the eye are the result of blunt trauma to the eyeball, or the transmission of energy when surrounding tissues are struck. At the time of injury, the eyeball's great elasticity permits a high degree of displacement of the intraocular structures when the energy of impact is suddenly dispersed throughout the closed ocular system. As a result, many different types of injury are associated with blunt trauma. The type sustained is often not obvious when the eye is first examined, however, and careful study and a thorough, prolonged follow-up are necessary.

A *black eye* is the result of hemorrhage and swelling of the eyelids. Hemorrhage beneath the conjunctiva may occur, and abrasion of the cornea can be recognized by a loss of the bright surface reflex. Hemorrhaging into the anterior chamber (hyphema), usually from tears of the

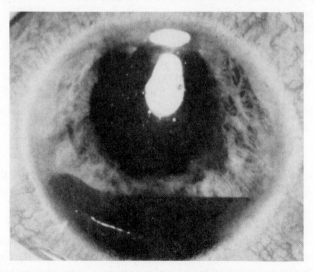

Fig. 19-9. Blood in lower part of anterior chamber often follows contusion of globe. Secondary glaucoma should be suspected.

ciliary body and iris, is a common and extremely serious injury (Fig. 19-9). Its complications include recurrent hemorrhage, secondary glaucoma, and blood-staining of the cornea with loss of vision. Damage to the outflow channels of the anterior chamber angle may result in chronic glaucoma years later.

Any patient with an injury severe enough to cause intraocular hemorrhage should be admitted to the hospital, sedated, and put at absolute bed rest for five to seven days with both eyes patched to minimize the chance of recurrent bleeding.

Traumatic iritis, indicated by cells and flare in the anterior chamber on slit-lamp examination, may follow blunt trauma. It should be treated with topical cycloplegics, and an ophthalmologist should be consulted for further evaluation and follow-up. The root of the iris may rupture, causing an extraperipheral pupil, known as an iridodialysis, or the sphincter muscle of the pupil may rupture, causing the pupil to dilate, sometimes permanently.

Damage to the lens capsule may cause a cataract to form years later. Blunt trauma may also cause a partial or complete dislocation of the lens.

Hemorrhage into the vitreous body can result from blunt trauma in association with damage to the peripheral retina, which can lead to retinal detachment. Patients with vitreous hemorrhage should be placed at bed rest. This allows the blood to settle so that the peripheral retina can be examined by indirect ophthalmoscopy and scleral depression. In this way, retinal tears or detachments can be detected.

Rupture of the choroid may occur at the posterior pole of the eye. It appears as a crescent-shaped, white area where a segment of sclera is visible through the rupture. If the macular area is affected, vision will be impaired.

Extensive edema of the retina, often associated with retinal hemorrhage, may be a contrecoup effect. The macular region of the retina will have a pale or white, edematous appearance. Cystoid macular degeneration or a macular hole may form later and cause permanent impairment of vision.

Rupture of the eyeball may occur if the force of the blunt injury is great enough. The most common sites of rupture are the limbus, the equator, and around the optic nerve. There may be extrusion of the ocular contents anteriorly or beneath the conjunctiva. The eye may be mushily soft and there may be massive hemorrhage into the vitreous body. A severe injury of this nature must be treated like any other penetrating ocular trauma, that is, by surgical repair in the operating room with the patient under general anesthesia. The eye must be protected with a sterile dressing and metal shield prior to surgery.

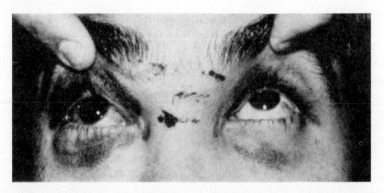

Fig. 19-10. Blowout fracture of right orbit. Note limitation of ability to look up with right eye. This causes diplopia on upward gaze.

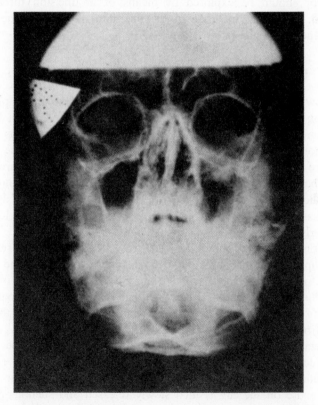

Fig. 19-11. Water's view showing blowout fracture of left orbital floor. Left maxillary sinus is clouded superiorly because of herniation of orbital contents through bony defect.

11

Blowout Fracture

A blow directly on the globe from the front can cause the intraorbital pressure to increase sharply. The orbital floor, which is one of the weakest parts of the orbit, can then be pushed down into the maxillary sinus, and the orbital contents may herniate into the opening. The inferior rectus and inferior oblique muscles may be incarcerated at the fracture site, with resultant diplopia when the patient looks up or down (Fig. 19-10). There is limited upward and downward movement of the eye when tested by forced duction with forceps under topical anesthesia. Enophthalmos may not become apparent until after the orbital hemorrhage and edema have subsided. The fracture site is demonstrated best on x-ray with the Water's view or by laminograms of the orbital floor (Fig. 19-11). When a fracture is present and there is entrapment of the muscles, or when the cause of the vertical diplopia is in doubt, the orbital floor should be explored by means of an incision through the lower lid. This must be done in the operating room with the patient under general anesthesia.

Protection of the Eyes of a Comatose Patient

In view of the increasing popularity of contact lenses, the physician must look for them when examining a comatose patient. When blinking reflexes are absent, as in the unconscious patient, a contact lens will not move enough to keep the tears circulating between it and the cornea, and there may be permanent corneal damage if the lenses are left in place. They can be very difficult to see, but if the cornea is illuminated from oblique angles with a penlight, a reflection from the edge of a contact lens should be visible, or a shadow may be cast by the lens onto the underlying iris (Fig. 19-12).

If a contact lens is found on the cornea, the safest way to remove it is by simple irrigation. With the patient supine, turn the head toward the side to be irrigated and separate the lids. Irrigate gently with sterile saline solution from the nasal side, and the lens will simply float out of the eye. To remove the other contact lens, turn the head to the other side and repeat the irrigation.

If irrigation is unsuccessful, try to remove the contact lenses by the rubber suction cup method. Wet a small contact lens suction cup with sterile saline solution and place it gently on the center of the contact lens. Pressure on the cup is then slowly released and suction will form so that the lens can be lifted from the eye. Great care must be exercised in applying the suction cup to the contact lens; rough handling can result in permanent scarring of the cornea.

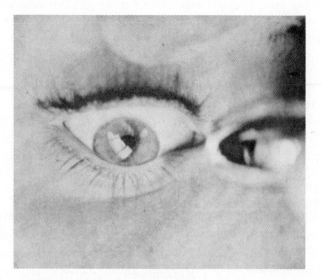

Fig. 19-12. Oblique illumination reveals corneal contact lens. Note curved shadow of edge of lens cast on underlying iris.

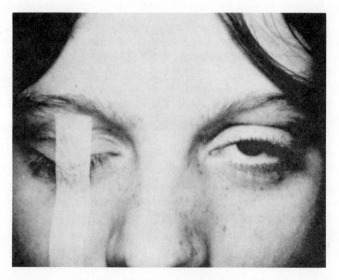

Fig. 19-13. Eye care in comatose patient. Apply sterile bland eye ointment and tape lids shut to protect cornea from desiccation.

When the preceding methods fail, or in an extreme emergency, the contact lenses can be moved temporarily onto the sclera. Gently push the lower lid against the bottom edge of the contact lens. This will slide the lens off the cornea and onto the bulbar conjunctiva where it can rest safely until an ophthalmologist can remove it. Make a note on the chart that the contact lens is still in the eye, and make every effort to have it removed as soon as possible.

Another traumatizing situation that is often ignored in the comatose patient is exposure of the cornea when the eye is left open and there is no blinking reflex. The cornea can be permanently damaged if it becomes dry and scarring supervenes. Management includes irrigating the cornea with sterile saline solution, applying a sterile bland eye ointment, and taping the lids shut to protect the corneal surface (Fig. 19-13). In prolonged coma, it may be necessary to suture the eyelids together by means of a tarsorrhaphy until the patient regains consciousness.

References

Behrendt, T. 1957. Experimental secondary effects of topical anesthesia on the cornea. *Amer. J. Ophth.*, 44:74.

Brown, S. I. 1972. Treatment of the alkali burned cornea. *Amer. J. Ophth.*, 74:316.

Cox, M., Schepens, C., and Freeman, H. 1966. Retinal detachment due to ocular contusion. *Arch. Ophth.*, 76:678.

Duke-Elder, W. S. 1972. Injuries, mechanical and non-mechanical, in *System of Ophthalmology*, Vol. XIV, Parts 1 and 2. St. Louis, C. V. Mosby Co.

Havener, W. H. 1966. Anesthesia, in *Ocular Pharmacology*. St. Louis, C. V. Mosby Co., p. 38.

Havener, W. H. 1971. Diagnosis and management of eye injury, in *Synopsis of Ophthalmology*, 3rd ed. St. Louis, C. V. Mosby Co., p. 219.

Meyer, R. F., and Sweet, E. R. 1973. Chemical injuries of the eye. *J. Amer. Coll. Emerg. Phys.*, 2:194.

Newell, F. W. 1969. Injuries of the eye, in *Ophthalmology, Principles and Concepts*. St. Louis, C. V. Mosby Co., p. 335.

Scheie, H. G., and Albert, D. A. 1969. Ocular injuries, in *Adler's Textbook of Ophthalmology*, 8th ed. Philadelphia, W. B. Saunders Co., p. 361.

Tenzel, R. R. 1970. Trauma and burns. *Internat. Ophth. Clin.*, 10:55.

Vaughan, D., Asbury, T., and Cook, R. 1971. Trauma, in *General Ophthalmology*, 6th ed. Los Altos, Ca., Lange Medical Publishers, p. 225.

Wolter, J. 1963. Coup-contrecoup mechanism of ocular injuries. *Amer. J. Ophth.*, 56:785.

Acknowledgement is hereby given to Mrs. P. Thygeson for her many hours of editorial assistance.

20

Patterns of Thoracic Trauma

Joe D. Morris

Recognition of the significance of thoracic trauma is based on knowledge of thoracic anatomy and a basic understanding of cardiopulmonary physiology. Because it contains the heart and lungs, the chest is intimately involved in the vital mechanics of respiration and circulation. This system is the basis of oxygen transport, on which life is dependent. Any significant thoracic trauma that interferes with the system, therefore, is life-threatening.

The thorax, in simplest terms, is the portion of the torso between the neck and the diaphragm. The skeleton of the thorax is overlaid by various heavy muscles, most of which contribute to movement of the shoulder girdle. The bony thorax is bounded in back by a staunch column of 12 dorsal vertebrae and in front by the breast bone, or sternum, which consists of the manubrium gladius (body), and xiphoid. These structures are joined by 12 ribs on each side. Beginning with the topmost first rib, which is short, the ribs increase progressively in length to the tenth rib, which is the longest; this arrangement gives the thorax the appearance of a truncated cone. The apex, or inlet, of the thorax provides passage for the anatomic structures of the neck into the mediastinum, but the base of the thorax is limited by the diaphragm.

Nature has provided the thoracic skeleton as a bony fortress for the vital structures of respiration—the heart and lungs. This protection is adequate against the natural forces of everyday life, it is not capable of withstanding the forces involved in highway vehicular accidents or in the explosive forces of missiles and other instruments of violence. Most cases of thoracic trauma seen in hospitals today have their etiology in the highway traffic accident. Testimony to the serious nature of such injuries is the 60% incidence of thoracic injuries among highway fatality victims.

The thorax is designed to provide the special function of pulmonary ventilation. Efficient ventilation is accomplished by rhythmically increasing and decreasing the intrathoracic volume, consequently increasing and decreasing the intrathoracic negativity. The pressure gradient provided between the atmosphere and the intrathoracic space inflates the lungs. Volume change during inspiration is created by the intercostal muscles raising the ribs slightly upward from the oblique to a more transverse position, thereby increasing the transverse diameter of the chest. Simultaneously, the diaphragm contracts, and the dome of the diaphragm is drawn downward, like a piston, to increase the vertical dimension of the intrathoracic space (Fig. 20-1). With relaxation of the inspiratory effort, the ribs descend to a more oblique position, and the dome of the diaphragm ascends. The negative intrathoracic pressure diminishes, and expiration occurs.

Any trauma that interferes with this normal cycle of events must interfere with ventilation. It follows, therefore, that treatment of thoracic injuries must be based on the restoration of normal intrathoracic physiology. This means that all treatment efforts must be directed to restoring ventilation and the oxygen transport system and eliminating or controlling all factors that would interfere with this system.

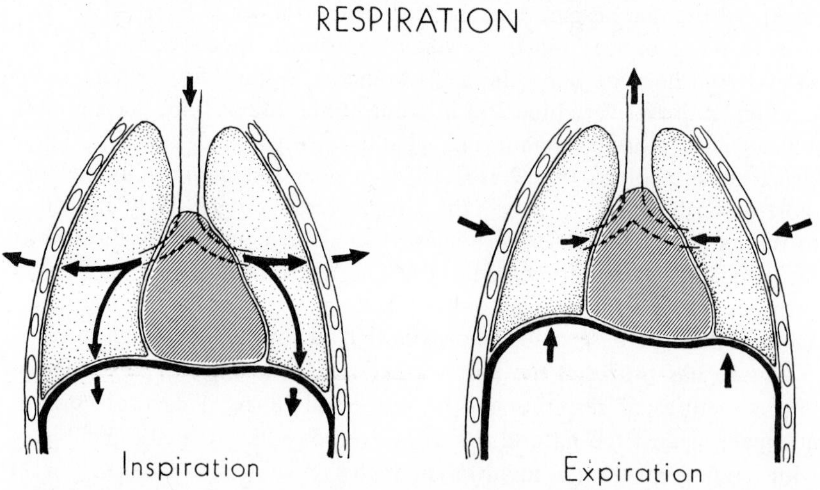

RESPIRATION

Inspiration   Expiration

Fig. 20-1. The mechanical basis of pulmonary ventilation is an alternating increase and decrease in intrathoracic volume. An increase in thoracic volume is accomplished by an increase in the transverse diameter of the thorax and descent of the diaphragm. The consequent increase in intrathoracic negativity produces inspiration. Narrowing of the chest diameter and ascent of the diaphragm reduce intrathoracic negativity and produce expiration.

Closed Chest Injury

A closed chest injury is usually the result of blunt force and occurs without perforation or penetration of the chest wall. Serious visceral injuries can be the result of such trauma, however.

Injuries of the Chest Wall. The most common chest wall injury is the rib fracture, most often involving the middle and lower ribs. Single rib fractures usually are not serious and do not pose treatment problems, aside from control of pain. The intact ribs on both sides of the fractured part provide excellent alignment and splinting.

Multiple and segmental rib fractures frequently result in unstable areas of the chest wall. When such instability is pronounced, these areas move counter to the normal chest wall movement—inward on inspiration and outward on expiration (Fig. 20-2). This abnormal state is called paradoxical or flail chest wall movement. It impairs the efficiency of ventilation and coughing, thereby hampering the elimination of tracheobronchial secretions and further impairing ventilation. Uncontrollable paradoxical chest wall movement is extremely painful and is comparable to repeated movement of any unsplinted fracture. Shock may ensue and may be augmented by further impairment of ventilation and hypoxia.

Treatment of paradoxical chest consists of prompt stabilization of the flailing segment of the chest wall. This is most easily accomplished by

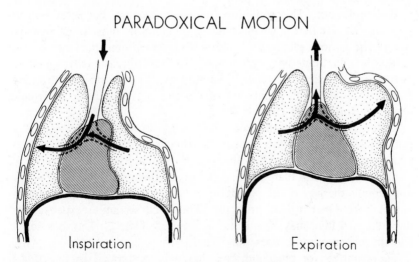

PARADOXICAL MOTION

Inspiration   Expiration

Fig. 20-2. Paradoxical or flail chest wall movement occurs as the result of multiple and segmental rib fractures. Unsupported areas of the chest wall move counter to normal direction. On inspiration the flail segment is drawn inward, and on expiration the segment is forced outward.

applying a pressure dressing with ample padding over the flailing segment. Firm manual pressure is effective until a specific solution is available. Maintaining fixation by splinting with a pressure pad for approximately five to ten days leads to the reestablishment of chest wall stability. Countertraction on the unstable segment can be applied by surgical fixation of traction to the underlying fragments; this keeps the flail segment in alignment with the surrounding chest wall.

Rib fractures on either side of the sternum may result in a paradoxical movement of the anterior chest wall. Traction immobilization of the sternum is often indicated in such circumstances. Perhaps the most effective means of controlling paradoxical movement of the chest wall is the use of endotracheal intubation or tracheostomy and positive pressure ventilation to align the unstable segment of the chest wall properly. This requires sophisticated respirator equipment and the constant presence of trained ventilator personnel. Such management should be reserved for serious chest wall injuries that cannot be managed adequately by the methods previously mentioned.

Control of the patient's pain is a major objective in any chest wall injury. Voluntary splinting of the chest wall and reluctance to breathe deeply to overcome impairment of ventilatory mechanics lead to poor ventilation and hypoxia. Narcotics must be used judiciously to avoid oversedation and suppression of respiration and the cough reflex. Intercostal nerve block is a safe and efficient method of improving respiratory mechanics impaired by pain.

Pneumothorax. This condition frequently accompanies chest wall injury and rib fracture. The mechanism of injury is most often penetration of the parietal pleura by a sharp rib fragment and puncture or laceration of the underlying pulmonary surface. Occasionally, pneumothorax occurs after chest trauma without evidence of rib fracture, suggesting that laceration or rupture of the lung surface can occur from a contusion force to the chest wall.

Treatment of pneumothorax should be governed by its severity. Oxygen inhalation allows the patient to compensate for most degrees of pneumothorax until specific therapy is available. Small degrees of pneumothorax—less than 20% collapse of the underlying lung—may not require therapy if the condition is not progressive and the contralateral lung is performing normally. Thoracentesis and reexpansion of the collapsed lung may be all that is required if the air leak has sealed and the pneumothorax does not recur.

Thoracentesis for pneumothorax should be performed by inserting a long 18-gauge needle in the second interspace in the midclavicular line. The technique consists of infiltrating the skin with 0.5 or 1.0% lidocaine with a No. 25 needle. Then an 18 gauge needle is advanced along the lower border of the interspace, infiltrating the tissues with lidocaine. When air is aspirated, the infiltrating syringe is removed and a three-way stopcock and 50-ml. syringe are attached to the needle through connecting tubing. The aspirated air can then be discharged through the side arm of the three-way stopcock. All air should be removed and the volume recorded.

Aspiration techniques for a hemothorax are essentially the same except that the aspiration is performed in the sixth or seventh interspace posterolaterally, and fluid and blood are removed rather than air.

Closed tube thoracostomy is performed for removal of air in the second interspace in the midclavicular line and for blood in the sixth or seventh interspace in the posteroaxillary line as for aspiration thoracentesis. The skin is more widely infiltrated. A small incision is made in the skin and a large Kelly clamp is tunneled to the pleura. A clear Argyle chest catheter with multiple holes near the end containing a radiopaque marker is then thrust into the pleural cavity. The distal end of the tube is clamped during this maneuver. The distal end of the tube

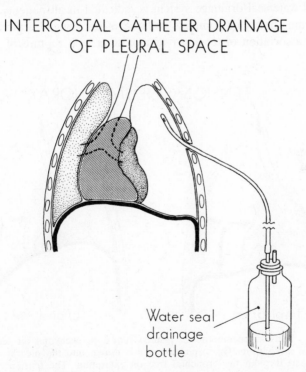

INTERCOSTAL CATHETER DRAINAGE
OF PLEURAL SPACE

Water seal
drainage
bottle

Fig. 20-3. Waterseal drainage of the pleural space provides reexpansion of the collapsed lung due to pneumothorax. Hemothorax also can be corrected by this technique. A low-pressure pump may be attached to the short tube to increase the mechanical efficiency of the system.

is then connected to an underwater seal or underwater suction system to evacuate the pleural space of air or blood.

If, by thoracentesis, it is apparent that a continuing air leak is present, as indicated by the removal of more than 3,000 ml. of air, intercostal tube and waterseal drainage should be performed (Fig. 20-3). *In any patient with pneumothorax who is to be submitted to anesthesia for an operation, thoracotomy tube and waterseal drainage of the pneumothorax should be established prior to the operation.*

Tension Pneumothorax. This condition results from a parenchymal air leak of the lung, acting as a one-way valve. Air in the pleural space is gradually increased with each inspiratory effort. The pressure on the side with the pneumothorax exceeds that of the opposite hemithorax, and the mediastinum is gradually shifted to the contralateral side, limiting ventilation and expansion of the intact lung (Fig. 20-4). The severe shift of the mediastinum and the increased pleural pressure interfere with venous return to the heart, and cardiogenic shock results. If progressive, this phenomenon is fatal. Immediate establishment of a tube and waterseal drainage system is indicated in all patients with tension pneumothorax or complete collapse of one lung. Furthermore, the frequent association of tension pneumothorax with rupture of the bron-

TENSION PNEUMOTHORAX

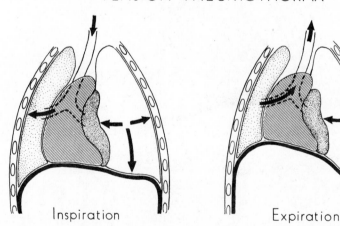

Inspiration   Expiration

Fig. 20-4. Tension pneumothorax results from a parenchymal air leak with a check valve mechanism. On inspiration, air is drawn into the pleural space, but it cannot exit through the bronchial tree on expiration. The tension completely collapses the lung on the involved side and presses the diaphragm downward. The mediastinum is progressively shifted toward the uninvolved side, compromising the intact lung. Return of venous blood to the heart is diminished, leading to cardiogenic shock.

chus should not be forgotten, and bronchoscopy should be performed if there is a persistent and large air leak.

Hemothorax. The accumulation of blood in the pleural space after chest wall injury is usually the result of bleeding from lacerated intercostal vessels at the site of rib fractures. Hemorrhage may also occur from injury to underlying lung parenchyma or vessels in the mediastinum.

Hemothorax has two major consequences: (1) loss of circulating blood volume into the pleural space, leading to shock, and (2) impairment of ventilation because of compression of the underlying lung. Treatment consists of prompt replacement of blood to restore the circulating volume and to avoid or correct shock. Thoracentesis or intercostal catheter and waterseal drainage restores the normal pleural space, permitting complete expansion of the underlying lung, and measurement of the rate of blood loss. Infrequently, continued loss of blood in a short period of time indicates the necessity for thoracotomy to control a persistent site of hemorrhage.

An unevacuated hemothorax resolves in time, but it may result in fibrothorax. The sequelae of thickened parietal and visceral pleura and adhesions decrease pulmonary chest wall compliance and restrict movement of the diaphragm, hampering ventilation.

Open Chest Injury

A penetrating or perforating injury of the chest wall produces serious breathing abnormalities. Extensive wounds not sealed by the chest wall musculature are called sucking wounds of the chest. Air rushes into the violated pleural space, collapsing the underlying lung. The flexible mediastinum is forced toward the contralateral hemithorax, compressing the opposite lung as well. On inspiratory effort, air rushes into the open chest as the thorax expands, competing with the volume of air that ordinarily inflates the lungs through the trachea (Fig. 20-5). The mediastinum shifts more sharply toward the intact hemithorax, reducing the normal inflation of the intact lung. On expiration, the mediastinum shifts back to its resting position, while air from the intact lung is expelled through the trachea (Fig. 20-5). The oscillating movement of the mediastinum with respiration is called mediastinal flutter.

If the opening of the chest wall defect is larger than the cross section of the tracheal airway, the lung on the same side as the injury will not inflate, and inflation of the contralateral lung, because of the mobile mediastinum, will be inadequate. Unchecked, the sucking wound of the chest results in violent hyperventilation, hypoxia, shock, and death. The

OPEN PNEUMOTHORAX

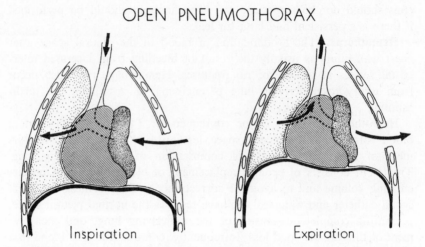

Inspiration   Expiration

Fig. 20-5. Traumatic interruption of continuity of the chest wall leads to communication of the pleural space with the atmosphere, creating a sucking chest wound. The to-and-fro shifting of the mediastinum with inspiratory and expiratory effort is called mediastinal flutter. Inefficient ventilation may be fatal.

first step in treatment is prompt mechanical closure of the sucking wound by application of a pressure dressing. A petroleum jelly gauze dressing is preferable if immediately available. Thoracentesis to evacuate trapped pleural air should be carried out as soon as possible. In the case of injury to the underlying lung, a continuous air leak may demand continuing thoracentesis until a pleural catheter and waterseal drainage system can be established.

Visceral Injuries

Visceral injury may occur in either closed or open chest trauma. In closed chest trauma, visceral injury is difficult to recognize. *Pulmonary contusion* is the most frequent visceral injury encountered, but its diagnosis is neither immediate nor apparent. Subsequent chest x-rays reveal an increasing opacification of the lung field at the site of injury, which represents posttraumatic inflammation. Edema, ecchymosis, and perivascular fluid loss into the interstitial space characterize the injury. The roentgenographic picture gradually resolves over a period of seven to ten days. Bronchial secretions are increased, and the airway must be cleared by coughing and intratracheal aspiration (Fig. 20-6).

Pulmonary laceration ordinarily produces a parenchymal lung leak and pneumothorax. Bleeding from the lung surface usually stops spon-

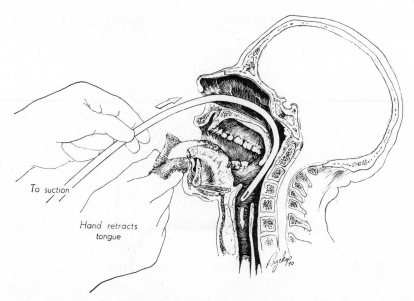

Fig. 20-6. Technique of intratracheal suction to remove tracheobronchial secretions that have accumulated because of inadequate coughing. A catheter is passed through the nasopharynx. Lingual traction brings the epiglottis forward to permit the catheter tip to pass through the glottis and into the trachea. Turning the head to either side steers the catheter into the opposite main stem bronchus.

taneously because of the low pulmonary artery pressure. Thoracotomy may be required to control significant hemorrhage due to laceration of a sizable branch of the pulmonary artery.

Bronchial and Tracheal Lacerations. Injuries to the major bronchi and trachea result from violent crushing forces applied swiftly. The nature of the injury may be a transverse fracture occurring between cartilaginous rings of the bronchus, producing an avulsion of either lung from the main stem bronchus. Mediastinal and subcutaneous emphysema appear promptly (Fig. 20-7), creating the dramatic appearance of the puffball man with swollen neck, face, and eyelids. The characteristic crinkling sensation of tissue paper beneath the skin on palpation is unmistakable to the examiner. The associated pneumothorax continues to leak large volumes of air on intercostal catheter tube drainage. Failure of the lung to reexpand after appropriate management makes the diagnosis further suspect. Bronchoscopy confirms the injury, and surgical repair is indicated as soon as the patient's general condition permits.

A transverse fracture with separation of the trachea demands emergency surgery to restore the unsatisfactory airway.

SUBCUTANEOUS EMPHYSEMA

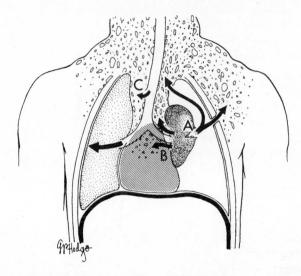

Fig. 20-7. Mediastinal and subcutaneous emphysema occur by the following mechanisms; A, laceration of visceral and parietal pleura permitting air in the pneumothorax to spread into the soft tissues of the chest wall and mediastinum, B, peripheral bronchial injury permitting the dissection of air retrograde along bronchial and vascular planes to the mediastinum (called interstitial emphysema); and C, rupture of trachea or main stem bronchus prompting severe mediastinal emphysema, with subsequent rupture of mediastinal pleura creating pneumothorax.

Partial tears of the bronchus and trachea occur without loss of airway or normal lumen. Conservative management is usually satisfactory in such situations. Bronchoscopy is indicated in all suspected cases of bronchial injury.

Myocardial Contusion. This type of contusion, almost exclusively an automobile steering column injury, is most often associated with closed chest trauma and multiple rib or sternal fractures. The diagnosis is confirmed by electrocardiographic ST and T wave changes, which may not be manifest until 24 hours after injury. Serum enzyme changes also occur in the presence of myocardial contusion. The treatment is conservative and is the same as that for myocardial infarction. Posttraumatic myocardial infarction has led to complications such as ventricular septal defect and papillary muscle dysfunction with tricuspid valve insufficiency.

Cardiac Tamponade. Perforating injury to the heart may result in bleeding into the pericardial sac. If such bleeding is ventricular or arterial in origin, tamponade will result. When the pressure of the blood

in the pericardium is greater than the venous pressure of blood returning to the heart, cardiac return ceases, and cardiac output decreases.
Shock and cardiac arrest result unless tamponade is relieved immediately. If pericardiocentesis does not provide permanent cardiovascular
stability, thoracotomy is indicated as soon as possible. Continuous
bleeding into the pericardial sac without severe tamponade indicates an
atrial tear and demands surgical exploration.

Rupture of Aorta and Major Vessels. Fifty percent of victims of
rupture of the aorta or other major vessels sustain the injury when they
are thrown out of a vehicle. A significant number are cycle riders. Rupture of the aorta occurs as the result of a severe decelerating force oc-
casioned by high-speed accidents involving collision with tree trunks,
bridge abutments, and approaching cars. Eight out of ten victims of

SITES OF AORTIC RUPTURE

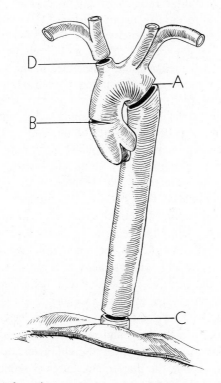

Fig. 20-8. Sites of aortic rupture in order of frequency: A, distal to left subclavian artery at the level of the ligamentum arteriosum; B, ascending aorta; C,
lower thoracic aorta above diaphragm; and D, avulsion of innominate artery
from aortic arch.

such accidents die at the scene before adequate medical attention is available.

The most common injury of this kind is total or partial disruption of the aorta, just distal to the left subclavian artery (Fig. 20-8). The relatively well immobilized arch of the aorta, with its major trunks extending into the neck and the upper extremities, stays firm while the inertia of the thoracic aorta, fixed only by the smaller intercostal arteries, permits a severe shearing force to be exerted at the junction of the arch and the descending thoracic aorta. A giant hematoma of the mediastinum surrounds the rupture site, and only the intact mediastinal pleura contains the aortic flow and channels it into the distal, open end of the aorta.

A pressure gradient between the upper and the lower extremity is frequently present. The diagnosis is suspected by the history and the x-ray evidence of a widened mediastinum. The diagnosis is confirmed by emergency aortography. Surgical correction should be carried out immediately, because fatal rupture of the mediastinal hematoma into the pleura eventually occurs in nearly all cases.[4] A small number may survive and develop an aortic aneurysm.

Avulsion of the major vessels of the arch presents a similar x-ray appearance of widened mediastinum. The pulse in the involved extremity is diminished or absent. Confirmation by aortography is indicated before repair is attempted. Repair requires use of an aortic bypass to provide blood flow to the kidneys and spinal cord while the aorta is cross-clamped above and below the site of the injury. Two methods of bypass are the ascending aorta to descending aorta polyvinyl tube shunt and the left atrial to femoral artery shunt employing a pump. Partial tears may be sutured directly. Total separation may require a short segment of aortic prosthesis to restore aortic continuity.

Injury to the Diaphragm. Traumatic rupture of the diaphragm occurs most often on the left side. The tear in the diaphragm may involve the muscular or the tendinous portion, or both, and may extend into the esophageal hiatus. The pressure gradient between the negative intrapleural space and the positive intraabdominal cavity favors the migration of the abdominal viscera into the thoracic cavity. Stomach, colon, omentum, and spleen are the most commonly involved organs. As the abdominal viscera crowd the lung and mediastinum, respiratory distress occurs. The diagnosis is established by the characteristic gastric and intestinal gas patterns above the diaphragm. Surgical reduction and repair of the hernia should be undertaken as soon as the patient's condition permits. Splenic rupture occurs frequently in association with rupture of the diaphragm.

Management of Thoracic Trauma

A fundamental principle in management of the accident victim is to maintain an awareness of priorities. A life-threatening thoracic injury may be overshadowed by the superficial and more dramatic trauma, which may totally occupy the attendant's attention. Injuries that threaten survival must be recognized and controlled before the attendant becomes engrossed in sophisticated x-ray studies and therapy of nonvital injuries. Since the traffic victim frequently suffers injuries to multiple organ systems, a comprehensive plan of management directing the coordination of involved medical specialties is essential to achieve maximal potential for the victim's survival and restoration. The general surgeon is usually best qualified to quarterback the team approach to multiple system trauma.

The objective of treating thoracic trauma is to restore function. Pain is a common denominator in chest injuries; it interferes with normal respiratory movements and discourages necessary coughing. Bronchial secretions accumulate and increase hypoventilation. Pain should be controlled by judicious use of analgesics and intercostal nerve blocks, when necessary.

Bronchial secretions, increased in all instances of thoracic trauma, demand constant attention from the medical and nursing staff caring for thoracic injuries. Although the lung fields may appear to be satisfactory in the initial chest X-rays, haziness and congestion usually follow after 24 to 36 hours. This may be due to posttraumatic edema and intrabronchial bleeding. The progressive increase in secretions may lead to scattered zones of atelectasis, and the clinical picture, when severe, has been called the wet lung syndrome. Long-term smokers normally have a much greater volume of bronchial secretions than do nonsmokers. An ineffectual cough following chest trauma allows these secretions to accumulate rapidly, leading to atelectasis and secondary infection. Smoker's bronchitis undoubtedly contributes significantly to the severity of the wet lung syndrome. Treatment consists of periodic intratracheal suctioning to remove the secretions when the patient's cough is inadequate. In severe circumstances, endotracheal intubation or tracheostomy is necessary to maintain a clear airway

Whereas tracheostomy was once considered necessary for ventilatory support beyond 72 hours, the newer oral endotracheal tubes with low pressure cuffs have been used for two- and three-week intervals without difficulty.

Two kinds of respirators provide ventilatory assistance: pressure cycled and volume cycled. The pressure cycled (volume variable) respirator is a normal lung ventilator and should be reserved for respiratory support in respiratory failure due to nonpulmonary cases, such as head injury and drug overdosage. The volume respirator, in contrast, can deliver a determined tidal volume despite changes in the patient's pulmonary compliance or airway resistance. Therefore, the volume respirator is preferred in thoracic trauma, when underlying lung injury, pulmonary contusion, or eventual wet lung syndrome are possibilities.

Intelligent respirator therapy is based on the routine use of properly timed blood gas determinations, including arterial oxygen tension, arterial carbon dioxide tension, and arterial pH. The scope of this text does not allow detailed discussion of this precise therapy, which has become a medical specialty in its own right.

Thoracentesis. A recent chest x-ray is important for reference in planning a thoracentesis. The only exception is a life-threatening tension pneumothorax, wherein there is no doubt as to the diagnosis and the side involved, and delay to gain roentgenographic confirmation might be hazardous to the patient. Thoracentesis is performed through the appropriate intercostal space with the aid of local infiltration of anesthesia. Aspiration of air to relieve a pneumothorax is best performed in the anterior second or third interspace, at the midclavicular line. Positioning of the patient in semi-Fowler's position with the torso slightly elevated provides a posterior and inferior shifting of the collapsed lung away from the site of thoracentesis, facilitating the procedure.

When thoracentesis is employed to aspirate a hemothorax, the procedure is elective rather than emergent. If the patient's injuries permit him to sit upright with support to his back, or to lean forward with his elbows braced on a pillow supported by the overbed table, ideal access is gained to the lower intercostal spaces posteriorly and laterally. The temptation to attempt thoracentesis at the lowest intercostal level possible may be a tactical error because of interference of the diaphragm with the aspirating needle. Blood clots, fibrin, and cellular sediment may obstruct the needle when thoracentesis is performed at the costophrenic angle. More consistent success in tapping for blood or an effusion is achieved at the level of the sixth interspace at the posterior or midaxillary line or of the eighth intercostal space posteriorly.

After the appropriate site for thoracentesis is selected, local anesthesia is achieved by raising a skin wheal with 1% lidocaine, using a 24-gauge needle. A 21-gauge needle is employed to infiltrate the layers of the chest wall down to the pleura. Care is taken to avoid intercostal vessels, infiltrating the inferior aspect of the intercostal space. A #11 scalpel blade is then employed to make a 3-mm. stab wound through the skin wheal. A 16- or 18-gauge short-beveled needle, attached to a 50-ml. syringe, is then passed through the cutaneous stab wound and into the pleural space, while negative pressure is applied to the syringe.

When the needle bevel enters the pleural space, air or fluid enters the syringe. The needle is advanced no further than 1 cm. into the pleural space, and a hemostat is applied to the shaft of the needle flush with the chest wall to immobilize the needle and avoid possible injury to the underlying lung.

Closed Thoracostomy Tube Drainage. Intercostal tube drainage of the thorax is indicated in tension pneumothorax, continuing pneumothorax due to persisting air leak from the lung, and progressive hemothorax.

Local anesthesia is obtained as for thoracentesis. A 2-cm. incision is made through the skin and superficial fascia. Muscle fibers are separated with a hemostat down to the pleura. A plastic catheter, stiffened by an appropriate sized mandril sharpened at its tip to provide a trocar, is then passed into the pleural space and the mandril is removed. Although No. 16 French catheter is adequate for pneumothorax, a larger size, up to No. 24 French, should be employed for hemothorax. The catheter should then be connected to a waterseal drainage system, which may be subjected to a negative pressure of 15 to 20 cm. of water. The catheter should project into the pleural space 5 to 10 cm. and be secured to the wound edges by a nonabsorbable suture.

Pericardiocentesis. This procedure is most easily performed through the subxiphoid area, with the patient supine and his head and torso elevated approximately 30 degrees from the horizontal. The heart rate and rhythm should be monitored by a bedside cardioscope. After local infiltration with 1% lidocaine, an 18-gauge needle attached to a 50-ml. syringe is introduced into the left paraxiphoid area at the angle between the xiphoid and the left costal margin. The needle is directed upward in the plane of the midline at an angle of 45 degrees until the pericardium is entered. Contact of the pericardiocentesis needle with the epicardium is manifested as a premature contraction on the cardioscope.

Aspiration of as little as 30 ml. of blood may result in dramatic improvement in the patient's blood pressure and cardiac output. If bleeding into the pericardial space continues, resulting in recurrence of the cardiac tamponade, formal surgical exploration of the pericardium and control of hemorrhage are indicated.

Conclusion

Pneumothorax and hemothorax are treated by the same principle: evacuation of air and blood from the pleural space to permit reexpansion of the underlying lung. This is accomplished most simply by thoracentesis. Intercostal catheter drainage may be necessary if air continues to leak from the lung, tension pneumothorax is present or thoracentesis fails to control a hemothorax adequately. Thoracotomy is infrequently required to control intrathoracic hemorrhage.

Paradoxical movement of the chest wall because of multiple and segmental rib fractures is controlled by a compression dressing or traction applied to the bony fragments of the flailing segment. Positive pressure breathing, maintained by a respirator applied to a tracheostomy tube, provides the most sophisticated and exacting control of the flailing chest wall. Respirator therapy is reserved for the more serious chest wall injuries.

Open or sucking wounds of the chest require immediate control by dressing until definitive surgical closure can be achieved. Consideration must include possible injury to the underlying lung and the resulting pneumothorax, which requires intercostal catheter and waterseal drainage.

Visceral injuries to the heart and lung, resulting from contusion, are treated conservatively. Cardiac tamponade, resulting from arterial or ventricular bleeding into the pericardium, demands immediate decompression. If pericardiocentesis fails to provide permanent relief, thoracotomy and surgical control of the intrapericardial hemorrhaging are indicated.

Rupture of the aorta or its major trunk requires skillful radiologic evaluation by aortography to localize the site of injury before mounting a surgical attack.

Bronchial and tracheal lacerations should be confirmed by bronchoscopy, and therapy may be conservative. Complete transection of the trachea is a serious emergency demanding immediate surgical repair to preserve the airway. Traumatic transection of the main stem bronchi requires intervention and surgical repair, which may be carried out on an elective basis.

Rupture of the diaphragm occurs most commonly on the left side and is recognized radiologically by the characteristic gastric and intestinal gas patterns above the elevated left diaphragm. A ruptured spleen may accompany a ruptured diaphragm. Treatment consists of return of the abdominal viscera to the proper position below the diaphragm and repair of the diaphragm.

Shock frequently accompanies major thoracic injuries and has its origin in a number of factors including blood volume loss, hemorrhage, pain, and hypoxia due to interference with the oxygen transport system. Treatment is based on restoring normal thoracic function to the oxygen transport system, relieving pain, and restoring blood volume. Blood loss may be concealed by hemorrhage into soft tissues at rib fracture sites. Hemothorax may be underestimated on the basis of a supine chest x-ray, in which the intrapleural blood volume is distributed over a broad area.

In summary, the proper management of thoracic trauma is governed by five fundamental principles:

1. Establishing and maintaining a proper airway
2. Restoring cardiopulmonary function
3. Controlling hemorrhage
4. Restoring blood volume
5. Controlling pain

References

1. Avery, E. E., Morch, E. T., and Benson, D. W. 1956. Critically crushed chests. *J. Thorac. Surg.,* 32:291.
2. Borrie, J. 1972. *Management of Emergencies in Thoracic Surgery.* New York, Appleton-Century-Crofts.
3. Johnson, J., MacVaugh, H., III, and Waldhausen, J. A. (eds.). 1970. *Surgery of the Chest.* Chicago, Yearbook Medical Publishers.
4. Kirsh, M. M., et al. 1970. Repair of acute traumatic rupture of the aorta without extra-corporeal criculation. *Ann. Thorac. Surg.,* 10:227–236.
5. Nealon, T. F., Jr. 1969. In *Surgery of the Chest,* J. H. Gibbon, D. C. Sabiston, and F. C. Spencer (eds.). Philadelphia, W. B. Saunders Co. pp. 168 and 182.

21

Intraabdominal Injuries

Charles F. Frey

Injuries to the abdomen may be penetrating or blunt. Penetrating injuries caused by stab wounds or low velocity missiles create little tissue damage, whereas shotgun and high velocity missiles cause extensive tissue destruction. The less the tissue destruction, the more favorable the prognosis. Blunt injuries are caused by crushing or shearing forces. An example is intraabdominal viscera that are crushed between the rigid spine posteriorly and an impinging anterior force, such as a tree trunk or a steering post of a car. Likewise, the aorta and other major intraabdominal vessels may be sheared at points of fixation. Treatment of blunt injury is often difficult and the prognosis guarded because tissue damage is usually extensive.

The pattern of abdominal injury resulting from blunt trauma is different from that of penetrating trauma. Organs most frequently injured in blunt trauma are the solid viscera, spleen, liver, and kidneys, followed in frequency by the hollow viscera, intestines, and bladder, and most infrequently the mesentery, pancreas, and diaphragm.[1] In penetrating trauma the hollow viscera and the intestines are most frequently injured, followed by the liver, spleen, and pancreas.[2-6] In either blunt or penetrating abdominal injury, the abdominal wall, retroperitoneum, mesentery, or diaphragm may also be injured. The two major threats to life in abdominal injuries are hemorrhage and infection.

The diagnosis and localization of organ injury in the abdomen may be exceedingly difficult, particularly in the case of blunt trauma. The problem of diagnosis is compounded when the patient is unconscious from head injury and is unable to indicate pain associated with his injuries.[7] Treatment of intraabdominal injury is complicated by the frequency of multiple organ injuries, particularly in blunt trauma, for which the motor vehicle is largely responsible. Before operation it is often impossible to know which intraabdominal organs are injured.

328

Abdominal and pelvic injuries are seen less frequently than are injuries to the head, limbs, or chest and account for only about 11% of all accident injuries.[8] They are life-threatening, however, and while they may not always be the major cause of death, they are seen in about 43% of fatal accident victims.[9]

The occurrence of associated injuries in intraabdominal or extraabdominal organs increases the mortality rate. Motor vehicular accidents, regardless of whether the victim is the driver, a passenger, or a pedestrian, have the highest incidence of associated injuries. In the Heidelberg study, 73% of patients with abdominal trauma had associated injuries when the accident was traffic-related as compared to 40% when it was associated with sports and the home. In patients with abdominal injuries secondary to the motor vehicle and who were dead on arrival at the hospital, 97% had associated extraabdominal injuries.[8]

Diagnosis

The history and circumstances of injury may be difficult to obtain because the patient is unconscious or intoxicated. If the patient is unconscious and has physical findings compatible with shock, it should be assumed that the cause of shock is blood loss and not intracranial injury. Wilson and co-workers found the association of head and abdominal injury to have a mortality rate four times greater than that of abdominal injury alone. Often abdominal injury was not recognized until autopsy.[7] It has been found that 60 to 75% of those injured in motor vehicular accidents, regardless of whether they are drivers, passengers, or pedestrians, are intoxicated.[10] Drunkenness is also a factor in many cases of assault; in a report by Hopson and associates, 87% of 297 patients with stab wounds of the abdomen were found to have been drinking.[2]

In the intoxicated or unconscious patient, the ambulance attendant, particularly if he is well trained, may be able to give helpful information the patient is unable to provide to the physician in the emergency department regarding the body areas subjected to trauma. Sometimes physicians will not deign to talk to ambulance attendants, which deprives the physician of information useful in the treatment of his patients. The ambulance attendant, now known as the emergency medical technician, should be viewed as a vital part of the medical team. He can provide the physician with information regarding the patient's position in the car, whether he was ejected from the vehicle, whether there were objects inside or outside the car which the patient might have struck, alterations in vital signs, or neurologic change that may enable

DIAGNOSIS

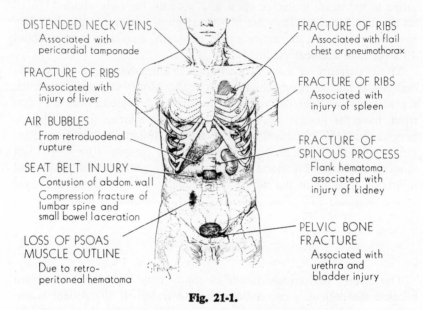

DISTENDED NECK VEINS
Associated with
pericardial tamponade

FRACTURE OF RIBS
Associated with
injury of liver

AIR BUBBLES
From retroduodenal
rupture

SEAT BELT INJURY
Contusion of abdom. wall
Compression fracture of
lumbar spine and
small bowel laceration

LOSS OF PSOAS
MUSCLE OUTLINE
Due to retro-
peritoneal hematoma

FRACTURE OF RIBS
Associated with flail
chest or pneumothorax

FRACTURE OF RIBS
Associated with
injury of spleen

FRACTURE OF
SPINOUS PROCESS
Flank hematoma,
associated with
injury of kidney

PELVIC BONE
FRACTURE
Associated with
urethra and
bladder injury

Fig. 21-1.

the physician to focus his diagnostic skills on the appropriate body area and hasten definitive therapy. The physician also needs to know what kind of resuscitation was required at the scene of accident or in transit to the hospital.

Physical examination of the conscious patient in conjunction with the history often provides the clinician with sufficient information to establish the likelihood of intraabdominal injury. Evidence of internal hemorrhage in the absence of external bleeding may be manifested by symptoms of shock, abdominal guarding, the presence of an intraabdominal mass, or fractures of the lower ribs overlying the spleen or liver (Fig. 21-1).

Signs of peritoneal irritation, such as guarding, tenderness, or rebound tenderness, may be produced by hemoperitoneum or peritonitis secondary to leakage of intestinal contents following laceration of a hollow viscus. Hemoperitoneum may result from lacerations of major vessels or intraabdominal organs. The presence or absence of bowel sounds is an inconsistent and unreliable indicator of hemoperitoneum or leakage of intestinal contents. Auscultation of bowel sounds above the diaphragm, however, indicates diaphragmatic rupture with displacement of the hollow viscera into the chest. Entrance and exit wounds are clues to the trajectory of missiles. In patients with penetrating wounds, the back, perineum, rectum, and vagina should be carefully inspected.

Examination of the unconscious or intoxicated patient is a difficult and demanding challenge for the clinician, who must exercise fully his diagnostic acumen to avoid error. Frequently, the signs and symptoms of intraabdominal injury so easily elicited in the conscious patient are absent or obscured in the patient who is comatose from head trauma or alcoholic intoxication. When confronted with the injured comatose patient, the clinician should selectively consider the complete range of available laboratory techniques that are necessary to rule out or establish the diagnosis of intraabdominal injury. These techniques include the monitoring of vital signs, a complete blood count, urinalysis, central venous pressure and hourly urine output, serum amylase and blood alcohol levels, peritoneal lavage, flat plate and upright films of the abdomen, cystourethrography, intravenous pyelography, arteriography, and abdominal scan.

Monitoring of Vital Signs and Initial Resuscitation. In the absence of visible external blood loss, the presence of shock (in the patient comatose from injury) should suggest an associated intraabdominal or intrathoracic injury. Regardless of whether the blood loss is from an intraabdominal or an intrathoracic source, its rate may be assessed by frequent observations of the vital signs, including the blood pressure, pulse and respiration, central venous pressure, and urinary output.

When there is rapid blood loss from a lacerated intraabdominal vessel or organ, hypotension, tachycardia, and hyperventilation result. These signs develop when approximately one-third of the total blood volume, or 1,000 ml. of blood, has been lost in the 70-kg. adult. There is a lag period of 6 to 12 hours between rapid blood loss and equilibration of intravascular plasma and red cell ratios reflected in the hematocrit. The hematocrit, therefore, is not an accurate index of rapid blood loss. When blood loss occurs more gradually over 24 to 48 hours as with some intrasplenic, intrahepatic, or retroperitoneal hematomas, vital signs may initially remain stable. Under these circumstances, a decreasing hematocrit is evidence of blood loss.

White Blood Cell Count. The white blood cell count may be elevated as a result not only of infection or peritonitis, such as that associated with leakage of intestinal contents from a bowel laceration, but also from an intraabdominal or retroperitoneal hematoma.

Urinalysis. The urinalysis is an essential part of any examination following blunt abdominal trauma. Microscopic or gross hematuria may be an indication of injury to the kidney, bladder, ureter, or urethra. Gross and microscopic hematuria may be absent, however, in 10 to 30% of patients with significant injury to the kidney and lower urinary tract.[11]

Central Venous Pressure and Hourly Urine Output. The central venous pressure can be measured by introducing a catheter through the subclavian or internal jugular vein and passing it proximally until it is in the superior vena cava (Fig. 21-2). The height of the water column when the catheter is above the right atrium is the central venous pressure. Normal central venous pressure is between 4 and 10 cm. saline. The technique of introducing the catheter through the subclavian vein is illustrated in the chapter on shock.

The central venous pressure measurement can be helpful in distinguishing between shock from blood loss and that from myocardial failure. The central venous pressure is high in myocardial failure and low in hypovolemia from blood loss (see chapter on shock). The central venous pressure can also be used as a guide to prevent overload during fluid replacement. Replacement of fluid after the central venous pressure reaches 12 to 16 cm. of saline is inadvisable without a careful evaluation of the patient. The Swan-Ganz balloon-tipped, flow guided catheter is an improvement on the central venous pressure catheter. The central venous pressure measures right ventricular function and systemic venous resistance. Left ventricular failure and pulmonary venous congestion may be present, however, when the central venous pressure is normal. The flow guided pulmonary arterial catheter provides a

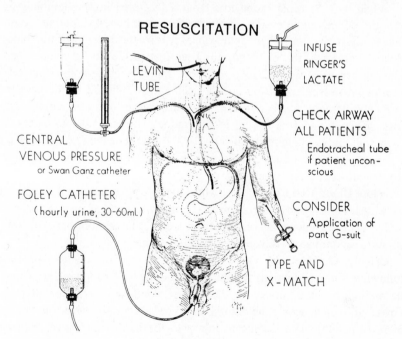

RESUSCITATION

LEVIN TUBE

INFUSE RINGER'S LACTATE

CHECK AIRWAY ALL PATIENTS
Endotracheal tube if patient unconscious

CENTRAL VENOUS PRESSURE
or Swan Ganz catheter

FOLEY CATHETER
(hourly urine, 30-60ml.)

CONSIDER
Application of pant G-suit

TYPE AND X-MATCH

Fig. 21-2.

reliable means of obtaining the mean left atrial pressure by measurement of the mean pulmonary artery "occluded" pressure.

In the absence of pelvic fractures, placement of a Foley catheter in the urinary bladder is a simple method of obtaining a urine specimen and initiating measurement of the hourly urine output (Fig. 21-2). An hourly urine output of 30 to 60 ml. provides a rough index of the adequacy of fluid replacement and renal function. More accurate assessments of renal function by paraaminohippuric acid and inulin clearance require special conditions and are not applicable to the usual emergency department setting.

Serum Amylase. Amylase is an enzyme synthesized within the acinar cells of the pancreas. This and other pancreatic enzymes are normally secreted into the pancreatic ductal system. Amylase aids in the hydrolysis of starch. When the pancreatic ductal system becomes obstructed, as it can following a contusion or transection of the ductal system, the amylase molecule may pass through interacinus clefts or through the lacerated end of the duct and into the interstitial space or interstitium of the gland. The amylase deposited in the interstitium of the pancreas is mobilized into the blood through venous capillaries or lymphatic vessels, augmenting normal blood levels. Elevated levels of serum amylase, therefore, may be an indication of pancreatic injury. The serum amylase may be increased as soon as five or six hours or as late as 48 hours following injury.[12]

Clinical decisions regarding operation should not be based on a single serum amylase determination. Serial determinations ought to be obtained from all patients in whom an intraabdominal injury is suspected. Persistently or increasingly elevated serum amylase levels following blunt abdominal trauma are an indication for celiotomy.[12]

Blood Alcohol. The blood alcohol level should be determined in all comatose patients in order to identify the etiology of the loss of consciousness. When this important determination is made for medical reasons, there is no need for the physician to be concerned about any possible legal consequence of his actions.

Abdominal Tap or Peritoneal Lavage. Hemoperitoneum, the result of intraabdominal bleeding from a lacerated intraabdominal vessel or organ, is cause for immediate operation. The presence of blood within the abdominal cavity is one of the most reliable signs of intraabdominal injury.

Several techniques have been advised to ascertain the presence or absence of hemorrhage within the abdominal cavity. Historically, the technique as first conceived involved passage of a sterile 18- or 20-gauge needle into the abdominal cavity. A syringe was then attached and aspiration performed. Return of blood or bloody fluid was considered a positive tap, indicating intraabdominal hemorrhage and need for prompt operation.[13] This technique was not always reliable. Sometimes the tap was negative in the presence of active intraabdominal hemorrhage in an area distant from the site of the tap in as many as 40% of patients.

In spite of insistent warnings to the contrary, many clinicians were misled into a false sense of security by a negative tap. To improve the accuracy of an abdominal tap, Wilson and co-workers recommended increasing the number of sites tapped to four.[7] Tapping all four quadrants of the abdomen increased the percentage of positive taps by 18 to 30% in patients with intraabdominal hemorrhage. A study by Yurko and Williams utilizing the four-quadrant tap in patients with blunt abdominal trauma indicated a diagnostic accuracy of 90%.[14] Other authors did not have as much success with the technique and reported an accuracy of 78%.[15]

The danger of significant unrecognized intraabdominal hemorrhage (in spite of a negative tap) led surgeons to modify the technique. Root and associates and then Veith and his co-workers reported the use of peritoneal lavage as an improved method for recognizing significant intraabdominal injury (Fig. 21-3).[16,17] A liter of Hartmann's solution is introduced into the peritoneal cavity through a peritoneal lavage catheter if initial aspiration does not return blood. The patient is then tilted so that the fluid is distributed throughout the abdomen. The pa-

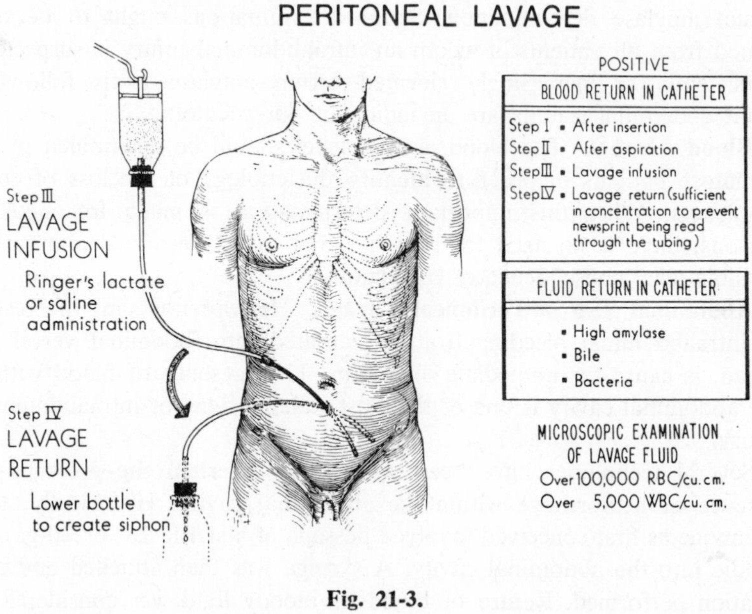

PERITONEAL LAVAGE

Step III
LAVAGE
INFUSION
Ringer's lactate
or saline
administration

Step IV
LAVAGE
RETURN
Lower bottle
to create siphon

POSITIVE

BLOOD RETURN IN CATHETER
Step I • After insertion
Step II • After aspiration
Step III • Lavage infusion
Step IV • Lavage return (sufficient in concentration to prevent newsprint being read through the tubing)

FLUID RETURN IN CATHETER
• High amylase
• Bile
• Bacteria

MICROSCOPIC EXAMINATION
OF LAVAGE FLUID
Over 100,000 RBC/cu. cm.
Over   5,000 WBC/cu. cm.

Fig. 21-3.

tient and the lavage catheter are then positioned so that the intraabdominal fluid is siphoned back through the dialysis catheter.

Flat Plate and Upright Films of the Abdomen. When the patient is stable following initial resuscitation, time should be taken for radiographic examination, including chest x-rays. Plain and upright or decubitus films of the abdomen may demonstrate the presence of free air beneath the diaphragm or lateral wall, thereby providing evidence of a ruptured hollow viscus. Although peritonitis does not present the immediate threat to life that massive hemorrhage does, the longer the gastrointestinal or colonic contents drain into the abdominal cavity, the greater the risk of fatality. A hollow viscus that has ruptured is an indication for operation, the objective of which is to close the perforation or divert colonic contents from further soilage of the peritoneal cavity. On the plain and upright film particular attention needs to be given to the possibility of retroperitoneal rupture of the duodenum, which is manifested by stippling or a soap bubble appearance of extralumenal air in the right upper quadrant. Late diagnosis of this injury makes repair difficult because of necrosis, edema, and infection. The necrosis and cellulitis of the duodenum and retroperitoneal tissues resulting from retroperitoneal duodenal rupture is a life-threatening injury with a mortality rate approaching 70%.[18]

Foreign bodies such as bullets or swallowed objects may be localized by radiographs. Diaphragmatic rupture may be confirmed if intraabdominal organs appear in the chest. Loss of the psoas muscle outline on the plain film may be an indication of an overlying retroperitoneal hematoma (Fig. 21-1). Lower rib fracture seen on plain film or chest x-ray of the patient's right side suggests the possibility of hepatic injury, and on the left it suggests splenic injury (Fig. 21-1). Enlargement of the spleen, medial displacement of the stomach, and indentation of the greater curvature of the stomach are signs of splenic rupture. Fracture of the spinous processes may indicate renal injury (Fig. 21-1). Seat belt injuries often include compression of the anterior lips of the lumbar spine and splenic and intestinal lacerations (Fig. 21-1).

Cystourethrography, Intravenous Pyelography, and Arteriography. Inability to void or hematuria in the presence of fractures of the pubic rami is an indication for a cystourethrogram to determine the patency of the urethra and the integrity of the bladder. Whenever renal injury is suspected, an intravenous pyelogram or arteriogram should be obtained to demonstrate the functional status of both kidneys. Nonfunction of the kidney on the injured side could indicate massive injury or renal artery thrombosis; lack of function on the uninjured side could indicate congenital absence. Arteriography, now widely used in major trauma centers, has proven its usefulness as an adjunct in the diagnosis of intraabdominal injury, because through its use the precise nature and location oí the injury often can be determined.[19]

Selective arteriography also permits the clinician to identify injuries to the aorta, spleen, liver, and kidney (Fig. 21-4). The seriousness and extent of injury may also be assessed by angiography and influence the surgeon's plan of operation. The decision to resect a liver lobe, for example, may be influenced by the information derived from the arteriogram, *i.e.,* pseudoaneurysm, intrahepatic hematoma, thrombosis, or transection of the hepatic artery. Features characteristic of injury that are demonstrable on arteriography include occlusion of major vessels, intimal tears of major vessels, extravasation of contrast material, arteriovenous fistulas, rate of venous filling, and stretching of vessels about hematomas.[19,20]

Features of specific organ injury on selective celiac or superior mesenteric arteriography include the following: *hepatic*—pseudoaneurysm or occlusion of hepatic artery or major branches, extravasation of contrast material into hematomas, stretched vessels, and filling defects secondary to intrahepatic hematomas; *renal*—nonfunction, nonfilling of the renal arteries and major branches, and extravasation of contrast material.

SELECTIVE ARTERIOGRAPHY

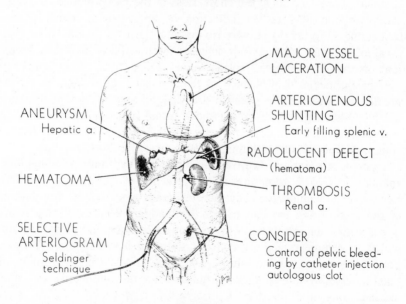

Fig. 21-4.

Initial Management of the Acutely Injured

Treatment of the acutely injured patient must be initiated at the scene of the accident and continued during transit to the hospital. A number of authors have estimated that 18 to 25% of patients die unnecessarily as a result of failure to initiate endotracheal intubation or intravenous fluid therapy or to relieve tension pneumothorax at the scene of accident or in transit to the hospital.[4,21] A sophisticated emergency medical service system has been instituted in Jacksonville, Florida. Waters and Wells reported that 20% of those who would previously have died from accidents are now being salvaged.[22]

New technological developments may further improve the care of the acutely injured patient. The modern G-suit of shock pants may also reduce the mortality rate among patients in hypovolemic shock from intraabdominal hemorrhage. Kaplan and co-workers report a marked decrease in the mortality rate from intraabdominal hemorrhage when the G-suit is applied by the emergency medical technician at the scene of accident and worn until operation.[23]

Standard practice in resuscitation of the acutely injured patient should include reports to the emergency department physician by the emergency medical technician regarding the mechanism and circumstances of injury, body areas that are or may be injured, estimated magnitude of the forces causing injury, treatment initiated during pick up and transport of the patient to the hospital, and neurologic or vital sign changes.

Abdominal wounds resulting in evisceration of intestinal contents should be covered with a sterile dressing and the patient should receive nothing by mouth. Without the use of a general anesthetic or muscle relaxant it is virtually impossible to return the hollow viscera to the abdominal cavity. Attempts to do so may only injure the intestine and result in further contamination.

After the patient's arrival at the hospital, the delay in initiating definitive therapy depends on the nature of the patient's injuries and the time spent in examination, resuscitation, and completion of diagnostic procedures. Advanced planning and frequent practice increase the efficiency of this phase of management. In truth, hospitals in which many acutely injured patients are treated have a better management record than do those in which only an occasional patient with abdominal injuries is received. In the early 1960s, Von Wagoner found that one-sixth of all soldiers injured while on leave and brought to civilian hospitals in the Southwest died unnecessarily after arrival at the hospital.[24] These figures were reconfirmed in 1972 by Gertner and associates who compared the results of treatment in hospitals in the city and the suburbs of Baltimore.[25] They found the mortality rate associated with treatment of intraabdominal injuries in suburban Baltimore hospitals to be much greater than that in large city hospitals. Suburban hospitals received far fewer patients with intraabdominal injuries than did city hospitals.

Maintenance of the airway and control of hemorrhage receive top priority in the patient with multiple injuries. These basic rules need reiteration because they are frequently ignored in actual practice, to the detriment of the patient.

Penetrating Trauma

In penetrating trauma the decision to operate is made easy by the dictum that all missile wounds of the abdomen be explored. Nance and co-workers, at Charity Hospital, challenged this well entrenched belief in a report describing the results of the expectant treatment of a well selected group of patients with low velocity missile wounds.[26]

Most surgeons feel that the likelihood of intraabdominal injury to a hollow viscus or vascular structure following penetrating trauma from a gunshot wound is sufficiently great that all such patients should be subjected to celiotomy.[27] When the gunshot wound is from a low velocity missile, symptoms of peritoneal irritation following penetration of a hollow viscus may initially be minimal. Free air and associated findings of peritonitis, characterized by fever, abdominal muscle guarding and tenderness, and an elevated white blood cell count, may not develop for 24 to 48 hours after injury. By this time infection is well established, making the prognosis less favorable.

Shotgun discharges at close or point blank range (10 to 20 ft.), even though of low velocity (1,000 to 1,300 ft. per second), create massive tissue destruction because of the cumulative effect of hundreds of pellets concentrated in a close pattern. When the discharge is directed at the abdomen, wide debridement, including abdominal wall skin, muscle, and fascia as well as underlying intraabdominal structures, is necessary.[28] Because of the extensive tissue injury associated with close range shotgun wounds, the mortality rate is twice that of low velocity gunshot wounds.[29]

High velocity gunshot wounds have a high mortality rate because of associated extensive tissue necrosis. Military weapons are in the high velocity category, and muzzle velocities range from 2,500 to 3,500 ft. per second. Increases in velocity triple the kinetic energy released in the tissues, which move outward at right angles to the bullet trajectory as it penetrates. A ballooning cavity is formed along the course of the bullet in soft tissue; it later collapses and sucks in clothing and other foreign bodies from the exit wound.

Unlike the injuries resulting from low velocity missile wounds in which the tissue damaged is that struck by the missile, in high velocity injuries, organs (including bone and blood vessels) that are untouched by the missile may be disrupted, shattered, or thrombosed.

Abdominal stab wounds made by a pick or knife cause little tissue necrosis. Many such wounds never penetrate the full thickness of the abdominal wall, or if they do, may not cause injury. Even when intraabdominal injury occurs, often no treatment is required at operation. Traditionally, it was believed necessary to explore all stab wounds by celiotomy. The high rate of negative explorations (25 to 60%), however, caused some surgeons to try to discriminate between patients with significant injury and those who could be observed expectantly.

Shafton and more recently Nance and associates have advocated celiotomy for abdominal stab wounds only in the presence of abdominal tenderness, rigidity, blood loss, free air, or gastrointestinal bleeding.[26,30] In Shafton's series the mortality rate was 7.37% in the group that was explored and 0.5% in the group that was unexplored. The author did not believe that any deaths could be attributed to his policy of expectant observation of patients with stab wounds in the absence of physical signs of peritoneal irritation or hemorrhage. In order to reduce further the number of unnecessary celiotomies and to identify quickly the patients at risk whose physical signs are equivocal or who initially have few signs of injury, other diagnostic procedures have been recommended by some authors.

Exploration of the stab wound is recommended by McClelland and co-workers to determine if the abdominal wall fascia has been violated.[31] Cornell and associates perform a sinogram by inserting a catheter and injecting contrast material.[32] The catheter is held in place and retrograde leakage of contrast material is prevented by a purse-string suture. Lateral abdominal x-rays are taken. Celiotomy is performed if contrast material enters the abdominal cavity. Clinical indications for celiotomy include peritonitis, free air, and evidence of hemorrhage (shock or hematuria).

Some acceptable methods for handling the patient with penetrating trauma are outlined in Figure 21-5. The ideal method of management is one in which no intraabdominal injuries are overlooked and no unnecessary celiotomies performed.

12

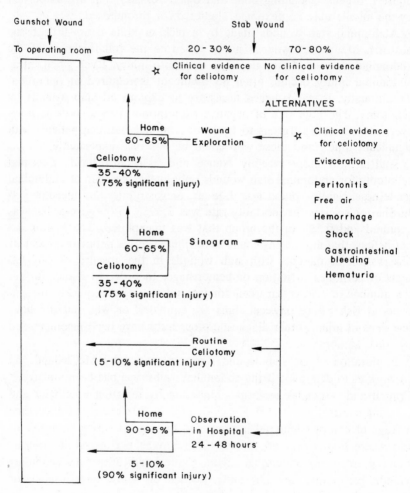

Fig. 21-5.

Blunt Trauma

Patients with hypotension, tachycardia, cold clammy skin, and evidence of peritoneal irritation in the absence of multiple long bone fractures or of external signs of blood loss or bleeding into the chest should be assumed to have bleeding into the abdominal cavity or retroperitoneal space. After typing, cross matching, and withdrawing blood for blood gas and laboratory determinations, maintaining the airway, inserting a Foley catheter and a large bore intracatheter, and administering Ringer's lactate, patients who do not respond or respond only transiently to Ringer's lactate should be transported to the operating room after a chest x-ray and flat upright or lateral decubitus films of the abdomen have been taken. Time used for numerous x-rays and blood studies only delays celiotomy.

The necessity for rushing the patient to the operating room with minimal workup, however, is infrequent. Whenever possible, time should be taken to evaluate the patient who is unconscious, has equivocal or questionable abdominal findings, or is stabilized after administration of Ringer's lactate. There also is usually time for peritoneal lavage. If the lavage is positive, there is at least a 75% chance of a significant intraabdominal injury, and celiotomy should be promptly undertaken.[33]

Peritoneal lavage is performed by introducing a peritoneal dialysis catheter through a midline infraumbilical incision by use of a trocar. The abdomen is prepared and the bladder emptied; a local anesthetic is then injected into the skin and the trocar is introduced through a small stab incision. The catheter is then aspirated. If the return is bloody, the tap is positive. If the return is negative, 1,000 ml. of Ringer's lactate solution or saline is introduced by gravity flow. The patient is moved from side to side. The bottle then is placed on the floor and the peritoneal fluid allowed to siphon out. The lavage is not considered to be positive unless the fluid in the tubing is sufficiently opaque that newsprint cannot be read through it (Fig. 21-6). Patients in whom the lavage is negative or traces of blood are seen in the lavage return should be observed and further diagnostic studies pursued if injury is still suspected. If the patient's vital signs or laboratory indices alter while under observation, lavage may be repeated and other diagnostic studies such as arteriography initiated, or celiotomy performed, depending on the individual circumstances.

The steps to be followed in the management of the patient with blunt trauma are diagrammed in Figure 21-7 and outlined in Table 21-1.

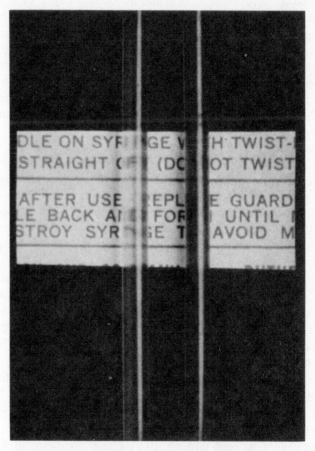

Fig. 21-6. The results of peritoneal lavage are considered to be positive only if the fluid in the tubing is sufficiently opaque that newsprint cannot be read through it (right). A negative result is shown at the left.

TRIAGE IN THE EMERGENCY DEPARTMENT

BLUNT TRAUMA

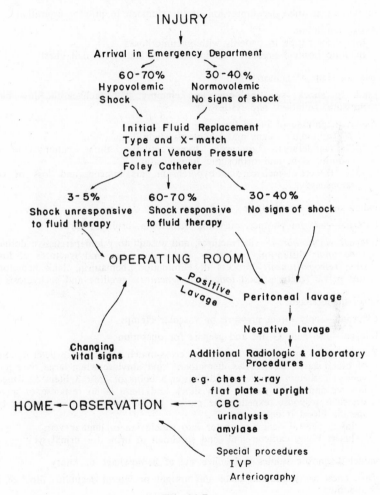

INJURY

Arrival in Emergency Department

60-70%
Hypovolemic
Shock

30-40%
Normovolemic
No signs of shock

Initial Fluid Replacement
Type and X-match
Central Venous Pressure
Foley Catheter

3-5%
Shock unresponsive
to fluid therapy

60-70%
Shock responsive
to fluid therapy

30-40%
No signs of shock

OPERATING ROOM

Positive Lavage

Peritoneal lavage

Negative lavage

Changing
vital signs

Additional Radiologic & laboratory
Procedures

e.g. chest x-ray
flat plate & upright

HOME←OBSERVATION ←— CBC
urinalysis
amylase

Special procedures
I V P
Arteriography

Fig. 21-7.

Table 21-1. Management of Blunt Trauma by the Emergency Department Physician

---

Check airway, lungs, and ventilation

Maintain airway with nasal or endotracheal intubation when obstruction or secretions threaten patency of a low resistance airway, *e.g.,* in patients who are at risk, who have facial fractures, and who are semiconscious or unconscious from head injury, alcohol, or other drugs

Initiate Levin tube decompression of the stomach to prevent aspiration

Assist ventilation
Insert chest tube in patients with pneumothorax
Institute positive pressure ventilation in patients with flail chest

Check for signs of hemorrhage

Look for shock—sweating, cold and clammy skin, tachycardia, low blood pressure, agitation, and restlessness

Assess magnitude of blood loss
15% (minimal)—signs and symptoms slight
30% (moderate)—tachycardia, hyperventilation, thirst, pallor, cold and clammy skin, and orthostatic hypotension
45% (severe)—tachycardia, hypotension, air hunger, and loss of consciousness

Localize signs of hemorrhage

External—arterial pumper, pulsating hematoma, bruit, or thrill

Internal—*hemothorax*: rib fractures, and auscultatory and percussive dullness; *abdominal*: distention, tenderness, peritoneal signs, and fractures of lower ribs; *retroperitoneal*: process of elimination, hematuria, flank hematoma, and pelvic fractures; and *long bone fracture*: swelling and ecchymosis

Control hemorrhage

External—apply direct pressure or vascular clamps

Internal—use pant G-suit and prepare for operation

Volume replacement—draw, type, and cross-match blood; make determinations of blood gases, electrolytes, hematocrit, and amylase when large bore intravenous catheters are placed, administer a bolus of 2 or 3 liters of Ringer's lactate, and if the patient is in shock and there is no response or a very transient response, expedite the patient to the operating room, giving type specific blood if necessary
Insert central venous catheter into subclavian or jugular vein
Insert Foley catheter and send specimen of urine for urinalysis

Conduct diagnostic studies to localize site of hemorrhage or injury

Take chest x-ray and flat plate and upright or lateral decubitus films of the abdomen.

Institute peritoneal lavage
Insert dialysis catheter and check fluid for presence of blood
Infuse 1,000 ml. of Ringer's lactate; tilt or roll patient and then place infusion bottle on floor for siphon effect; return of blood sufficiently concentrated that newsprint cannot be read through the tubing indicates positive lavage

---

Table 21-1.—Continued

Control infection
  Initiate tetanus prophylaxis
  Administer broad-spectrum antibiotics if injury to hollow viscus or liver is
    suspected

Conduct complete history and physical examination to identify and assess all
  associated injuries

Management of patient with a positive lavage
  When lavage is positive and the patient's vital signs are unstable, the safest
    course is to take the patient to the operating room. There is no need for
    further special studies to identify the specific intraabdominal organ injured
    because this will be better determined at operation
  When lavage is positive and the patient is stable, the patient accompanied by
    a physician may go to the radiology department for chest x-ray, flat plate
    and upright films of the abdomen, and other appropriate studies of sus-
    pected associated injuries before going to the operating room
  When the lavage is negative, the patient may be taken to the radiology de-
    partment for chest x-ray, flat plate and upright films of the abdomen, ap-
    propriate studies for suspected associated injury, and special studies, e.g.,
    arteriograms, cystourethrograms, and intravenous and retrograde pyelograms
  In the patient with multiple trauma, the steps to be taken in the history,
    physical examination, diagnosis, and resuscitation can be identified and de-
    scribed and priorities assigned. Many of these steps must be initiated and
    performed concomitantly in patients with life-threatening injuries resulting
    in compression of the airway and exsanguinating hemorrhage

Spleen

The spleen is the organ most often injured in blunt abdominal
trauma.[1,34,35] Splenic injury is the fifth or sixth most frequent injury
associated with penetrating abdominal trauma (Table 21-2).[26,36] Not-

Table 21-2. Incidence of Splenic Injury in Abdominal Trauma

	Patients with Abdominal Injuries (number)	Patients with Splenic Injuries (number)	(percent)	Rank
Starkloff, 1953[15]				
Blunt trauma	102	28	27.0	1
Penetrating trauma	206	12	5.8	6
Welch and Giddings, 1950[35]				
Combined trauma	200	38	1.9	2
Pridgen, 1967[36]				
Penetrating trauma	776	60	7.7	5
DiVincenti, 1968[1]				
Blunt trauma	430	267	62.0	1

withstanding the technical ease of splenectomy for the trained surgeon or the absence of noticeable loss of function resulting from the spleen's removal in most patients, 10% of all patients with splenic injury die. When trauma to other organs is associated with splenic injury, the mortality rate approaches 20%.[34,37-41]

Diagnosis. Splenic rupture causes a spectrum of injuries ranging from a small capsular tear and minimal blood loss to total anatomic disruption associated with brisk hemorrhage (Fig. 21-8B and D). Sometimes with splenic injury the capsule initially remains intact and contains an expanding hematoma (Fig. 21-8C). Progressive enlargement of the hematoma within the splenic pulp leading to capsular rupture and hem-

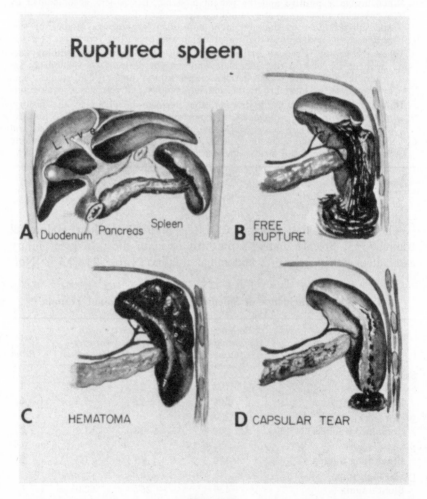

Fig. 21-8.

orrhage 36 to 48 or more hours after injury is called delayed rupture of the spleen and accounts for 20 to 30% of all splenic injuries (Table 21-3).[42] Seventy-five percent of delayed ruptures of the spleen occur within one week of injury, but some may appear clinically for the first time months after injury. A higher mortality rate is associated with delayed than with early rupture of the spleen.[42] The patient with delayed rupture who may have already left the hospital must be rushed back and prepared for an emergency splenectomy.

The incidence and the concept of what has been called delayed rupture of the spleen has recently been challenged. The use of peritoneal lavage in assessing intraabdominal injury after blunt trauma has markedly reduced the number of patients with delayed rupture of the spleen to between 1 and 5%. Most cases of what has been called delayed rupture of the spleen, therefore, may not be a delay in rupture but rather a delay in recognition of injury.

In any instance in which there is a clinical suspicion of splenic rupture following a negative lavage, or a lavage returning less than 20 ml. of blood per liter, a femoral percutaneous selective splenic arteriogram may be performed. On arteriography, a splenic hematoma appears as a radiolucent defect within the spleen during the capillary phase as well as moderate opacification of the pulp and early filling of the splenic vein due to macroscopic acquired arteriovenous fistulas.[19] Progression of an intrasplenic hematoma to final rupture may be related to these acquired arteriovenous fistulas. Occasionally in splenic injury only the capsule surrounding the spleen is torn (Fig. 21-8D). The rate and clinical significance of such bleeding from superficial lacerations is unknown. The steps to be taken by the emergency department physician in the man-

Table 21-3. Splenic Injury

	No. of Patients	Penetrating Trauma	Blunt Trauma	Delayed Rupture	Mortality Rate (percent)
Willox, 1953–1963[37]	103	3	100	19	17
Byrne, 1936–1946[38]	101	25	76	14	16.8
Terry, to 1956[39]	102	49	53	11	24.5
Sizer, 1954–1965[42]	52	—	—	12	10
Cloutier, 1937–1957[40]	43	5	36	30 (24 hrs.)	25
Shirkey, 1946–1962[41]	189	125	64	19	22
DiVincenti, 1951–1956[1]	267	—	267	—	28

Table 21-4. **Management of Splenic Injury by the Emergency Department Physician**

Remember that the spleen is the intraabdominal organ most frequently injured in blunt trauma

Look for diagnostic clues
    Left shoulder pain (Kehr's sign)
    Left upper quadrant tenderness, spasm, or guarding
    Fractured lower left ribs
    Positive peritoneal lavage—an indication for celiotomy
    Elevated white blood cell count
    Displacement of stomach medially on flat films
    Shock—presence depends on amount of blood loss

Beware of delayed rupture from contained hematoma
    If peritoneal lavage is negative and clinical suspicion of splenic injury persists, arteriography is indicated

Resuscitate patient
    Type and cross-match blood
    Administer Ringer's lactate solution
    Measure central venous pressure
    Consider administering broad-spectrum antibiotics
    Measure central venous pressure
    Insert Foley catheter
    Apply pants G-suit

Look for indications to operate
    Shock—lack of response to fluid replacement
    Positive lavage
    Peritoneal signs
    Positive findings on arteriography

Be cognizant of late complications after hospital discharge
    Delayed splenic rupture
    Intravascular coagulopathy from thrombocytosis following splenectomy

agement of the patient with suspected splenic injury are outlined in Table 21-4.

Treatment. Until information to the contrary becomes available, all splenic injuries, including superficial capsular tears, should be treated promptly by splenectomy. The technique is relatively simple in the absence of portal hypertension, multiple adhesions, or an extremely large spleen. The splenocolic and gastrosplenic ligaments are divided; the gastrosplenic ligament, which contains the short gastric vessels, must be individually ligated. The splenic pedicle is exposed. It is usually convenient to mobilize the spleen from its bed posterolaterally, thereby bringing the hilus containing the vascular pedicle anteriorly into the field so that the splenic artery and then the splenic vein can be easily ligated. Mobilization of the spleen by freeing its attachments posterolaterally is an important measure in assuring control of the splenic pedicle and preventing or controlling hemorrhage from the spleen. It used to be thought that drainage of the splenic bed was essential. Most authors now report that this is associated with an increased incidence of intraabdominal abscess, and reserve drainage for patients having associated injuries to a hollow viscus or pancreas.[43]

Following splenectomy, thrombocytosis may occur. Disseminated intravascular thrombosis following splenectomy is an infrequent but lethal complication. If the platelet count exceeds one million, intravenous or intramuscular heparin or anticoagulant therapy should be instituted. The platelet count seldom reaches one million until a week postsplenectomy. Once heparin therapy is instituted, it should be continued until the platelet count decreases to below a million (usually within six weeks of injury). Coumadin derivatives have no effect on platelet adhesiveness and therefore are of no value in the prevention of thrombosis from thrombocytosis. Because of their effect on platelet adhesiveness, aspirin derivatives theoretically offer protection against postsplenectomy thrombocytosis, but there is no well controlled study to substantiate this possibility.

Liver

The liver plays an important role in the metabolism of fat, carbohydrates, and proteins and is essential to life. It is the first or second most frequently injured organ in penetrating trauma and the third or fourth most commonly injured in blunt trauma to the abdomen (Tables 21-5 and 21-6).[44-52]

Table 21-5. Liver Trauma

	Penetrating Trauma			Blunt Trauma	
	No. of Patients	No. of Patients	Mortality Rate (percent)	No. of Patients	Mortality Rate (percent)
Balasegaram, 1961–1968[44]	35	—	—	35	16
Crosthwaith, 1939–1968[45]	640	573	14.3	67	44.8
Atik, 1942–1959[46]	309	201	15	108	55
McClelland, 1953–1963[47]	259	228	10	31	26
DiVincenti, 1951–1966[1]	102	—	—	50	49
Longmire, 1949–1962[48]	90	35	14	55	37
Shrock, 1960–1966[49]	61	41	5	20	65
Kindling, 1961–1966[50]	303	262	6.9	41	31.7
Frey, 1956–1970[54]	178	51	15.8	127	29.6

Table 21-6. Blunt Hepatic Trauma

	Automobile			Other	
	Total No. of Patients	No. of Patients	Mortality Rate (percent)	No. of Patients	Mortality Rate (percent)
Balasegaram, 1961–1968[44]	35	32	16	3	—
Shafton, 1950–1959[51]	38	26	57	12	50
Longmire, 1949–1961[48]	55	45	—	10	—
Baker, 1955–1964[52]*	58	41	17	13	46
Schrock, 1960–1966[49]	20	—	—	—	—
Kindling[50]	41	34	35.3	7	14.3
Frey[54]	127	98	31	—	—

* Did not include anyone dying in less than 12 hours after operation.

Penetrating injuries include wounds from knives, picks, screwdrivers, and other sharp objects, shrapnel, and firearms. The mortality rate of penetrating wounds of the liver depends largely on the wounding agent, injury to major vessels, and the number of other abdominal organs injured. When the wounding agent is a knife or low velocity missile, the mortality and complication rates tend to be low (Table 21-5). In stab wounds of the liver, hemorrhage is often inconsequential and repair is not required; other abdominal organs and major vessels also are less likely to be injured. High velocity or shotgun projectiles are much more likely to produce devastating wounds of the liver with extensive destruction and massive hemorrhage, as well as a high incidence of injury to other abdominal organs. Penetrating wounds of the liver with entry through the abdominal wall may also follow a trajectory leading to penetration of the diaphragm. Conversely, penetrating wounds with entry through the thorax may produce intraabdominal injury. The combination of hepatic wounds with those of the biliary tract, duodenum, pancreas, or colon are particularly lethal.

Kindling and co-workers reported only four deaths in a group of 193 patients with stab wounds.[50] All four deaths (2.1%) were attributed to bleeding from associated injuries of other organs or large vessels. The complication rate following stab or low velocity missile wounds was 9%.

Hepatic injuries from blunt abdominal trauma are serious. Thirteen of the 41 patients (31%) with blunt hepatic injury in Kindling and associates' report died as a result of blunt injury to the liver.[50] These deaths were attributed directly to the hepatic injury.

Ordinarily the two lobes of the liver are well protected from blunt injury by the rib cage, but when massive forces such as those developed

Crush injury of liver

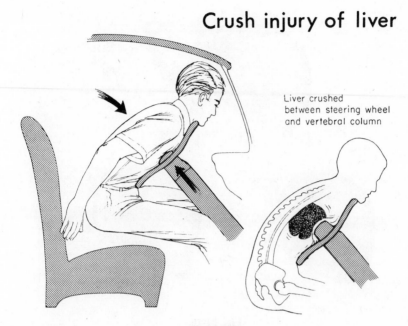

Liver crushed
between steering wheel
and vertebral column

Fig. 21-9.

during vehicular accidents compress the rib cage against the vertebral column, the liver may be crushed between them (Fig. 21-9).

The energy directly applied to the liver of primates that is necessary to produce a fracture was measured by Trollope and co-workers[53] and found to be much less than the energy necessary to produce an hepatic fracture when the force was transmitted to the liver through the abdominal wall. Data from several hundred impact studies performed on squirrel and Rhesus monkeys were used to develop a formula for predicting the severity of injury in relation to the impacting force, contact areas, duration of impact, and size of the test animal.

$$\text{Estimated Severity Index} = \text{Log} \frac{fr2}{m\sqrt{a}}$$

$$f = \text{force of impact}$$
$$r = \text{duration of impact}$$
$$m = \text{mass of animal}$$
$$a = \text{contact area}$$

Depending on the energy on impact with the liver, it may be fractured or shattered. Hemorrhage may be profuse from a liver that has been crushed or shattered. In patients in whom an entire hepatic lobe has

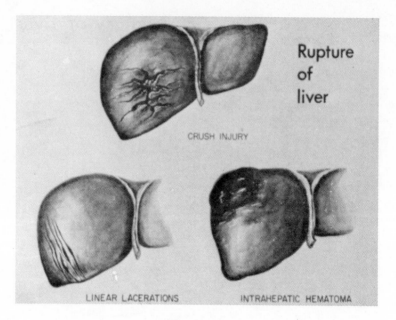

Fig. 21-10.

been crushed, the mortality rate is high because of the accompanying hemorrhage, which may be massive (Fig. 21-10). Technical difficulties in controlling hemorrhage are sometimes encountered at operation, particularly if there are associated injuries of the hepatic veins and inferior vena cava.[54]

Of all the causes of blunt hepatic injury, the automobile is the most frequent, producing more than 75% of all hepatic injuries from blunt forces, including those from falls, assaults, and blasts (Table 21-6).[52]

Death from hemorrhage following hepatic injury due to a vehicular accident may occur at the scene of the accident and in transit to the hospital as well as in the hospital. Because of improvements in transport and resuscitation, there has been a steady decrease in the number of patients dying at the scene of the accident and in transit to the hospital.[54] In 1946, Castren reported that 63% of 166 patients died before reaching the hospital.[55] Mills in 1961 and Hanna and associates in 1965 reported that 50% reached the hospital alive.[56,57] Hellstrom studied the spectrum of 192 fatal hepatic injuries caused by the automobile during the 24-year period between 1939 and 1963.[58] Sixty deaths occurred at the scene of accident or in transit to the hospital, 65 occurred within 12 hours after hospital admission, and 67 occurred later during hospitalization.

The time involved in transportation to the hospital in a suburban community was reduced from 45 to 90 minutes between 1956 and 1965 to 25 minutes between 1966 and 1970. Similarly, the time required to move a patient with hepatic injury from the emergency department to the operating room decreased from an average of 206 minutes between 1955 and 1960 to 140 minutes between 1965 to 1970.[54]

Prognosis. The presence of shock (systolic blood pressure less than 80 mm. Hg) in patients admitted to the emergency department with hepatic trauma is correlated with either the extent of hepatic injury or the severity of associated injuries. In fact, in the series of hepatic injuries from blunt trauma reported by Frey and associates, there were no deaths between 1966 and 1970 in patients without evidence of shock in the emergency department.[54] Likewise, there were no deaths from the hepatic injury itself in patients during the same period unless the liver showed the classic "burst" pattern or multiple lacerations more than

Table 21-7. Management of Hepatic Injury by the Emergency Department Physician

---

Remember that the liver is frequently injured in both blunt and penetrating trauma

Look for diagnostic clues
    Right shoulder pain
    Right upper quadrant tenderness, spasm, or guarding
    Shock—present or absent depending on amount of blood loss; when deep and unrelieved by Ringer's lactate, immediate operation is indicated
    Fractured lower right ribs
    Peritoneal lavage—positive result is an indication for operation
    Signs of peritonitis in the absence of significant blood loss—may indicate a bile leak from injury to the liver, biliary ductal system, or gallbladder

If peritoneal lavage is negative and clinical suspicion of injury persists, arteriography is indicated

Resuscitate patient
    Type and cross-match blood
    Administer Ringer's lactate intravenously
    Measure central venous pressure
    Insert Foley catheter
    Apply pants G-suit
    Consider administering broad-spectrum antibiotics

Look for indications to operate
    Shock—lack of response to fluid replacement
    Positive lavage
    Peritoneal signs
    Positive findings on arteriography

Be cognizant of late complications of unrecognized injury
    Hepatic artery or branch pseudoaneurysm
    Hepatic arteriovenous fistula
    Hypertension

---

4 cm. in depth and more than 5 cm. in length. The in-hospital mortality rate of hepatic injury from blunt and penetrating trauma, including the most extensive hepatic injuries, has been progressively reduced over the years.

The steps to be taken by the emergency department physician in the management of the patient with suspected hepatic injury are outlined in Table 21-7.

Treatment. The principles of therapy are similar for penetrating and blunt hepatic injury and include the following: (1) control of hemorrhage; (2) debridement of devitalized hepatic tissue, including hepatic lobectomy if necessary; (3) external drainage of the hepatic injury; and (4) T-tube decompression of the biliary ductal system for patients with serious hepatic injury requiring lobectomy, or involving multiple deep lacerations or a large intrahepatic hematoma.[54]

Control of Hemorrhage and Debridement of Devitalized Tissue. At the time of operation, the injured liver may have ceased bleeding, or only a few sutures may be required to prevent further hemorrhage from a stab wound or superficial laceration. If the laceration is deep, but the hepatic segment on each side is viable, and hemorrhage is a problem along the face of the cut, hemostasis may be achieved by suture ligature, metal clips, or compression of the hepatic tissues 1 cm. from the edge of the laceration by insertion of parallel sutures with 5-inch curved, blunt hepatic needles.[59]

Control of active hemorrhage from multiple, deep hepatic lacerations or a crush injury of an hepatic lobe or segment is a formidable problem for the surgeon. At operation, hemorrhage from the injured liver may be controlled temporarily by clamping the portal triad (the Pringle maneuver). The portal triad may be safely clamped for 30 minutes in the normovolemic patient, but the time should be shorter in patients in shock.

Devitalized or amputated hepatic tissue is removed. Multiple mattress sutures are placed 1 cm. from the lacerated surface, compressing the hepatic tissue and reducing blood loss from the surface of the laceration. Large bleeding vessels and bile ducts should be individually ligated. Hepatic lobectomy is a form of debridement and is indicated when a lobe has been devitalized as a result of a crush injury or interruption of its blood supply. The penalty for not debriding devitalized hepatic tissue is infections, abscesses, biliary fistulas, and recurrent hemorrhage.

The technique of lobectomy is based on a knowledge of the arterial and venous blood supply, as described by Quattlebaum.[60] The line of resection between the right and left lobes is the gallbladder fossa. Lobectomy is performed by ligating the appropriate branch of the hepatic artery, portal vein, and bile ducts supplying the lobe to be amputated. The hepatic veins draining the lobe are then ligated prior to resection. Large mattress sutures are then placed on each side of the proposed incision to reduce blood loss. However, formal hepatic lobectomy is seldom required. Usually, the line of resection is defined by the site of fracture, even though this may include most of a lobe.

Madding and Kennedy as well as Mays have advocated hepatic artery ligation or lobe dearterialization as a less time-consuming, life-threatening procedure than lobectomy for control of hemorrhage.[61,62] Sixty percent of the hepatic blood flow is derived from the portal blood supply, and the risk of hepatic necrosis is reported to be small. Concomitant shock, fever, and infections of the biliary tract, however, may predispose the patient to hepatic necrosis and a fatal outcome following hepatic artery ligation, according to Brittain and co-workers.[63] Antibiotics are believed to help prevent hepatic necrosis following dearterialization of the liver, but their efficacy in man has not been proven.

Most deaths from hemorrhage in patients with hepatic injury result from lacerations of the hepatic veins and vena cava. Such patients are invariably in shock in the emergency department.[54] Concomitant resuscitation and operation are essential for survival. At operation, the area of injury can be packed and the chest opened through the fifth or sixth interspace by teeing the incision if the abdomen was explored through a subcostal incision or by extending a midline incision up over the right costal margin. Some surgeons, however, prefer a sternal splitting incision. A large bore 25-mm. siliconized catheter with a side vent designed to open intraartrially is inserted through the wall of the right atrium, or through the atrial appendage if a sternal splitting incision has been used, and on into the inferior vena cava. Tourniquet ligatures are passed about the inferior vena cava and inlying catheter supradiaphragmatically, intrapericardially, and distally above the renal veins. With the blood from the inferior vena cava bypassing the liver through the internal shunt and with the portal triad clamped, lacerations in the hepatic veins and inferior vena cava can be oversewn without further blood loss and with vision of the operative site unobscured by blood.[64-67] Siliconization of the tubing makes total body heparinization unnecessary.

Attempts to close lacerations of the hepatic vein and inferior vena cava without diverting the vena caval flow usually fail because the subdiaphragmatic attachments of the inferior vena cava prevent collapse of the cava and inhibit side clamping of the cava with vascular clamps. Accurate application of the vascular clamp is further hindered by massive life-threatening hemorrhage issuing from the vena cava and obscuring the operative field.

Yellin and associates recommend cross-clamping the inferior vena cava at the level of the diaphragm and above the renal vessels.[68] Technically, cross clamping the inferior vena cava at the diaphragm is easier than side clamping. These authorities also clamp the portal triad and the aorta.

The necessity for excising all devitalized hepatic tissue can be documented by reviewing the failures that resulted from the practice continued to the mid 1960s of packing hepatic wounds with lap pads, Gelfoam, and Oxycel to control hemorrhage. The course of patients with major hepatic injuries treated by packing was often complicated by recurrent hemorrhage, intrahepatic and intraabdominal abscesses, and biliary fistulas, resulting from discontinuity of the biliary ductal system and nonperfused necrotic liver.[54]

External Drainage. External drains should be inserted following debridement of devitalized hepatic tissue, including lobectomy, to remove potential collections of blood or bile.

T-tube Decompression of the Biliary Ductal System. The procedure of T-tube decompression of the biliary ductal system following hepatic injury, which was originally recommended by Merendino and associates,[69] is not necessary except in the severe hepatic injury. More recently, Lucas recommended discontinuing the practice of utilizing T-tube drainage of the common duct in hepatic trauma.[70] He reported instances of inadvertent removal of the T-tube, difficulty with placement, and iatrogenic injury of the biliary ductal system, and he attributed some of the complications of hepatic injury, e.g., stress ulcers, intraabdominal abscesses, and biliary fistula, to the use of the T-tube.

Advocates of T-tube decompression of the biliary tract in severe hepatic injury have found it useful during and following operation.[54] The intraoperative injection of saline or methylene blue through the T-tube helps in the identification of transected bile ducts on the cut liver surface.[71] Ligation of the transected bile ducts reduces the likelihood of bile leakage and some of its sequelae, such as bile peritonitis, biliary fistula, and intraabdominal abscess. Decompression of the biliary tract can be achieved by placing the T-tube to low bubble suction. The T-tube can also be utilized in the evaluation of postoperative jaundice and the source of hematobilia. The incidence of abscesses, stress ulcers, and biliary fistulas in patients with and without T-tubes and with hepatic injuries of similar severity were identical in Frey's experience and therefore believed to be coincidental.[54]

Injuries of the Extrahepatic Biliary Tract, Associated Structures, and Gallbladder. Often the patient with either hepatic artery or portal vein injury does not survive to reach the operating room, but if he does, hemorrhage can often be controlled initially by the Pringle maneuver until vascular clamps can be applied to the injured vessels. After careful dissection and exposure of the injured vessel proximal and distal to the site of injury, repair can be effected with fine cardiovascular suture.

Injuries of the common, proper, and lobar branches of the hepatic artery should be repaired if possible with end-to-end anastomosis or autogenous saphenous vein if the defect is appreciable. The sentiment for repair of the hepatic artery is based on uncertainty as to the safety of ligating the hepatic artery in the presence of shock.[63] Portal vein injuries can be repaired after application of vascular clamps or Fogarty balloon catheter tamponade. In the event that repair is impossible, the portal vein may be ligated; conversely, the superior mesenteric vein may not be ligated.[72]

Injury to the extrahepatic biliary tract and gallbladder in the absence of associated injuries often appears as bile peritonitis. Sometimes there is a delay in the diagnosis of a bile leak in the absence of infection. Injury to the gallbladder is treated by cholecystectomy. Common duct injuries are repaired by end-to-end anastomosis, choledochoduodenostomy, or choledochojejunostomy, depending on the nature of the injury and degree of inflammation in the periductal tissues.

Kidneys

The kidneys are essential to life. Satisfactory renal function can be maintained, however, with only one of these paired organs. If one kidney is damaged, it therefore may be removed and survival of the patient assured if the other kidney functions normally.

The kidneys, like the liver, are well protected by the rib cage and further insulated from injury by the surrounding fat pad encompassed by Gerota's fascia. In spite of the seemingly impregnable position of the kidneys, renal injuries are the second or third most common injuries in the abdominal cavity as a result of blunt trauma (25%)[1,34] and sixth and seventh as a result of penetrating trauma (5 to 7%).[1,21,36] Renal injuries account for half of all injuries to the genitourinary tract.[73]

Preexisting renal disease, such as hydronephrosis or pyelonephritis, makes the kidneys more susceptible to injury.

Renal injuries from blunt trauma can be divided into three general types: (1) parenchymal tears associated with perinephric hematuria; (2) parenchymal tears with hemorrhage into the collecting system; and (3) crush injuries.

Most blunt injuries of the kidneys do not require surgery. Penetrating injuries involving the kidneys should be examined at operation.

Diagnosis. Flank pain is experienced by 80% of all patients with renal injury. The pain may be colicky because of the passage of blood clots. Hematuria is an important indication of renal injury, even if it is transient or intermittent. Blood clots can obstruct the egress of blood or urine from the upper urinary tract and may result in anuria and renal damage. On the other hand, severe injury to the urinary tract, including the kidney, bladder, ureter, or urethra, can occur in the absence of hematuria, particularly in injuries to the lower urinary tract, in which case gross hematuria may be absent in 50% of patients.[73,74]

Other clues to genitourinary tract injury that can be demonstrated on plain films of the abdomen include fractures of the lower ribs posteriorly and inferiorly and of the transverse processes in the thoracolumbar region, and loss of the psoas shadow. Intravenous pyelograms or arteriograms ought to be obtained in all patients with suspected renal injury. The status of renal function on the injured and the uninjured side and whether there is extravasation of contrast material must be known by the surgeon in his management of the patient with renal trauma and should be obtained by the emergency department physician. Retrograde pyelography may be utilized to examine the anatomy of the injury in more detail, but it should not be performed unless injury to the lower part of the urinary tract is ruled out. Selective arteriography has proven to be an effective technique for assessing the nature and severity of renal injury. Any patient with nonfunction on intravenous pyelography, extravasation of urine, or signs of continuing blood loss or late onset of hypertension should be subjected to arteriography.[75-77]

Treatment. Indications for operation include all patients with penetrating renal injuries. Following blunt trauma, operation is indicated when there is evidence of continuing hemorrhage into an extensive perinephric hematoma, parenchymal destruction, extension of the renal fracture into the collecting system, extrarenal extravasation of contrast material, or thrombosis or avulsion of the renal artery or its major branches as evidenced by nonfunction or continuing hemorrhage. Recurrent hemorrhage, regardless of whether perinephric or in the form of hematuria, is another indication for nephrectomy. The steps to be taken by the emergency department physician in the management of the patient with suspected upper urinary tract injury are outlined in Table 21-8.

The management of renal trauma has undergone major changes in the past 10 years.[74] There has been an increased tendency by urologists to preserve the injured kidney or to save part of it as long as there is a reasonable expectation of maintaining some renal function. Hematuria and retroperitoneal hematoma about the kidney are not in themselves indications for nephrectomy. Major or critical injuries are those with a perinephric pulsating hematoma, parenchymal destruction, fracture extension into the collecting system, and marked extravasation of contrast

Table 21-8. Management of Upper Urinary Tract Injury by the Emergency Department Physician

---

Remember that the kidney is the third most frequently injured abdominal organ as a result of blunt trauma

Look for diagnostic clues
 Flank pain—often colicky
 Fractured lower ribs
 Preexisting hydronephrosis or pyelonephritis predisposing to injury
 Hematuria, which may not always be present, even in significant injury
 Peritoneal lavage—may be negative in significant injury
 Shock—present or absent depending on amount of blood loss
 Fractures of transverse processes of second, third, and fourth lumbar vertebrae
 Loss of psoas shadow on flat film
 Intravenous pyelography is useful in assessing function of injured and uninjured kidney
 Selective arteriography and retrograde pyelography are useful in assessing the nature and severity of injury

Resuscitate patient
 Type and cross-match blood
 Administer Ringer's lactate intravenously
 Measure central venous pressure
 Insert Foley catheter
 Apply pants G-suit
 Administer broad-spectrum antibiotics

Look for indications to operate
 Penetrating renal injury
 Blunt trauma
 Continuing hemorrhage
 Large perinephric hematoma
 Parenchymal destruction
 Extension of renal fracture into collecting system
 Extrarenal extravasation of contrast material
 Thrombosis or avulsion of renal arteries
 Evidence of recurrent hemorrhage

---

material. When a portion of the kidney has been devitalized by pulpifaction, or a laceration interrupting its blood supply, the remainder of the kidney is worth preserving if it shows function. Partial nephrectomy with excision of the devitalized and hypoxic tissues is essential to prevent late onset of hypertension. If the entire kidney is fragmented and shows no sign of function, nephrectomy should be performed, particularly if hematuria is brisk and life-threatening.

Renal artery thrombosis or avulsion may result from trauma in which the kidney itself is uninjured. Prompt operative intervention with thrombectomy or revascularization may salvage the kidney. Patients with extensive renal injuries, particularly those involving the renal artery and its major branches, should be followed closely for several years because of the possible development of renal hypertension, which is said to occur in 6% of patients undergoing vascular repair.[78] Recently investigators reported that continued hemorrhage in the presence of normal renal function can be controlled by injection of autologous clot treated with epsilon aminocaproic acid, thus making operation unnecessary.[79] Principles of surgical management of renal injuries are similar to those for management of hepatic injuries.

1. Prevention of life-threatening hemorrhage by first gaining central control of the renovascular pedicle before attempting to open a retroperitoneal hematoma.
2. Debridement of all devascularized tissue, including the entire kidney if it has undergone pulpifaction.
3. External extraperitoneal drainage of the operative area.
4. Closure of the collecting system if lacerated.
5. Determination of the status of the contralateral kidney prior to nephrectomy. Otherwise the patient may be left with no kidney.

Ureter

Ureteral injuries usually result from penetrating trauma and, fortunately, are relatively uncommon. Flank pain or fever that is otherwise unexplained may be the only clue to injury. Hematuria may be absent, particularly if the ureter is totally transected. Untreated ureteral injuries may result in "death of the kidney," and late repair may be impossible because of the development of a retroperitoneal phlegmon and necrosis of an extensive length of ureter.

Intravenous and retrograde pyelography should be performed to establish the diagnosis and site of injury before operative intervention. The transected ureter should be repaired by end-to-end anastomosis whenever possible. If long segments of the ureter have been destroyed, it may be necessary to resort to ureteroileostomy or ureterosigmoidostomy diversion because a successful repair depends on an anastomosis with no tension and mucosa-to-mucosa apposition.

Urinary Bladder

Bladder trauma constitutes 15% of all genitourinary injuries and often occurs secondary to motor vehicular accidents. In Brosman's experience, 86% of bladder injuries were secondary to blunt trauma and 14% due to penetrating injury.[80] Injury is more severe if the bladder is full at the time of the accident.[80] Fractures of the pubic rami in conjunction with bladder injury are frequent. Extraperitoneal rupture is more frequent than intraperitoneal or combined intraperitoneal and extraperitoneal rupture of the bladder. Retroperitoneal urinary extravasation may be manifested by swelling of the anterior abdominal wall, scrotum, buttocks, or perineum. Because of associated injuries to the pelvic bone, iliac veins, and their tributaries, blood loss may be profuse and accompanied by shock.

On attempts to void, the patient may be aware of increased pain if bladder rupture is extraperitoneal. Voiding may be impossible if the rupture is intraperitoneal.

The diagnosis of bladder rupture is made by cystography. The bladder contour is often distorted by the extravasation of blood and urine compressing the bladder. Because of the high incidence of associated urethral injury, the injection of contrast material (Renografin) into the bladder should be done via the urethra rather than by insertion of a catheter into the bladder.

At operation the intraperitoneal bladder laceration should be closed and suprapubic cystotomy drainage instituted in addition to drainage of the prevesical space.

Urethra

About 10% of all genitourinary injuries involve the urethra. Most urethral injuries occur in males who are involved in motor vehicular accidents, and they are usually associated with pelvic fractures[81] and frequently with rectosigmoid laceration. Many urethral injuries are in the bulbomembranous portion and result from crushing or disruption associated with fractures of the pubic arch. Urethral injuries may be accompanied by a large hematoma on the anterior abdominal wall suprapubically, or with dissection into the scrotum because of disruption of the periprostatic venous plexus. On physical examination the prostate may not be palpable if the urethra has been totally transected above the urogenital diaphragm. Diagnosis of the urethral injury is established by cystourethrography and one must avoid insertion of a catheter, which can create through the disrupted urethra a false passage and result in increased destruction.

Treatment of urethral injuries has not been very satisfactory because of a high incidence of stricture and incontinence. Suprapubic drainage initially followed by a two-stage urethroplasty has been popularized recently. The steps to be observed by the emergency department physician in the management of the patient with suspected lower urinary tract injury are outlined in Table 21-9.

Table 21-9.   Management of Lower Urinary Tract Injuries by the Emergency Department Physician

Look for diagnostic clues
  Pelvic fractures—often associated with these injuries
  Shock—may or may not be present depending on blood loss and urine extravasation
  Peritoneal signs—present in intraperitoneal rupture
  Extraperitoneal signs—swelling of anterior abdominal wall, scrotum, buttocks, or perineum may occur if rupture is extraperitoneal
  Voiding may or may not be difficult
  Prostate may not be palpable in urethral injuries
  Hematuria—significant if present, but may not be seen with severe injury
  Intravenous pyelogram identifies site and often nature of injury; cystourethrogram determines integrity of urethra and bladder

Resuscitate patient
  Type and cross-match blood
  Administer Ringer's lactate intravenously
  Measure central venous pressure
  Insert Foley catheter
  Administer broad-spectrum antibiotics

Look for indications to operate
  Injury to ureters, bladder, or urethra

Be cognizant of late complications
  Stricture and incontinence—common following urethral injuries

Pancreas

The pancreas is both an endocrine and an exocrine organ. As an exocrine organ, it produces enzymes that help to digest fat, protein, and carbohydrates. The endocrine function of the pancreas takes place in the islet tissue, the site of insulin and glucagon production. The pancreas can be totally removed if injured, and life is maintained if the patient receives appropriate exogenous insulin and pancreatic enzyme replacement therapy. The pancreas is located retroperitoneally and is not frequently injured. Although hemorrhage is the greatest threat to life following injury to the spleen, liver, and kidneys, this is not the case in pancreatic injuries unless there is an additional associated major vessel injury.

The mortality rate associated with pancreatic injuries as reported over the last 10 years varies between 15 and 55% with an average of 20%.[12,82-84] The pancreas is the powder keg of the abdomen. If one of the major pancreatic ducts is disrupted, potent enzymes are released into the interstitium of the pancreas. If these enzymes are activated by enterokinase in duodenal juice or by bacterial infection, they (in combination with duodenal juice) can digest the pancreas and surrounding tissue, including the patient's skin if there is a cutaneous fistula. Injuries to

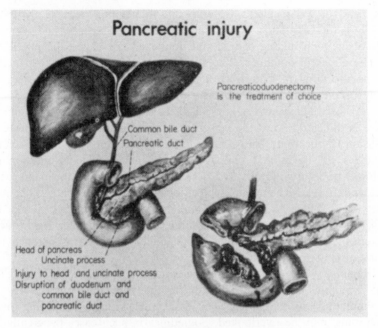

Fig. 21-11.

Pancreatic injury

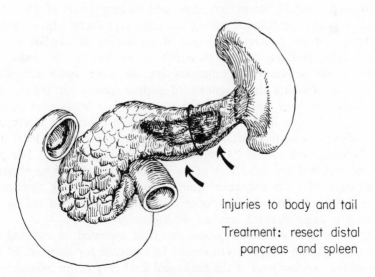

Fig. 21-12.

the head of the pancreas are truly life-threatening because they may result in the disruption of the duodenum and pancreatic and common bile ducts, with mixing of bile and duodenal and pancreatic juices.[12]

The vertebral column is like the hub of a wheel with the pancreas wrapped around it. The head of the pancreas is on the right side, the body of the gland is in the center of the abdomen, and the tail is on the left side. The pancreas is most likely to be injured if the impinging force is directed toward the vertebral column. At the time of a head-on collision, if the right side of the abdomen is anterior, the head of the pancreas will be injured (Fig. 21-11); if the left side is anterior, the tail will be injured (Fig. 12-12). The parenchyma of the pancreas is soft and friable. The nonmuscular ductal system, by contrast, is relatively rigid. When an impinging blunt force crushes some portion of the pancreas against the vertebral column, the more brittle, rigid ductal system often is disrupted, while the pancreatic vasculature, parenchyma, and capsule remain intact.

Diagnosis. The diagnosis of pancreatic injuries can be difficult. Clinical symptoms attributable directly to the pancreatic injury may be minimal and, in the absence of associated injuries producing overt symptoms, may be overlooked. Sometimes in such cases pancreatic injury is unrecognized for weeks or months until the development of upper abdominal pain, ileus distention, low-grade fever, weight loss or a mass brings attention to a pseudocyst or pancreatic ascites.

To prevent a pancreatic injury from being overlooked, serial amylase determinations should be obtained routinely in all patients with blunt abdominal injury.[12] Serum peritoneal and urinary levels of pancreatic amylase reflect the balance among the degree of ductal obstruction or disruption of the pancreas, the rate of production of amylase by the acinar cells, and the rate of clearance of amylase by the kidneys.[85] Serial serum amylase determinations are the most useful laboratory tests in establishing the diagnosis of serious pancreatic injury. The serum amylase level may be elevated as early as six hours after pancreatic injury.[12] Even in the presence of extensive pancreatic injury and total disruption of the ductal system, however, the amylase level may not become elevated for 24 to 48 hours following injury.[12] For this reason, repeated determinations of the amylase level should be obtained in all cases of blunt abdominal trauma. Conversely, in the absence of other indications for celiotomy, operation should not be initiated on the basis of a single elevated amylase determination.

At the time of peritoneal lavage, any fluid aspirated on entering the abdomen and the lavage return should be analyzed for amylase. Elevation of the amylase level of the peritoneal fluid may be an indication of pancreatic injury. Pancreatic ductal obstruction or disruption leads to interstitial edema, which if marked may result in a weeping of the pancreatic fluid through the intact capsule of the pancreas and into the peritoneal cavity. Similarly, if there is a ductal disruption with an outpouring of pancreatic enzymes into the peritoneal cavity, the amylase level of the peritoneal fluid will become elevated. The level of pancreatic enzymes in peritoneal fluid may be elevated, however, in the absence of pancreatic injury if a laceration of the stomach or duodenum permits discharge of intestinal contents into the peritoneal cavity. The one- or two-hour excretion of amylase may also prove useful in detecting pancreatic inflammation when serum levels are not elevated.[86] Greater than normal amounts of amylase may enter the blood but not elevate serum amylase levels as long as the renal clearance of amylase is not exceeded.

A contusion involving the parenchyma of the pancreas is not a serious injury if the ductal system is not disrupted.[87] A potentially lethal ductal disruption, however, may masquerade as an innocent-appearing hematoma. Such injuries may easily be overlooked at operation.[12] The steps to be followed by the emergency department physician in the management of the patient with suspected pancreatic injury are outlined in Table 21-10.

Table 21-10. Management of Pancreatic Injuries by the Emergency Department Physician

Look for diagnostic clues
  Epigastric and back pain
  Duodenal or splenic injuries, with which pancreatic injuries are often associated
  Ileus
  Serial determinations of serum amylase
  Peritoneal lavage—amylase level may be higher than in serum
  Urinary amylase—two hour
  Shock—usually not caused by pancreatic injury, but may be due to associated injuries
  Arteriography—usually not helpful in diagnosis

Resuscitate patient
  Type and cross-match blood
  Administer Ringer's lactate intravenously
  Measure central venous pressure
  Insert Foley catheter
  Administer broad-spectrum antibiotics

Look for indications to operate
  Positive lavage
  Elevation of serum amylase on progressive determinations
  Peritoneal signs

Be cognizant of late complications
  Overlooked injury
  Pseudocyst
  Fistula
  Pancreatic insufficiency following resection of 80 to 90% of pancreas

Complications of Unrecognized Pancreatic Injury. Complications following either undiagnosed or unrecognized disruption of the pancreatic ductal system include necrotizing pancreatitis frequently progressing to abscess formation, intraabdominal hemorrhage, pseudocyst formation, pancreatic ascites, prolonged ileus, and pancreatic fistulas. Pancreaticocutaneous fistula is a common complication of pancreatic ductal disruption that is unrecognized at celiotomy in which the upper part of the abdominal cavity has been drained. In Bach and Frey's experience with 44 patients with pancreatic injury, there were 19 patients in whom the pancreas was examined at operation and simple drainage instituted.[12] The seriousness of the injury was not appreciated in 12 of 19 patients as determined by subsequent complications. All 12 patients had major pancreatic injuries with transections of the pancreatic duct. One patient died before a second operation could be performed. Eleven of the 19 patients required reoperation, and three of them died.[12]

In order to avoid overlooking a major injury of the pancreatic ductal system at operation, several steps are recommended. All pancreatic hematomas should be explored or a pancreatogram obtained in order to ascertain if the ductal system is intact. A pancreatogram can be obtained either by cannulating the pancreatic duct through the ampulla of Vater or by taking it retrograde through the transected duct after excision of the tail of the pancreas. Pressure of the injection containing contrast material should not exceed 30 cm. H_2O because of the risk of initiating pancreatitis. Delay in surgical intervention and definitive repair of a pancreatic injury increases the technical difficulties at operation resulting from inflammation and reduces the chances for a successful result.

Treatment. For injuries of the neck, body, and tail of the pancreas (Fig. 21-12), we favor distal pancreatectomy, which can be performed quickly with minimal morbidity and mortality rates. Of 20 patients with pancreatic injury who were treated by distal pancreatectomy in the University of Michigan experience, 19 survived.[12] The only death occurred in a patient who had undergone operation previously, and in whom a massive pancreatic abscess was found at operation. One of the 19 surviving patients required tolbutamide; none needed insulin.

For injuries of the body and tail of the pancreas, some surgeons have advocated procedures involving anastomoses, usually of intestine with pancreas, which are more time-consuming and inherently dangerous than is distal resection. These procedures include end-to-end suture of the pancreas with primary repair of the pancreatic ductal system.[88] Letton and Wilson advocate Roux-en-Y jejunal drainage of the distal segment of the pancreas with closure of the proximal end.[89] Jones and

Shires recommend Roux-en-Y jejunal drainage of the proximal and distal ends of the divided pancreas.[90]

We do not advocate these measures because of the additional operative time required to fashion multiple anastomoses and the possibility of an anastomotic leak (25%) of small intestinal contents, which contain bacteria and pancreatic juice. Resection of as much as the distal 80% of the pancreas is seldom associated with exocrine and endocrine insufficiency. Preservation of the distal transected segment of pancreas, if representing less than 80% of the gland, therefore should not be given a high priority in the treatment of pancreatic injury.

Injuries to the head of the pancreas in which the major duct has been transected, which would require distal resection of more than 80% of the gland, and in which the duodenum and common bile duct are intact can be treated by Roux-en-Y pancreaticojejunostomy sewn over the site of injury.[91] Under these circumstances the risk of pancreatic insufficiency from a distal resection of more than 80% of the pancreas is high enough that the 25% risk of anastomotic leak from Roux-en-Y pancreaticojejunostomy is worth accepting.

Injuries to the head of the pancreas, especially when associated with injury to the duodenum and common bile duct, present a complex challenge to the surgeon (Fig. 21-11). Such injuries are reported to be associated with a mortality rate of 73%, but it has been reduced by pancreaticoduodenectomy. This procedure has been performed on five patients at the University of Michigan Medical Center and affiliated hospitals, and four have survived.[12] Pancreaticoduodenectomy should be performed when there is extensive damage or avulsion of the head of the pancreas associated with compromise of the blood supply to the duodenum or combined injuries involving the head of the pancreas, duodenum, and common bile duct. Operative treatment includes excision of the lacerated and contused duodenum, proximal pancreas, and distal common bile duct by pancreaticoduodenectomy and reestablishment of biliary, pancreatic, and gastrointestinal continuity by pancreaticojejunostomy, choledochojejunostomy, and gastrojejunostomy. A vagotomy should always be performed in association with pancreaticoduodenectomy to avoid the complication of postoperative stress ulcers and a symptomatic ulcer disease that has a high incidence following major pancreatic resection.

Penetrating injuries of the pancreas from stabbing or low velocity missiles can be treated by resection of the segment distal to the area of injury or by Penrose drainage if the ductal system is intact (as demonstrated by pancreatogram). We have encountered a number of patients with knife or low velocity missile wounds of the inferior vena cava posterior to the pancreas in which the missile pierced the superior mesenteric vein and overlying pancreas. In such instances, after closing the anterior and posterior caval wounds, the superior mesenteric vein is exposed by left-to-right distal pancreatectomy and splenectomy, permitting direct access and control of hemorrhage from the superior mesenteric vein.

Stomach and Small Intestine

The hollow viscera of the abdomen, *e.g.,* stomach, duodenum, jejunum, ileum, large intestine, and bladder, are more frequently injured as a result of penetrating than of blunt trauma.[21,23,49]

Infection is the most frequent life-threatening consequence of injury to the hollow viscera. Release of the intraabdominal contents of the stomach, duodenum, jejunum, and bladder, which are chemically irritating and often have high bacterial counts, into the peritoneal cavity causes an intensive inflammatory response. Within 12 hours a bacterial peritonitis becomes established.

Diagnosis. The diagnosis of a perforated hollow viscus following trauma can often be established on the basis of the history and physical examination. Signs of peritoneal irritation characterized by muscle guarding, tenderness, and rebound tenderness are usually present shortly after injury. Tympany over the liver is a pathopneumonic indication of free air secondary to a perforated viscus. On laboratory examination the white blood cell count is usually elevated. Flat plate and upright or lateral decubitus films may demonstrate air under the diaphragm. Having the patient sit up or on his side for five minutes increases the accuracy of the examination. A Levin tube should be passed into the stomach shortly after the patient's admission. The presence of blood in the Levin drainage fluid following penetrating or blunt trauma is considered an indication of gastric or duodenal perforation until proved otherwise at operation.

Once the diagnosis of a perforated viscus is suspected or established, the patient should be prepared for surgery. At operation, highest priority should be given to the prevention of further soilage of the peritoneal cavity from the perforated viscus or anastomotic repair. When the abdomen is entered, the extent of injury should be completely assessed if immediate efforts to control hemorrhage are not required. Both anterior and posterior surfaces of the stomach need to be examined by opening the lesser sac if there is an anterior entrance wound. In the presence of periduodenal edema, crepitus, bile, or hematuria following blunt trauma, a Kocher maneuver should be performed to examine the posterior surface of the duodenum.

The small intestine and its mesentery should be closely inspected for viability, perforation, contusion, or hematoma. All mesenteric hematomas should be explored and bleeding vessels ligated. As a result of blunt trauma, the intestine may be sheared at points of fixation, such as the ligament of Treitz. Patients wearing seat belts are subject to lacerations of the small intestine if the belt is worn incorrectly above the iliac crest.[92] The presence of skin ecchymoses along the belt line indicates the possibility of underlying intestinal injury and often an associated flexion compression fracture of the anterior portion of the lumbar spine.[93] The intestine may be divided by compression when the anterior abdominal wall is pushed posteriorly against the vertebral column by the seat belt as the body is jackknifed forward. Although the incorrectly worn seat belt may be a contributing factor in injuries to intraabdominal organs, particularly the uterus of the pregnant female, seat belts save lives by preventing ejection from the vehicle. Ejection is associated with a very high mortality rate.[94]

Treatment. If injury to the stomach or small intestine results from a stab wound or low velocity missile injury, simple closure of the intestinal wound after debridement of all necrotic tissue suffices. In wounds of the small intestine and stomach created by high velocity missiles, those associated with extensive injury to the intestinal mesentery, those creating large intestinal defects whose closure would compromise the lumen, those causing crushed, infarcted, or necrotic bowel, or those causing multiple intestinal wounds, the intestine should be resected and gastrointestinal continuity reestablished by end-to-end anastomosis. The risk of intraabdominal infection and anastomotic leakage can be reduced by the initiation of broad-spectrum antibiotic coverage with agents such as clindamycin and gentamicin preoperatively in the emergency department. In all intestinal injuries, peritoneal soilage is inevitable and every attempt should be made to reduce the degree of contamination by thoroughly irrigating the abdominal cavity with copious amounts of saline solution during and at the end of the procedure.

The steps to be observed by the emergency department physician in the management of the patient with suspected injuries of the stomach and small intestine are outlined in Table 21-11.

Retroduodenal Rupture from Blunt Trauma. A high fatality rate is associated with unrecognized retroperitoneal rupture of the duodenum. The diagnosis of duodenal injury following blunt trauma mandates special attention by emergency department physicians. The flat plate and upright films of the abdomen should be closely examined for extraluminal air bubbles giving a stippled appearance in the right upper quadrant, which is pathognomonic of retroperitoneal rupture of the intestine.[18,95–97] At celiotomy the presence of crepitus, bile, edema, or

Table 21-11. Management of Injuries to the Stomach, Duodenum, and Small Intestine by the Emergency Department Physician

---

Look for diagnostic clues
    Seat belt trauma—ecchymosis along line of seat belt
    Abdominal pain
    Signs of peritoneal irritation—guarding, tenderness, or rebound tenderness
    Tympany over liver—sign of free air
    Elevated white blood cell count
    Fever
    Free air on upright film of the abdomen—a stippled effect may be produced
        because of small air bubbles in retroperitoneal tissues associated with retro-
        duodenal rupture
    Bloody Levin aspirate
    Compression fracture of anterior aspect of lumbar spine in seat belt users
    Peritoneal lavage—intestinal contents in aspirate or high bacterial and white
        blood cell counts in lavage return (may be negative in retroduodenal injury)

Resuscitate patient
    Type and cross-match blood
    Administer Ringer's lactate intravenously
    Measure central venous pressure
    Insert Foley catheter
    Administer broad-spectrum antibiotics, e.g., clindamycin and gentamicin
    Institute tetanus prophylaxis

Look for indications to operate
    Peritonitis
    Free air
    Retroduodenal air
    Positive lavage

Be cognizant of late complications
    Adhesions

---

hematoma around the duodenum is an indication for the surgeon to perform a Kocher maneuver and examine the posterior surface of the duodenum.[18,95–97] Simple, fresh lacerations may be closed by suture. Hematomas dissecting along muscular planes of the intestine may obstruct its lumen.

Treatment consists of the evacuation of blood clots and gastrostomy.[98,99] Large or ragged lacerations of the duodenum may be closed by jejunal patch as first proposed by Kobold and Thal.[100] Combined injuries involving the common bile duct, the head of the pancreas, and the duodenum have been discussed under injuries to the pancreas.

Large Intestine

The high concentration of bacteria in the intraluminal contents of the large intestine makes bacterial peritonitis a certainty in injuries to the colon. During World War II most colonic injuries were treated by proximal colostomy when feasible. This mode of therapy was successful in the management of military casualties and influenced the method of treatment of colonic injuries in civilian life. Civilian colonic injuries, however, tend to be less severe than those encountered in military casualties, because the velocity of the wounding missile and the associated tissue necrosis are usually less.

Although intestinal closure and proximal colostomy is still the standard procedure for sigmoidal and rectal perforations, some surgeons are now experimenting with primary colonic repair without protective colostomy for stab and low velocity missile wounds of the cecum and ascending and transverse colon.[101,102] In each case of colonic injury in which deviation from the standard method of treatment is proposed, the surgeon should carefully consider and weigh the effects of the wounding missile, the time between injury and operation, the age of the patient, the site of colonic injury, the degree of peritoneal soilage, and the associated injuries that influence the incidence of complications and survival. Deviation from the standard method of treatment has been associated with a higher incidence of intraabdominal complications, according to Chilimindris and associates.[103]

Cecum and Right Colon–Hepatic Flexure. Stab and low velocity missile wounds may be treated by closure or tube cecostomy.

Shotgun or high velocity missile wounds are best treated initially by resection, temporary proximal ileostomy, and distal mucous colonic fistula. The risk of anastomotic leak under these latter conditions is sufficiently great in the unprepped intestine and in the presence of bacterial peritonitis to make primary reanastomosis indefensible.

Transverse Colon and Splenic Flexure. Stab and low velocity missile wounds may be treated by primary closure, resection, and primary anastomosis. Wounds from high velocity missiles are best treated by resection or exteriorization. When resection is performed, most surgeons believe that a temporary proximal colostomy and distal mucous fistula are safer than reanastomosis.

Left Colon and Sigmoid. Stab and low velocity missile wounds are treated by closure and proximal colostomy. Shotgun and other high velocity missile wounds are best treated by resection, end colostomy, and mucous fistula. Reanastomosis is staged later in a second operative procedure. Four weeks later the colostomy may be closed in a third procedure.

Rectal Wounds. All rectal wounds should be closed either through the rectum or intraabdominally by freeing the intestine sufficiently below the peritoneal reflection to visualize the injury. The remainder of the rectum should be thoroughly examined digitally or by sigmoidoscopy above

13

Table 21-12.   Management of Injuries to the Large Intestine by the Emergency Department Physician

Look for diagnostic clues
  Abdominal pain
  Peritoneal signs
  Tympany over the liver—sign of free air
  Elevated white blood cell count
  Fever
  Rectosigmoid perforation on sigmoidoscopy
  Free air on upright films of the abdomen
  Peritoneal lavage—intestinal contents in aspirate or elevated white blood cell
    and bacterial counts in lavage return

Resuscitate patient
  Type and cross-match blood
  Administer Ringer's lactate intravenously
  Measure central venous pressure
  Insert Foley catheter
  Administer broad-spectrum antibiotics, *e.g.,* clindamycin and gentamicin
  Institute tetanus prophylaxis

Look for indications to operate
  Peritonitis
  Free air
  Positive lavage

Be cognizant of late complications
  Adhesions

and below the site of perforation to insure against a second overlooked entrance or exit wound.

After closure of the perforation, the retroperitoneal space should be drained externally. A completely diverting colostomy in the proximal transverse colon should then be performed, and it is imperative that the distal colon be irrigated free of feces. If the wound is below the peritoneal reflection and defies closure because of its size, external drainage of the retroperitoneal space is essential.[104] The steps to be taken by the emergency department physician in the management of the patient with suspected injury of the large intestine are outlined in Table 21-12.

Major Vessels

Hemorrhage from major vessels, including the aorta, inferior vena cava, and portal vein, can be brisk, and many patients with such injuries exsanguinate before reaching the hospital.

The pant G-suit[30] and intraaortic balloon tamponade[105] reduce intraabdominal blood loss from lacerations of major vessels. The pant G-suit covers the lower extremities and abdomen. The pressure suit, when inflated, increases the intraabdominal pressure, thereby decreasing intra-vascular and extravascular pressure difference. Blood loss, even from the aorta, is markedly reduced. Inclusion of the lower extremities in the pant suit also reduces the extent of venous pooling and in effect provides an autologous infusion.

Percutaneous transfemoral retrograde passage and inflation of the balloon catheter to the level of the diaphragm is another means of re-ducing blood loss from the abdominal aorta. Intraaortic balloon tam-ponade has reduced blood loss from the abdominal aorta in the dog and pig. Spinal cord injuries, however, are frequent when the balloon is ex-panded for more than 15 minutes. The danger is particularly marked if the animal has been hypotensive prior to expansion of the balloon.

If the patient with a major vessel laceration survives until he arrives at the hospital, the presence of shock and a distended abdomen will alert the emergency department physician to the possibility of hemor-rhage resulting from a major vessel injury. Prompt resuscitation and operation are required for survival and must be carried out concomi-tantly. At operation, control of the bleeding vessel should be obtained proximal and distal to the site of hemorrhage. Sometimes, the aorta or inferior vena cava may be completely transected and the nature of the injury obscured by a retroperitoneal hematoma. Exploration of hema-tomas without first gaining proximal and distal control of major vessels feeding the hematoma could lead to uncontrolled hemorrhage and death.

Uterus

The uterus in its nonpregnant state is well protected deep within the pelvic bony structure. During the last three months of pregnancy, how-ever, the uterus rises out of the pelvis and becomes an abdominal or-gan. When the uterus is located high in the abdomen, it is susceptible to injury, particularly by the seat belt. Severe injuries may result in loss of the fetus, uterine rupture, and massive hemorrhage. Hysterectomy is usually required in order to salvage the mother's life. Although the seat belt may cause injury to the fetus and to the uterus in the pregnant female, it may nevertheless be life-saving if it prevents a more serious injury, which is the likely result of ejection from the car.

Retroperitoneal Hematomas

The diagnosis of retroperitoneal hematoma in blunt trauma often appearing as hypovolemic shock from blood loss is in part one of exclusion. The diagnosis is considered after ruling out hemorrhage into the chest and abdomen. Hemorrhage into the abdomen may be hard to exclude, because in retroperitoneal hemorrhage, peritoneal lavage may or may not be positive, depending on whether the retroperitoneum remains intact. Arteriography may be helpful in ruling out major vessel injuries.

Penetrating wounds of the abdomen, flank, and back that may have transversed the retroperitoneum should be explored because of the danger of major vessel injury with exsanguinating hemorrhage. Late complications of overlooked injuries to major vessels include false aneurysms and arteriovenous fistulas.

Large amounts of blood (as much as 2 liters) may be confined in the retroperitoneal space of the 70-kg. adult without the appearance of overt localizing signs. In fact, according to McCarroll and co-workers, the most frequent unrecognized cause of death in pedestrians involved in motor vehicular accidents was exsanguination secondary to unrecognized retroperitoneal hemorrhage.[106] Signs and symptoms of retroperitoneal hematomas, such as back pain, ileus, or costovertebral angle tenderness, are nonspecific. Flank hematomas, when present, are diagnostic of retroperitoneal hematomas.

Flat plate and upright films of the abdomen in a patient with otherwise unexplained blood loss may show obliteration of the psoas shadow or fractures of the pelvis, transverse processes, and lumbar spine, all of which are diagnostic of retroperitoneal hematoma.

Recognition of the presence of a retroperitoneal hematoma in a patient subjected to blunt trauma is only the first step in his management. The nature and seriousness of the underlying injury creating the hematoma must then be assessed. In general, the higher and more central the retroperitoneal hematoma is situated in the abdomen, the more probable the need for operative intervention, exploration, and evacuation of the hematoma. All central hematomas in the upper abdomen should be explored because of the possibility of disruption of the aorta, inferior vena cava, superior mesenteric artery and vein, pancreatic ductal system, or duodenum. The possibility of rupture of the thoracic aorta superior to the diaphragm with dissection inferiorly into the abdomen should also be considered in the differential diagnosis of high, centrally located hematomas. Those located laterally in the upper abdomen are often associated with renal injury.

Not all hematomas overlying the kidney need be explored at operation. Exploration of hematomas that are nonpulsatile and not expanding in patients with normal pyelograms is meddlesome. Expanding or pulsatile hematomas should be explored, but only after first gaining proximal control of the vessels in the renal pedicle at the aorta and cava.[107]

Hematomas involving either the duodenum or the pancreas must be explored. Hematomas at the root of the mesentery may be an indication of injury to the superior mesenteric artery and vein and require exploration after gaining control of the aorta.

Pelvic hematomas are usually associated with pelvic fractures. In the presence of a negative lavage and the absence of evidence of continued hemorrhage, celiotomy is not necessary. In the presence of pelvic fractures, and signs of continued hemorrhage, the use of autologous clot treated with epsilon aminocaproic acid and injected into the bleeding artery demonstrated by arteriography provides an effective means of terminating hemorrhage.[108] If hemorrhage from a source in the pelvis unidentified by arteriography continues, operation will have to be undertaken. In the absence of evidence of expansion or pulsation, pelvic hematomas seen at operation should not be explored or evacuated. Expanding or pulsating hematomas must be explored. The iliac vessels should be exposed, and if no source of hemorrhage can be identified and hemorrhage continues, iliac artery ligation on the affected side or even bilaterally may have to be performed.[109] Because of numerous collateral vessels in the area, this is usually unsuccessful in terminating hemorrhage.

Under these desperate circumstances, alternatives may have to be considered. It may be necessary to divide the symphysis to obtain

Table 21-13. Management of Retroperitoneal Hematoma by the Emergency Department Physician

---

Look for diagnostic clues
  Shock—may be present depending on amount of blood loss
  Back pain
  Ileus
  Abdominal distention
    Costovertebral angle tenderness
    Flank hematomas
    Obliteration of psoas shadow—fracture of the pelvis, transverse process, and lumbar spine

Once the presence of a retroperitoneal hematoma is suspected, efforts should be directed at establishing the source of hemorrhage *e.g.,* kidney or major vessel

Resuscitate the patient
  Type and cross-match blood
  Administer Ringer's lactate intravenously
  Measure central venous pressure
  Insert Foley catheter
  Administer broad-spectrum antibiotics

Look for indications to operate
  Indications pointing to a specific organ, *e.g.,* kidney
  Continuing hemorrhage that is unresponsive to Ringer's lactate and whole blood replacement

---

better visualization of the pelvic vessels, or to pack the pelvis, close the abdomen, and then use arteriography to inject autologous clot if a source of bleeding can be identified. The steps to be observed by the emergency department physician in the management of the patient with suspected retroperitoneal hematoma are outlined in Table 21-13.

Prognosis for Injuries to Retroperitoneal and Intra-abdominal Organs

The prognosis for any injured patient is in part determined by the nature of the injury, the patient's constitution prior to injury, and the degree of planning for his care that the community has provided. The chance for survival of an injured patient, therefore, depends on the organ injured, the degree of injury to the organ, the number of associated injuries to other body areas, the age of the patient, the presence of preexisting disease, and the resuscitative measures undertaken at the scene of the accident and in transit to the hospital. The resuscitative efforts depend on advanced community planning to develop a complete emergency health service system, including provision for emergency medical technicians and well equipped vehicles with central dispatch and equipment for communication between the vehicle and the physician in the emergency department. An emergency medical service plan further insures that the acutely ill and injured patient is delivered to a hospital that has physician coverage in the emergency department night and day, as well as hospital back-up staff and facilities (such as x-ray technicians, operating crews, and surgical specialists), and a blood bank capable of providing 40 to 50 units of blood for the patient with multiple injuries.

References

1. DiVincenti, F. C., et al. 1968. Blunt abdominal trauma. *J. Trauma,* 8:1004–1013.
2. Hopson, W. B., Sherman, R. T., and Sanders, J. W. 1966. Stab wounds of the abdomen. *Amer. Surg.,* 32:213–218.
3. Perry, J. F., Jr. 1970. Blunt and penetrating abdominal injuries. *Curr. Probl. Surg.,* May Issue.
4. Stein, A., and Lissoos, I. 1968. Selective management of penetrating wounds of the abdomen. *J. Trauma,* 8:1014–1025.
5. Kazarian, K. K., et al. 1971. Stab wounds of the abdomen: an analysis of 500 patients. *Arch. Surg.,* 102:465–468.
6. Moss, L. K., Schmidt, F. E., and Creech, O. 1962. Analysis of 550 stab wounds of the abdomen. *Amer. Surg.,* 28:483–485.
7. Wilson, C. B., Vidrine, A., and Rives, J. D. 1965. Unrecognized abdominal trauma in patients with head injuries. *Ann. Surg.,* 161:608–613.
8. Goligher, E. 1962. Road accidents. Series Chirurgia #5, Documenta. Heidelberg, *Geirgy University Surgical Clinic.*

9. Frey, C. F., Huelke, D. F., and Gikas, P. W. 1969. Resuscitation and survival in motor vehicle accidents. *J. Trauma*, 9:292–310.
10. Waller, J. A. 1967. Drinking drivers and driving drinkers: the need for multiple approaches to accidents involving alcohol. Proceedings of Symposium on Prevention of the Highway Injury. Highway Safety Research Institute. Ann Arbor, University of Michigan, pp. 30–37.
11. Morehouse, D. D., and McKinnon, K. J. 1969. Urological injuries associated with pelvic fractures. *J. Trauma*, 9:479–496.
12. Bach, R. D., and Frey, C. F. 1971. The diagnosis and treatment of pancreatic trauma. *Amer. J. Surg.*, 121:20–29.
13. Drapanas, T., and McDonald, J. 1961. Peritoneal tap in abdominal surgery. *Surgery*, 50:742–746.
14. Yurko, A. A., and Williams, R. D. 1966. Needle paracentesis in blunt abdominal trauma. A critical analysis. *J. Trauma*, 6:194–200.
15. Orloff, M. J. 1966. *Abdominal Injuries—Early Management of Acute Trauma*, A. M. Nahum (ed.). St. Louis, C. V. Mosby Co.
16. Root, H. D., et al. 1965. Diagnostic peritoneal lavage. *Surgery*, 57:633–637.
17. Veith, F. J., et al. 1967. Diagnostic peritoneal lavage in acute abdominal disease. *Ann. Surg.*, 166:290–295.
18. Cocke, W. M., Jr., and Meyer, K. K. 1964. Retroperitoneal duodenal rupture. *Amer. J. Surg.*, 108:834–839.
19. Frey, C. F., et al. 1967. Use of arteriography in the diagnosis of acute gastrointestinal and traumatic intra-abdominal hemorrhage. *Amer. J. Surg.*, 113:137–148.
20. Lium, R. C., Jr., Gleilman, M. G., and Hunt, T. K. 1972. Angiography in patients with blunt trauma to the chest and abdomen. *Surg. Clin. N. Amer.*, 52:551–565.
21. Waller, J. A. 1969. Emergency health services in area of low population density. *JAMA*, 207:2255–2258.
22. Waters, J. M., Jr., and Wells, C. H. 1973. The effects of a modern emergency medical care system in reducing automobile crash deaths. *J. Trauma*, 13:645–647.
23. Kaplan, B. C., et al. 1973. The military anti-shock trouser in civilian prehospital emergency care. *J. Trauma*, 13:843–849.
24. Von Wagoner, F. H. 1961. A 3 year study of deaths following trauma. *J. Trauma*, 1:401–408.
25. Gertner, H. R., Jr., et al. 1972. Evaluation of the management of vehicular fatalities secondary to abdominal injury. *J. Trauma*, 12:425–431.
26. Nance, C., et al. 1974. Surgical judgment in the management of penetrating wounds of the abdomen. Experience with 2212 patients. *Ann. Surg.*, 179:639–647.
27. Steichen, F. M. 1967. Penetrating wounds of the chest and the abdomen. *Curr. Probl. Surg.*, August issue.
28. DeMuth, W. E., Jr. 1971. The mechanism of shotgun wounds. *J. Trauma*, 11:219–229.
29. Martin, J. B. 1971. The management of shotgun wounds. *J. Trauma*, 11:522–527.
30. Shafton, G. W. 1966. Selective conservatism in penetrating abdominal trauma. *Surgery*, 59:650–653.
31. McClelland, R. N., et al. 1966. Trauma to the abdomen, in *Care of the Trauma Patient*, G. Shires (ed.). New York, McGraw-Hill, p. 360.
32. Cornell, W. P., et al. 1967. A new non-operative technique for the diagnosis of penetrating injuries to the abdomen. *J. Trauma*, 7:307–314.
33. Olsen, W. R., and Hildreth, D. H. 1971. Abdominal paracentesis and peritoneal lavage in blunt abdominal trauma. *J. Trauma*, 11:824–829.
34. Griswold, R. A., and Collier, H. S. 1961. Blunt abdominal trauma. *Surg. Gynec. Obstet.*, 112:309–329.

35. Welch, C. E., and Giddings, W. P. 1950. Abdominal trauma. *Amer. J. Surg.,* 79:252–258.
36. Pridgen, J. E., et al. 1967. Penetrating wounds of the abdomen. *Ann. Surg.,* 165:901–907.
37. Willox, G. L. 1965. Non-penetrating injuries of abdomen causing rupture of the spleen. Report of 100 cases. *Arch. Surg.,* 90:498–502.
38. Byrne, R. V. 1950. Splenectomy for traumatic rupture with intra-abdominal hemorrhage. Report of 101 cases. *Arch. Surg.,* 61:273–285.
39. Terry, J. H., Self, M. M., and Howard, J. M. 1956. Injuries of the spleen. *Surgery,* 40:615–639.
40. Cloutier, L. C., and Zaepfel, F. M. 1958. Traumatic rupture of the spleen. *Surg. Gynec. Obstet.,* 107:749–752.
41. Shirkey, A. L., et al. 1964. Surgical management of splenic injuries. *Amer. J. Surg.,* 108:630–635.
42. Sizer, J. S., Wayne, E. R., and Frederick, P. L. 1966. Delayed rupture of the spleen. *Arch. Surg.,* 92:362–366.
43. Daoud, F. S., Fischer, D. C., and Hefner, C. D. 1966. Complications following a splenectomy with special emphasis on drainage. *Arch. Surg.,* 92:32–34.
44. Balasegaram, M. 1969. Blunt injuries to the liver. *Ann. Surg.,* 169:544–550.
45. Crosthwaith, R. W., et al. 1962. The surgical management of 640 consecutive liver injuries in civilian practice. *Surg. Gynec. Obstet.,* 114:650–654.
46. Atik, M., et al. 1966. Hepatectomy for severe liver injury. *Arch. Surg.,* 92:636–642.
47. McClelland, R. N., and Shires, T. 1965. Management of liver trauma in 259 consecutive patients. *Ann. Surg.,* 161:248–257.
48. Longmire, W. P., Jr. 1965. Hepatic surgery. Trauma, tumors, and cysts. *Ann. Surg.,* 161:1–14.
49. Schrock, T., Blaisdell, W., and Mathewson, C. 1968. Management of blunt trauma to the liver and hepatic veins. *Arch. Surg.,* 96:698–704.
50. Kindling, P. H., Wilson, R. F., and Walt, A. J. 1969. Hepatic trauma with particular reference to blunt injury. *J. Trauma,* 9:17–26.
51. Shafton, G. W., Gleidman, M. L., and Coppelletti, R. R. 1963. Injuries to the liver: a review of 111 cases. *J. Trauma,* 3:63–75.
52. Baker, R. J., Taxman, P., and Freeark, R. J. 1966. An assessment of management of non-penetrating liver injuries. *Arch. Surg.,* 84–91.
53. Trollope, M. L., et al. 1973. The mechanism of injury in blunt abdominal trauma. *J. Trauma,* 13:962–970.
54. Frey, C. F., et al. 1973. A fifteen-year experience with automotive hepatic trauma. *J. Trauma,* 13:1039–1049.
55. Castren, P. 1946. Uber Subkutane Leberrisse Und das Hepatorenale Syndron. *Acta Chir. Scand.,* Supp. 105.
56. Mills, R. H. B. 1961. The problem of closed liver injuries. *Gut,* 2:267–276.
57. Hanna, W. A., Bell, D. M., and Cochran, W. 1965. Liver injuries in Northern Ireland. *Brit. J. Surg.,* 52:99–106.
58. Hellstrom, G. 1966. Lesions associated with closed liver injury: a clinical study of 192 fatal cases. *Acta Chir. Scand.,* 131:460–475.
59. Frey, C. F. 1966. A method of liver hemostasis. *Surg. Gynec. Obstet.,* 123:1322–1325.
60. Quattlebaum, J. K., and Quattlebaum, J. K., Jr. 1959. Technique of hepatic lobectomy. *Ann. Surg.,* 149:648–651.
61. Madding, G. F., and Kennedy, P. A. 1972. Hepatic artery ligation. *Surg. Clin. N. Amer.,* 52:719–728.
62. Mays, E. T. 1972. Lobar dearterialization for exsanguinating wounds of the liver. *J. Trauma,* 12:397–407.
63. Brittain, R. S., et al. 1964. Accidental hepatic artery ligation in human. *Amer. J. Surg.,* 107: 822–832.

64. Albo, D., et al. 1969. Massive liver trauma involving the suprarenal vena cava. *Amer. J. Surg.,* 118:960–963.
65. Bricker, D. L., et al. 1971. Surgical management of injuries to the vena cava: changing patterns of injury and newer techniques of repair. *J. Trauma,* 11:725–731.
66. Brown, R. S., et al. 1971. Temporary internal vascular shunt for retro-hepatic vena cava injury. *J. Trauma,* 11:736–737.
67. Shrock, T., Blaisdell, F. W., and Mathewson, C. 1968. Management of blunt trauma to the liver and hepatic veins. *Arch. Surg.,* 96:698–704.
68. Yellin, A. E., Chaffee, C. B., and Donovan, A. J. 1971. Vascular isolation in treatment of juxta hepatic venous injuries. *Arch. Surg.,* 102:566–573.
69. Merendino, K. A., Dillard, D. A., and Cammock, E. E. 1963. The concept of surgical biliary decompression in the management of liver trauma. *Surg. Gynec. Obstet.,* 117:285–293.
70. Lucas, C. E., and Walt, A. J. 1970. Critical decisions in liver trauma. *Arch. Surg.,* 101:277–283.
71. Dow, R., and Thompson, N. 1968. Bile stasis after hepatic resection. *Surg. Gynec. Obstet.,* 127:1075–1078.
72. Child, C. G., III. 1964. *Liver and Portal Hypertension.* Philadelphia W. B. Saunders Co., p. 23.
73. Waterhouse, K., and Grass, M. 1969. Trauma to the genitourinary tract: a 5-year experience with 251 cases. *J. Urol.,* 101:241–246.
74. Tynberg, P. L. H., et al. 1973. The management of renal injuries coincident with penetrating wounds of the abdomen. *J. Trauma,* 13:502–508.
75. Lucey, D. T., Smith, M. J. V., and Koontz, W. W., Jr. 1972. Modern trends in the management of urologic trauma. *J. Urol.,* 107:641–646.
76. Morse, T. S., and Harris, B. H. 1973. Non-penetrating renal vascular injuries. *J. Trauma,* 13:497–501.
77. Banowsky, L. H., Wofel, D. A., and Lackner, L. H. 1970. Consideration in diagnosis and management of renal trauma. *J. Trauma,* 10:587–597.
78. Zimmerman, S. J., and Radding, R. S. 1961. Hypertension due to trauma of the kidney. *New Eng. J. Med.,* 264:238–240.
79. Reuter, S. Personal communication.
80. Brosman, H. S., and Fay, R. 1973. Diagnosis and management of bladder trauma. *J. Trauma,* 13:687–694.
81. Reynolds, B. M., Balsano, N. A., and Reynolds, F. X. 1973. Pelvic fractures. *J. Trauma,* 13:1011–1014.
82. Sturim, H. S. 1966. The surgical management of pancreatic injuries. *Surg. Gynec. Obstet.,* 122:133–140.
83. Wilson, R. F., et al. 1967. Pancreatic trauma. *J. Trauma,* 7:643–651.
84. Northrup, W. R., III., and Simmons, R. L. 1972. Pancreatic trauma: a review. *Surgery,* 71:27–43.
85. Thistlethwaite, J. R., and Hill, R. P. 1952. Serum amylase levels in experimental pancreatitis. *Surgery,* 31:495–501.
86. Gambill, E. E., and Mason, H. L. 1963. One hour value for urinary amylase in 96 patients with pancreatitis. *JAMA,* 186:24–28.
87. Kerry, R. L., and Glas, W. W. 1962. Traumatic injuries of the pancreas and duodenum. *Arch. Surg.,* 85:813–816.
88. Pellegrine, J. N., and Stein, I. J. 1961. Complete severance of the pancreas and its treatment with repair of the main pancreatic duct of Wirsung. *Amer. J. Surg.,* 101:707–710.
89. Letton, A. H., and Wilson, J. P. 1959. Traumatic severance of pancreas treated by Roux-Y anastomosis. *Surg. Gynec. Obstet.,* 109:473–478.
90. Jones, R. C., and Shires, G. T. 1965. The management of pancreatic injuries. *Arch. Surg.,* 90:502–508.
91. Freeark, R. J., et al. 1965. Traumatic disruption of the head of the pancreas. *Arch. Surg.,* 91:5–13.

92. Schneider, R. C., et al. 1968. Lap seat belt injuries: the treatment of the fortunate survivor. *Michigan Med.,* 67:171–186.
93. Steckler, R. M., Epstein, J. A., and Epstein, B. S. 1969. Seat belt trauma to the lumbar spine: an unusual manifestation of the seat belt syndrome. *J. Trauma,* 9:508–513.
94. Tourin, B., and Garrett, J. W. 1960. *Safety Belt Effectiveness in Rural California Automobile Accidents: A Comparison of Injuries to Users and Non-Users of Safety Belts.* New York, Cornell University.
95. Roman, E., Silva, Y. L., and Lucas C. 1971. Management of blunt duodenal injury. *Surg. Gynec. Obstet.,* 132:7–14.
96. Cleveland, H. C., and Waddell, W. R. 1963. Retroperitoneal rupture of the duodenum due to non-penetrating trauma. *Surg. Clin. N. Amer.,* 43:413–431.
97. Donovan, A. J., and Hagen, W. E. 1966. Traumatic perforation of duodenum. *Amer. J. Surg.,* 111:341–350.
98. Bailey, W. C., and Akers, D. R. 1965. Traumatic intramural hematoma of the duodenum in children. *Amer. J. Surg.,* 110:695–703.
99. Moore, S. W., and Erlandson, M. E. 1963. Intramural hematoma of the duodenum. *Ann. Surg.,* 157:798–809.
100. Kobold, E. E., and Thal, A. P. 1963. A simple method for the management of experimental wounds of the duodenum. *Surg. Gynec. Obstet.,* 116:340–344.
101. Roof, W. R., Morris, G. C., Jr., and DeBakey, M. E. 1960. Management of perforating injuries to the colon in civilian practice. *Amer. J. Surg.,* 99:641–645.
102. Wolma, F. J., and Williford, F., III. 1965. Treatment of injuries to the colon. *Amer. J. Surg.,* 110:772–775.
103. Chilimindris, C., et al. 1971. A critical review of management of right colon injuries. *J. Trauma,* 11:651–660.
104. Trunkey, D., Hays, R. J., and Shires, T. G. 1973. Management of rectal trauma. *J. Trauma,* 13:411–415.
105. Berkoff, H., Carpenter, E. W., and Frey, C. F. 1971. Evaluation of balloon tamponade of the abdominal aorta. An adjunct to the treatment of hemorrhagic shock. *J. Surg. Res.,* 11:496–500.
106. McCarroll, J. R., et al. 1962. Fatal pedestrian automotive accidents. *JAMA,* 180:127–133.
107. Orloff, M. J., and Charters, A. C. 1972. Injuries of the small bowel and mesentery and retroperitoneal hematoma. *Surg. Clin. N. Amer.,* 52:729–734.
108. Starzl, T. E., et al. 1963. Penetrating injuries of the inferior vena cava. *Surg. Clin. N. Amer.,* 43:387–400.
109. Ravdin, I. S., and Ellison, E. H. 1964. Hypogastric artery ligation in acute pelvic trauma. *Surgery,* 56:601–602.

22

Obstetric and Gynecologic Emergencies

Bruce A. Work, Jr.

When female patients are seen in the emergency department initial decisions must be made regarding the orientation of their problems. As with all other areas of concern, the question of urgency of the patient's condition and its priority for investigation must be answered. This chapter deals only with problems of an emergency nature that focus on the female generative tract. It is also appreciated that patients are not seen as diagnoses, but rather as a series of problems. Discussing the subject from this viewpoint would lead to considerable redundancy, however, for this reason the orientation will be to the etiologic entities.

Female patients appear in the emergency department with symptoms that are referable to the generative tract. These include pain, fever, vaginal discharge, vaginal bleeding or other menstrual irregularities, peritoneal signs, and the presence of masses on examination. In addition to presenting symptoms, the patient's history must be sought with particular emphasis on her menstrual cycle. This should include the frequency of her periods, the average duration, the estimated amount of flow, and the occurrence of dysmenorrhea.

No attempt will be made to be all-inclusive in discussing these entities, but rather consideration will be given to the conditions that are true emergencies and the appropriate actions that should be taken in the emergency department.

Imminent Delivery

One of the most obvious and yet most threatening situations for emergency department personnel is imminent delivery. The physiologic termination of the second stage of labor should not be cause for panic and referred care. It is inappropriate to try to deter imminent delivery; past efforts to do so have produced extremely unsatisfactory results. The patient who appears in the delivery room at the termination of her second stage of labor, ready to deliver her infant, must be allowed to do so. The emergency physician's task is twofold. The first objective is to provide for a controlled delivery, which benefits both mother and infant by preventing lacerations and a traumatic birth. The second task is to provide for appropriate maintenance of the baby with particular attention to its airway.

The first task, controlled delivery, requires only a determined effort to control the egress of the fetal head from the birth canal. This can be done with bare hands, sterile gloves, or a sterile towel. Consideration of episiotomy in such circumstances generally depends on the availability of appropriate instruments. The delivery is better performed in the emergency department than in an elevator enroute to the delivery room.

The second consideration that must be remembered is the infant's airway. The most important needs of the immediate newborn are airway maintenance and oxygenation as reflected by the heart rate. The immediate attention to the infant's airway requires suction of the oral pharynx with a soft rubber syringe, such as an otic syringe. Oropharyngeal suction, which is available in emergency departments, can be used in lieu of rubber bulb suction.

The adequacy of oxygenation is indicated by the heart rate, which should be between 100 and 160 beats per minute. An excessively fast rate may indicate moderate asphyxia, and bradycardia is indicative of severe asphyxia. The heart rate is more accurately assessed by use of a stethoscope than by palpation. The heart rate is perhaps the most significant parameter to be evaluated.

Table 22-1. The Apgar Scoring Method

Sign	0	1	2
Heart rate	Absent	< 100	> 100
Respiratory effort	Absent	$<$ Low	Good
Muscle tone	Limp	Some flexion	Active
Response to stimulation of nose and mouth	None	Grimace	Cough or sneeze
Color	Blue or pale	Body pink; extremities blue	Completely pink

Each sign is scored and totaled at both 1 and 5 minutes of life.

Apgar included these signs in the scoring method she devised in 1953 for evaluating the newborn (Table 22-1). Five signs—heart rate, respiratory effort, muscle tone, reflex irritability, and color—are assessed at one and five minutes of life. The one-minute Apgar score correlates primarily with immediate delivery trauma. The five-minute Apgar score appears to have correlative significance with neurologic status at 1 year of age.

Sophisticated resuscitative efforts should probably not be undertaken in the emergency department, but rather deferred until later. Cleaning of the infant's airway and possibly intubation of the trachea should be considered. The importance of maintaining the airway and ensuring adequate oxygenation until additional help can be obtained cannot be overstressed.

Prolapsed Umbilical Cord

Perhaps the next most significant obstetric problem to be considered in the emergency department is the prolapsed umbilical cord. Several factors dictate the speed of response of emergency department personnel. If the fetus is alive and mature and the cord is prolapsed, immediate cesarean section is the treatment of choice. In this instance the patient is transported directly to the operating room without delay. If the mother comes from home with a prolapsed cord, ruptured membranes, and subsequent fetal demise, the response of the emergency personnel is less urgent. In the event of fetal demise or extreme prematurity, referral to the obstetric department for vaginal delivery is in order.

Presentation of the umbilical cord with intact membranes permits obstetric consultation prior to emergency intervention.

Premature Rupture of Membranes

Premature rupture of membranes can be defined as rupture of the amniotic sac prior to labor or before 34 weeks of gestation. The approach to the patient with premature rupture of membranes depends entirely on the duration of the pregnancy and the subsequent fetal maturity. The initial consideration of the emergency department physician is documentation of the rupture.

Near term, the amniotic fluid is alkaline, contains approximately 2 mg. of creatinine per 100 ml., and has a fernlike appearance on gross and microscopic examination. When the membranes rupture, the amniotic fluid contains sebaceous material that stains orange with 1% Nile blue sulfate; this is definitive proof of rupture of the membranes. Visualization of copious amounts of amniotic fluid from the cervical os certainly is a significant factor.

Management of the patient with premature rupture of membranes depends on the gestational age of the fetus. If the patient is at term, not in labor, and has only progressive leakage from the ruptured membranes, she can be admitted for induction of labor. This patient is often sent home for observation by her private physician. Why wait, however, for a major complication? The risk of fetal and maternal infection is not clear at this time.

The patient who has both a premature termination of the pregnancy and premature rupture of membranes, but is not in labor, is the ideal candidate for sepsis. In this situation, the emergency department physician should consider the only safe course of action, which is to admit the patient for observation and consultation to consider termination of the pregnancy. The question of discharge of the patient for observation at home is a particularly difficult one. The data regarding appropriate management of such patients are incomplete. The patient's socioeconomic status and reliability must be taken into account. Decisions regarding discharge for home care versus hospitalization require individual consideration. If there is any question, hospitalization is the conservative approach.

Premature Labor

Premature labor is a different and difficult situation. It is defined as labor prior to 34 weeks of gestation. This has been considered the pivotal time in gestation because many infants born between 34 weeks of gestation and term range from 1,800 to more than 2,000 grams at birth. These babies can often tolerate extrauterine life satisfactorily.

The distinction between premature labor and false labor must be made when such a patient appears in the emergency facility. Objective evidence of change in the cervix and station of the presenting part represents progression of labor rather than false labor. Ambulating the patient for an hour or two may enable one to differentiate between these two conditions.

The patient in progressive labor prior to 34 weeks should be admitted to the delivery unit for further consideration. This condition should be carefully differentiated from incompetent cervix, the treatment of which is entirely different from that of premature labor.

The etiology of premature labor should be seriously considered before a therapeutic program is undertaken. Classic symptoms of various diseases are well known, including those of abruptio placentae, a condition that is encountered all too often. The difficulty is encountered in patients in whom the classic symptoms of abruption and painful hemorrhaging of dark red blood in the third trimester are not seen. Premature labor is the diagnosis when no other symptoms are apparent.

The extent of abruption cannot be controlled with therapy. The effect on the fetus depends on the pathologic process. Treatment then is realized, in effect, by the mother and secondarily the fetus. The etiology of premature labor must be considered because the therapy can have major effects on the mother's circulatory status. In contrast to patients in early idiopathic premature labor, in whom termination of the labor is contemplated, stimulation of labor should be considered in patients with abruption to terminate the pregnancy rapidly and thereby decrease the risk of complications.

Serious abruption of the placenta, which is characterized by progressive abdominal pain, dark red vaginal bleeding, shock, disseminated intravascular coagulation, and fetal demise, must be considered a true obstetric emergency. These patients should be admitted to the obstetric department promptly. It is advantageous to have blood samples drawn for studies of the hematocrit, fibrinogen, fibrin split products, thrombin clotting time, and any other studies that might be warranted, such as the platelet count.

Incompetent Cervix

The diagnosis of incompetent cervix is based on progressive examinations of the patient. If a patient is examined for a reason other than labor, speculum examination of the cervix may reveal it to be painlessly but progressively dilating more than 2 or 3 cm. When the history is taken, this patient may mention a similar progressive but painless cervical dilatation during a previous pregnancy, with delivery of an immature infant in the second trimester of pregnancy that did not survive. If the occurrence is repeated, the diagnosis is incompetent cervix, which warrants immediate surgical therapy, with uterine cervix circlage being the procedure of choice. This procedure should be performed after premature rupture of membranes, abruptio placentae, and other causes of the premature dilatation have been ruled out. Such a patient obviously requires immediate hospitalization.

Sepsis

The most common and serious septic process affecting the nonlaboring pregnant patient is pyelonephritis. Pregnancy creates the ideal situation for the development of pyelonephritis, with mechanical and hormonal stasis of urinary outflow from the kidney and frequently with the substrate of bacteriuria. Under these conditions, patients in the second trimester of pregnancy commonly develop a classic triad of fever, costovertebral angle pain, and bacteriuria. The diagnosis is not difficult, but consideration of the therapy is important.

Pyelonephritis occurring during pregnancy should not be treated on an out-patient basis. A patient with pyelonephritis must be hospitalized because prompt and vigorous treatment is required.

Therapy consists of in-hospital bed rest, adequate parenteral antibiotics after appropriate cultures (including blood and urine) have been taken, and intravenous fluids to replace fluids lost because of high fever and inadequate intake. Vigorous therapy should bring prompt response in two or three days. If the patient's fever is not controlled, the likelihood of premature labor and septic shock is increased. The pregnant patient with pyelonephritis should not undergo excretory pyelography unless a urinary calculus is being considered in the diagnosis. In this case the radiologist should be consulted and special techniques utilized to minimize x-ray exposure and provide the necessary information with the least number of films. With careful timing of injection and film sequence, a minimum of one film may be possible.

The most important thing for the emergency department physician to remember is that these patients must be hospitalized.

The second significant septic process to be considered is chorioamnionitis, generally occurring late in pregnancy. In any patient in premature labor, chorioamnionitis should be considered as a possible cause. Fever, purulent cervical discharge, and uterine tenderness all point to a diagnosis of chorioamnionitis. Again prompt treatment is required in order to treat both mother and fetus satisfactorily. Hospitalization of the patient followed by administration of parenteral antibiotics and prompt emptying of the uterus is mandatory. Any patient with a septic process may manifest septic shock, and in the pregnant patient, chorioamnionitis can also be the etiology. Aggressive management is mandatory.

A third septic process is septic abortion, occurring either as a result of induced abortion or during spontaneous abortion. Diagnosis is based, first, on a history of an abortive process with bleeding and uterine cramping followed by abdominal pain. On examination, the cervix may reflect trauma if the patient has had an induced abortion. Fever exceeding 101° F and possibly a leukocytosis greater than 16,000 per cubic millimeter with a significant shift to the left may be present. Uterine tenderness is generally noted. Abdominal needle marks may indicate previous instillation of hypertonic solution to induce abortion. Pelvic examination usually reveals an open cervix with a purulent discharge and necrotic tissue in the vagina or at the cervical os.

Any patient with septic abortion is a candidate for septic shock. All studies required in the management of septic abortion should be done on admission and therefore should frequently be started in the emergency department. Hematologic studies include hematocrit, or hemoglobin, and white cell count with differential. Blood cultures should be taken for both anaerobes and aerobes. Liver function studies with specific reference to bilirubin may give important base line information and indicate a patient in early hemolysis.

Coagulation studies, including thrombin clotting time, fibrinogen, prothombin time, and fibrin split products, provide information about the patient's status and may allow early diagnosis of disseminated intravascular coagulation. These patients often require general anesthesia or have a significant cardiac abnormality. Chest x-ray examination should be undertaken to look for foreign bodies and evidence of free air, indicating visceral perforation of the gastrointestinal tract or uterus. Occasionally clostridial involvement can be gleaned from the abdominal x-ray if gas is apparent in the myometrium.

In addition to blood cultures, cervical cultures should be taken and a gram stain of the cervical smear made before therapy is initiated. Urinalysis can readily be obtained; hemoglobinuria is an indication of a possible hemolytic state.

Therapy for septic abortion centers on evacuation of the infected process. These patients must be hospitalized. Dilatation and curettage, suction curettage, hysterotomy, or hysterectomy may be required as circumstances warrant. Patients frequently need large amounts of fluids to combat septic shock; large caliber intravenous routes, therefore, must be established promptly. Central venous pressure monitoring also is essential in these patients. Administration of parenteral antibiotics, which is to precede the definitive surgical procedure, is frequently initiated in the emergency department. Corticosteroid therapy has been recommended in the treatment of septic shock secondary to septic abortion.

Trauma

Trauma in the pregnant patient is usually the result of a vehicular accident with force directed to the abdomen. In the first half of pregnancy, the primary concern is for disruption of the uterus as a perforated viscus and bleeding and loss of the fetus. The possibility of the uterus receiving the shock must be considered in managing trauma patients. Peritoneal lavage for blunt trauma is necessary in the pregnant patient as in the nonpregnant patient. Perforation by bone fragments from dislocated pelvic fractures must be kept in mind. During the second half of pregnancy, rupture of the uterus is also considered. In addition, abruptio placentae caused by blunt trauma but without loss of integrity of the uterine wall may be a cause for significant shock and fetal demise that requires emptying the uterus. Lower abdominal ecchymoses may be significant findings.

Straddle injuries and insertion of foreign bodies into the vagina may cause various forms of vaginal and vulvar lacerations. Appropriate surgical repair is necessary.

Salpingo-oophoritis

Acute. The most common gynecologic complaint seen in the emergency department is probably acute salpingo-oophoritis, which is characterized by bilateral lower abdominal pain without uterine tenderness. The patient may have had a fever as high as 103° F, and usually there is a vaginal discharge that may contain gram-negtive intracellular and extracellular diplococci. The patient may have lower abdominal peritoneal signs if the inflammatory process is severe enough, and this finding may be the deciding factor in when to hospitalize the patient. On examination, rarely is a mass felt during the acute stage. Therapy on an outpatient basis consists of an appropriate penicillin type of medication. Hospitalization, parenteral antibiotics, and intravenous fluids may all be required in treating the more severe case.

Chronic. Chronic salpingo-oophoritis has many manifestations. Because of the aggressive use of antibiotic therapy for many inflammatory processes, chronic salpingo-oophoritis may, in fact, occur less frequently now than in previous decades. A patient with chronic salpingo-oophoritis may experience an acute exacerbation, which must be handled as such. These patients, in contrast to those with acute salpingo-oophoritis, may actually have palpable pelvic masses.

The most severe form of chronic salpingo-oophoritis is tubo-ovarian abscess, which is also the most advanced form of the chronic condition. Marked systemic toxicity with severe pain is the outstanding clinical sign, and may be accompanied by nausea, vomiting, and frequently chills. Abdominal signs are present, with marked pelvic tenderness, a temperature frequently exceeding 101° F, and in contrast to the other conditions, both upper and lower abdominal peritoneal irritation. Bowel sounds are decreased and occasionally diarrhea is present. These patients may also be in septic shock at the time they are seen, and rapid, vigorous therapy is necessary.

Some authorities have reported a mortality rate as high as 50% in patients in whom surgery is not undertaken within 12 hours of rupture of the tubo-ovarian abscess. When rupture occurs, the patient must be considered a candidate for immediate pelvic extirpative surgery, which includes the uterus, oviducts and ovaries. Patients in whom chronic salpingo-oophoritis is not manifested as tubo-ovarian abscess do not usually require immediate surgery, although they may require hospitalization prior to surgery. Appropriate antibiotic and fluid therapy is essential prior to surgery for tubo-ovarian abscess.

Ectopic Pregnancy

The patient with an ectopic pregnancy may have the classic symptoms of amenorrhea, pain, and bleeding that is abnormal for the menstrual cycle. These patients frequently have atypical histories; any patient with abnormal bleeding and pain, therefore, must be considered as possibly having an ectopic pregnancy until proven otherwise. A confusing history of bleeding, discomfort, and atypical signs and symptoms may obscure the diagnosis. Evaluation by laparoscopy, culdoscopy, or colpotomy is generally necessary.

Ruptured Uterus

A patient with a ruptured uterus usually gives a history of trauma. The likelihood of a ruptured uterus in a nonpregnant patient is extremely rare, although it has been noted.

Degenerating Fibroid

The patient with a degenerating fibroid exhibits pain as her only symptom and may have knowledge of leiomyomas on previous pelvic examinations. The difficulty with leiomyomas is the confusion with more severe or acute problems.

Ovarian Lesions

Lesions of the ovary, when seen in the emergency department, may have the symptoms of cysts. It should be noted that an alteration of the normal physiology with variations in the patient's menstrual cycle may occur with physiologic or follicular cysts. Patients may experience pain at midcycle, which requires only symptomatic treatment. If the cyst enlarges significantly, torsion must be considered. In this case the diagnosis is made by palpation of a mass approximately 5 cm. in diameter. Active therapy for these lesions is required only when there is torsion of a cyst or there are abdominal findings of active bleeding.

Benign ovarian neoplasms may be discovered as coincidental findings. The benign cystic teratoma, or "dermoid," accounts for approximately 10% of the neoplasms of the genital tract and rarely causes acute symptoms. It may be found anterior to the uterus, which may be a clue to its etiology, and is of interest in that it is bilateral in approximately 25% of patients.

Mucinous cystadenomas represent approximately 40% of the gynecologic neoplasms of the genital tract and may appear as torsion or rupture, but acute symptoms are rarely seen.

Malignant ovarian neoplasms that have undergone metastasis or local spread are seen in the emergency department. Pain, bleeding into the abdomen, intestinal obstruction, and ascites may all be late manifestations of malignant ovarian neoplasms, and appropriate supportive therapy on either an in-patient or out-patient basis is indicated.

Rape

The emergency department physician may be called upon to perform examinations to ascertain whether a patient has had intercourse. Determining whether or not a patient has been raped is a legal rather than a medical decision. Determining whether a patient has had intercourse and the degree of force involved may well fall within the purview of the emergency department physician. On the other hand, hospital policy may dictate that all patients undergoing examination for rape must be seen by gynecologists.

A careful history should be taken, and one should attempt to ascertain as carefully as possible all the facts that can be related by the patient and record these as accurately as possible. A careful general physical examination should be then conducted and include close inspection of the patient's clothes. Tears, dirt, or blood in the wearing apparel is pertinent information. These garments should be examined, retained as legal evidence, and properly labeled so that they can be identified in court if necessary. The undergarments should also be examined for tears, fresh dirt, blood, or body secretions. The underpants should be retained for examination for sperm by washing with normal saline solution and also for ascertaining acid phosphatase by biochemical assay. Frequently law enforcement agencies request these garments as legal evidence.

The disrobed patient should be given a complete examination because other parts of her body besides the genital tract may have suffered violence. Marks about the head and neck and evidence of violence by instruments such as knives should be noted. If the patient relates that a particular bruise has been present for several days, this should be noted in her record.

Some patients are brought to the emergency department for examination at the request of the parents or guardians. In this case, the patient was away from home for an extended period of time and when local authorities were notified, they suggested that the patient be examined by a physician. In this patient, the history should be taken very carefully and her willingness to undergo gynecologic examination ascertained. If the patient does not wish to be examined, no coercion should be used. Although the legal guardians may insist upon the examination, the patient cannot be forced to undergo it.

During examination of the genitalia, particular note should be made of the presence of ecchymoses, lacerations, or other evidence of trauma to the external genitalia and vagina. Upon careful sterile speculum examination of the vagina and cervix, any secretion in the posterior vagina may be aspirated and, if necessary, sterile normal saline solution can be used to irrigate the posterior vaginal fornix. This material should be examined microscopically for the presence of sperm. The slides should be permanently identified, by glass etching, with the date and the names of the patient and the physician. Determination of whether the sperm is motile or immobile is as important as is the detection of sperm in the vagina. Appropriate smears and culture for gonococcus should also be obtained.

The patient must be appropriately counseled and an appropriate menstrual history obtained. If she is believed to be in the luteal phase or near ovulation, administration of diethylstilbestrol (with informed consent) can be prescribed to induce menses as an emergency procedure. The dosage is 50 mg. daily for 5 days, following which withdrawal bleeding occurs. The patient must be informed that she will probably be extremely nauseated by the medication but that the discomfort of the menstrual period thus induced outweighs the risk of pregnancy. Careful documentation of all this data is essential for the patient's care and for the medicolegal record in the event of subsequent litigation.

References

1. Abramson, H. (ed.). 1973. *Resuscitation of the Newborn Infant,* 3rd ed. St. Louis, C. V. Mosby Co.
2. Apgar, V. 1953. Proposal for a new method of evaluation of the newborn infant. *Anesth. Analg.,* 32:260.
3. Behrman, S. J., and Gosling, J. R. G. 1966. *Fundamentals of Gynecology,* 2nd ed. New York, Oxford University Press.
4. Novak, E. R., and Woodruff, J. D. 1972. *Gynecologic and Obstetric Pathology,* 7th ed. Philadelphia, W. B. Saunders Co.
5. Willson, J. R., Beecham, C. T., and Carrington, E. R. 1975. *Obstetrics and Gynecology,* 5th ed. St. Louis, C. V. Mosby Co.

23

Pediatric Emergencies

David Allan

The key to good management of pediatric emergencies is, first, organ support when indicated, then the establishment of the primary diagnosis, and last, but far from least, the institution of appropriate therapy in a timely manner. It cannot be overemphasized that the response to certain pediatric emergencies, such as diaphragmatic hernia, neonatal lobar emphysema, and neonatal hypoglycemia, must be extremely fast.

In pediatric emergencies, iatrogenic psychological trauma should be minimized. The child must be managed as a whole human being.

For convenience, pediatric emergencies can be classified as being surgical and medical. Other classifications, such as by age—neonatal, infant, child, and teenager—are also useful.

Surgical Emergencies

Some of the most important emergencies are those in the newborn. These patients may arrive in the emergency department following transfer from other hospitals by air or land. The following preparations must be made in advance of transfer to provide for the newborn's needs during transit and after arrival in the emergency department. Direct transfer to the newborn nursery obviates the need for admission to the emergency department. Specific preoperative and postoperative care depends on the patient, but in general the following considerations apply to all surgical problems of the newborn.

Newborn infants, especially those underweight, have difficulty maintaining body temperature. It therefore must be monitored continuously and the environmental temperature controlled to make up for any deficiency. In addition, temperature should be monitored in all children for the diagnosis and treatment of malignant hyperthermia.

The small airways of neonates and children are susceptible to obstructive secretions. Adequate humidification is essential for the scavenging mechanisms: ciliary activity, milking of the bronchioles, and the cough reflex.

If the patient's own humidification system is bypassed by an endotracheal tube or tracheostomy, it is essential that an artificial humidification system be employed. The humidification system in the standard incubator may have to be supplemented by a heated humidifier or an ultrasonic nebulizer.

Pure oxygen can be administered in an emergency until the patient is resuscitated and a diagnosis is established. Then the guidelines of the neonatal committee of the American Academy of Pediatrics should be followed. Oxygen should be administered at the lowest possible concentration for the shortest possible time to achieve the desired effect. The cerebral P_aO_2 should not exceed 100 mm. Hg. The F_IO_2 must be monitored continuously. In this manner, oxygen toxicity, retrolental fibroplasia, and bronchomalacia are usually avoided.

In a standard incubator, an F_IO_2 of 60% can be achieved. This can be augmented by the use of halos. When 100% oxygen is required, a closed system using a bag, mask, tracheostomy, or endotracheal tube is necessary.

The preceding needs are met by an intensive care incubator. Provisions for warmth must be made, however, during x-ray studies and procedures such as cut downs (by radiant heat lamps) and during transportation (transportation incubators).

The need for antibiotics is debatable, but they should be used when indicated by past experience with certain diseases. Preparations should also anticipate the need for 0.5 to 1 mg. of vitamin K, a gastric tube, nasopharyngeal suctioning, blood typing and cross-matching, and upper extremity cut-down.

Respiratory Insufficiency

This condition is diagnosed in the classic clinical manner—by observation; for example, one determines the respiratory rate, looks for stridor and color, and palpates the oropharynx, as for subcutaneous emphysema. A catheter can be placed through the nares and into the stomach to check for obstruction. The vocal cords should always be inspected by direct laryngoscopy. Auscultation is useful to determine diminished breath sounds.

Posteroanterior and lateral chest or neck x-rays are essential, and often a Lipiodol study of the esophagus is necessary along with bronchoscopy or esophagoscopy to discover esophageal abnormalities, such as vascular rings.

Blood gas analysis is necessary for definitive diagnosis of respiratory insufficiency and for differentiation between the components hypoxemia and hypoventilation. The treatment of hypoxemia is oxygen administration and the treatment of hypoventilation is ventilation. Blood gas analysis is also essential for monitoring the therapeutics of respiratory insufficiency.

Obstructive Lesions

Choanal atresia is diagnosed if the infant is not cyanotic when he cries. This distinguishes atresia from the "blue baby" cardiac defects. The diagnosis is confirmed by the inability to pass a catheter through the nares. In an emergency, an oropharyngeal airway is taped in place. Tracheostomy is seldom necessary.

Pierre-Robin syndrome consists of a micromandible and a midline cleft palate with the tongue enlarging to fill the void. Treatment requires fixing the tongue forward with a stitch and nursing the baby in the prone position. A nasogastric tube is helpful and a gastrostomy tube may be necessary. Tracheostomy is seldom required.

A *thyroglossal duct cyst* at the base of the tongue may cause almost complete airway obstruction. The diagnosis is established by palpation of the lingual mass. Treatment consists first of aspiration and then marsupialization.

Bilateral cord paralysis is diagnosed by direct laryngoscopy. Tracheostomy is mandatory. Partial laryngeal webs are diagnosed in the same way and can usually be surgically removed. Rarer tumors of the larynx and surrounding area are managed primarily by establishing an adequate airway through endotracheal intubation.

Vascular rings, such as a double aortic arch, have caused significant airway obstruction in the newborn period. Trouble usually begins with the introduction of solids to the diet, and there are often repeated upper airway infections. The diagnosis is based on the indentation on the back wall of the esophagus as evidenced by a barium esophagogram.

Lesions that Displace Pulmonary Tissue

Pneumothorax is often found in infants who require vigorous resuscitation. If it is of minimal severity, no treatment is required, but if the lung is compressed and the mediastinum shifted, a size 10 or 12F catheter is inserted into the pleural cavity in the midaxillary line and connected to a water seal.

Diaphragmatic hernia is diagnosed when the infant has tachypnea, cyanosis, and a scaphoid abdomen. Usually there are no breath sounds on the left side of the chest. A chest x-ray shows the outlines of the intestines in the thorax. It may be necessary to augment oxygen administration with endotracheal intubation and mechanical ventilation. Early correction of the hernia is mandatory. Preoperative and postoperative care is monitored by blood gas analysis.

Esophageal Anomalies

Hypersalivation, choking on eating, and respiratory distress are symptomatic of esophageal anomalies. Esophagograms confirm the diagnosis. Air in the gastrointestinal tract is indicative of a fistula. If the diagnosis is made early and the lungs are clear, early correction is indicated. If atelectasis or pneumonitis is present, it should be treated first. A gastrostomy is performed, and then the atelectasis or pneumonitis is treated with antibiotics, oxygen, humidification, frequent direct laryngeal suctioning, and pulmonary physical therapy.

Congenital Heart Disease

Children with undiagnosed respiratory distress should be thoroughly examined for congenital heart disease.

Intestinal Obstruction

The signs of intestinal obstruction in the neonate are green or biliary vomiting, abdominal distention, and failure to pass a meconium stool in the first day of life. Any of these symptoms necessitates an upright x-ray of the abdomen, and the passage of a nasogastric tube to prevent vomiting and aspiration. Atresias of the small intestine are recognized by air fluid levels in the intestines. Treatment consists of decompression of the stomach by a nasogastric tube, and fluid and electrolyte replacement. Severe deficiencies in blood volume are treated with plasma plasmanate. Atresias are treated by resection and anastomosis.

Malrotation of the Midgut

This entity usually becomes apparent in the first week of life with biliary vomiting. The obstruction is usually only partial, and a barium swallow may be necessary to obtain the diagnosis. Volvulus accompanies malrotation, and if there is blood in the stool, an operation is urgently needed to prevent gangrene. The patient is prepared as for any intestinal obstruction. After repair of the malrotation and volvulus, a gastrostomy is performed to prevent gastric distention.

Hirschsprung's Disease

When a baby is distended and must have an enema to secure passage of meconium, Hirschsprung's disease is suspected. A plain x-ray of the abdomen shows multiple air fluid levels. A barium enema demonstrates the distal narrow colon, and the diagnosis is confirmed by the absence of ganglion cells in the biopsy of the rectal wall. Initial treatment is a colostomy at the distal limit of colon containing ganglion cells.

Imperforate Anus

The initial treatment is a diverting sigmoid colostomy. Multiple congenital defects are common. Frequently associated lesions are imperforate anus with tracheoesophageal fistula, malrotation with diaphragmatic hernias and omphaloceles, duodenal atresias with mongolism, and genetic urinary disease with Hirschsprung's disease and imperforate anus.

Pyloric Stenosis

Classically, pyloric stenosis is seen as projectile vomiting in the firstborn male at the age of 2 to 6 weeks, but it has occurred from 1 to 4 weeks in both males and females. Repeated physical examinations demonstrate the tumor. This avoids the danger of aspiration following x-rays of the abdomen in which contrast material is used. Fluids and electrolytes are replaced over 12 to 14 hours and the stenosis is corrected.

Intussusception

Intussusception occurs commonly at 6 months of age. The child pulls his knees up and cries with pain; then he relaxes. These paroxysms occur 15 to 20 minutes apart.

Vomiting is common, and a stool mixed with blood and mucus is usually passed in the first 12 hours. Prior to the development of abdominal distention, a sausage-shaped mass may be palpated. Upright x-rays of the abdomen show air fluid levels. During the first 24 hours, if the abdomen is neither distended nor tender, a barium enema is performed to reduce the intussusception. Otherwise, an operation is performed after replacement of fluids and electrolytes.

Incarcerated Hernia

A swollen, tender scrotum is usually diagnostic. Initial treatment includes sedation, placement in the Trendelenburg position, insertion of a nasogastric tube, and replacement of fluids and electrolytes. If the hernia is not reduced spontaneously in a few hours, operation is necessary.

Torsion of the Testicle

Diagnosis is made when the child cries out and has a swollen testicle. Immediate operation is mandatory.

Gastrointestinal Bleeding

In the neonate, small amounts of blood may be vomited or passed in the stool secondary to ingestion of maternal blood, as in hypoprothrombinemia. Gastric lavage and treatment with vitamin K are usually all that is necessary. Rarely is fresh whole blood required to replace a deficit blood volume and clotting factors. In older children, anal fissures result in blood in the stool. Treatment consists of the use of stool softeners and a soothing ointment. Polyps must be considered in the differential diagnosis. Polyps in the lower part of the tract are removed, but those in the upper part are left alone because they are inflammatory.

Massive bleeding dictates immediate insertion of a Levin tube to differentiate gastric from lower intestinal bleeding. The child's blood volume is stabilized before gastrointestinal x-rays are obtained to look for duodenal ulcers or esophageal varices.

Initial treatment for duodenal ulcers is blood replacement. If a concomitant disease, such as a tumor or a central nervous system lesion is found following blood loss equivalent to the patient's blood volume, operation is usually indicated.

The immediate treatment of esophageal varices is the use of Blakeman tube and blood replacement.

Bleeding from a Meckel's diverticulum is suspected when no other source of lower intestinal bleeding is discovered. The bleeding usually stops spontaneously.

Appendicitis

When a child has abdominal pain, appendicitis should always be included in the differential diagnosis. A detailed history and repeated examinations are aided by the differential blood count and urinalysis. The importance of repeated examination cannot be overemphasized. Anorexia, nausea, vomiting, and constipation are often present. Diagnosis is easy if the pain has the classic pattern—moving from the center of the abdomen to the right lower quadrant. A rectocecal appendicitis may simulate pyelonephritis. A rectal examination is mandatory. The differential diagnoses include viral enteritis associated with acute pharyngitis, acute pyelonephritis, lead poisoning, acute rheumatic fever, diabetic acidosis, pneumonia, meningitis, and allergic purpuras. Immediate operation is indicated following fluid and electrolyte replacement. Hyperthermic convulsions are avoided by lowering the temperature to 100° F.

Foreign Bodies

Gastrointestinal foreign bodies are usually passed spontaneously. Failure to do so necessitates location by x-ray with or without the aid of barium. When the foreign body is in the upper part of the tract, esophagoscopy or gastroscopy is performed to remove the object. Open operation is indicated for objects that may perforate the lower part of the tract.

Abdominal Trauma

The injured child is evaluated rapidly but systematically. An airway is established, the level of consciousness is determined, and the vital signs are evaluated. The head is palpated, the cervical region is examined for tenderness or instability, the extremities are examined, the pelvis is compressed, and then the abdomen is evaluated.

Repeated examinations may be necessary to diagnose abdominal trauma. If this is suspected on the basis of factors such as superficial bruises, tenderness, distention, pain, unexplained tachycardia, hematuria, or paralytic ileus, the hematocrit is measured and the blood is typed and cross-matched. A large catheter is placed in a vein for blood replacement, and a central venous catheter is inserted. Lactated Ringer's solution in 5% dextrose is administered through both catheters. A Levin tube is used for gastric lavage and left in place. A urethral catheter is inserted and the urine is examined for red cells. Blood transfusion is started when indicated.

The child is then x-rayed as atraumatically as possible. Flat and upright films of the chest and abdomen are always obtained. An intravenous pyelogram is indicated if there is flank tenderness or hematuria. If there is a pelvic fracture, a cystourethrogram is mandatory. If the findings are still equivocal, a paracentesis may be necessary.

The child is monitored continuously, with particular attention paid to serial hematocrits and the central venous pressure. Repeated examinations will detect delayed rupture of the spleen or retroperitoneal rupture of the duodenum.

Cardiopulmonary Resuscitation

Cardiopulmonary resuscitation is at times necessary in both surgical and medical pediatric emergencies. There should be a written protocol or guidelines for the response to cardiopulmonary insufficiency. An example is the one used at Children's Memorial Hospital, Chicago, Illinois.

Emergency Resuscitation Procedures

There is a very short interval between cessation of heart action and death. Unconsciousness occurs in less than 20 seconds and irreversible brain damage in three to four minutes.

In the event that the patient becomes suddenly unresponsive or is without pulse, blood pressure, or respiration, or is in any other life-threatening situation, the person discovering the condition, if it is a nurse, doctor, or medical student, must immediately obtain help and start resuscitation. Any other person discovering the situation must immediately call for appropriate help.

Obtain Help.

1. Call out to the nearest hospital employee to summon medical and auxiliary help and to notify the operator.

2. Dial the operator on the phone. She will answer immediately; tell her the location. She will then quickly notify the cardiac resuscitation team, each member of which carries a specially assigned pocket pager for the anesthesiologist, pediatric house staff, inhalation therapist, nursing supervisor, floating cardiothoracic resident, and cardiologist (day pager). Each pager will beep quickly and loudly and announce the cardiac arrest code and location. The anesthesiology, cardiology, and respiratory therapy offices should also be notified by the operator (8 A.M. to 5 P.M.).

Start Resuscitation.

Thump the patient's sternum once or twice sharply; then start external cardiac massage. Start mouth-to-mouth ventilation, and shift to the mask and bag as soon as equipment is available.

When help arrives, the emergency cart or box and defibrillation equipment are brought to the patient.

IF RESUSCITATION IS NOT EFFECTED IMMEDIATELY, CONTINUE VENTILATION AND EXTERNAL MASSAGE.

1. Connect the patient to the cardiac monitor as soon as feasible. Emergency cart monitors have needle electrodes attached to facilitate rapid insertion. Each lead is marked with the area of the body to which it is to be attached, *i.e.,* RA (right arm), LA (left arm), and C (common ground, used on either leg as a grounding lead).

2. Have intravenous or cut-down started as soon as possible.

3. If ventricular fibrillation is present, defibrillation through the closed chest is necessary. Apply electrode paste to the electrodes. Then place one defibrillator electrode on the anterior chest wall at the level of the apex and slightly left of the sternum, and the second electrode on the left anterior axillary line so that the current traverses the heart. Have everyone stand clear of the patient and give D.C. shock. The recommended energy settings are as follows:

> Infant: 20–60 joules (watt-seconds)
> Small child: 70–100 joules (watt-seconds)
> Large child: 100–200 joules (watt-seconds)

In the patient with a large heart, increased voltage may be required. Resume external massage immediately.

4. If defibrillation is unsuccessful or ventricular standstill persists, the heart may be anoxic or acidotic. Check the adequacy of ventilation and of external cardiac massage (femoral pulsations present with each cardiac massage). Provide base buffer for metabolic acidosis by giving $NaHCO_3$ slowly by intravenous injection. Use 2 or 3 ml. of bicarbonate solution per kilogram of body weight (45 mEq. in 50 ml.), and repeat at 10- to 15-minute intervals 3 or 4 times if needed.

5. If ventricular standstill is still present, administer intracardiac epinephrine. For a 1:10,000 dilution, mix 1 ampule of Adrenalin 1:1,000 with 9 ml. of saline or 5% dextrose solution. Inject 2 to 5 ml. and initiate extracardiac massage. If there is no response, it it important to provide a base buffer as soon as possible to combat metabolic acidosis.

Repeat intracardiac epinephrine and start intravenous administration at the rate of 0.5 μg. per kilogram per minute. (One ampule of Adrenalin equals 1 ml., 1 mg., or 1,000 μg.) For example, a 5-kg. child requires 2.5 μg. per minute. Put 1 ml., or 1,000 μg., of epinephrine in 100 ml. of 5% dextrose in water, which will then contain 10 μg. per milliliter. Adjust the intravenous drip to 15 drops per minute (0.25 ml. or 2.5 μg per minute).

6. Search for the cause of anoxia and cardiac arrest once resuscitation is effected. Look for hidden causes, such as pneumothorax or kinked respiratory tubes, as well as for obvious causes, such as hemorrhage or aspiration.

7. Discontinue resuscitative efforts after signs of death as indicated by the central nervous system and heart are seen (dilated,

fixed pupils and deterioration and disappearance of electrocardiographic activity). This decision is the responsibility of the senior physician present.

8. After resuscitation, consider transporting the patient to intensive care, if indicated, because cardiopulmonary arrest often recurs. Consider additional therapy, such as hypothermia and cortisone, as indicated by the status of the central nervous system.

9. After every arrest a resuscitation report should be completed. These reports should be periodically analyzed by the emergency department staff in order to improve their management of the infant or child with a cardiac arrest.

Resuscitative Equipment for the Emergency Department. Not all emergency departments need to have an exact duplicate of the staff and

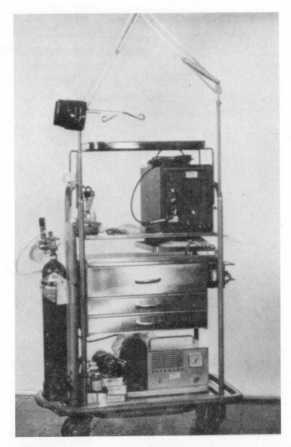

Fig. 23-1. Important features of a pediatric resuscitation cart. Because the pediatric patient's vessels are small, good light is necessary. A cut-down set is included, and all instruments are sterile because young patients, especially infants, are susceptible to infection.

facilities to care for a cardiac arrest in an infant or child as recommended in this chapter, but there must be close adherence to the principles of life support.

Emergency Cart. This should be a stainless steel cart designed to bring to the patient, rapidly and in complete form, all life support systems and drugs (Fig. 23-1). The cart should contain oxygen supply, resuscitation board, multiple adapter power panel, intravenous pole, quartz light, suction apparatus, electrocardiographic monitor, intravenous cut-down tray and solutions, adult and child size self-inflating breathing bags (Hope), work surface, and three drawers that can be opened from either side and that contain masks, airways, suction catheters, nasogastric tubes, medications, intubation equipment, and other necessities.

Emergency Box. Each box should be a tackle box with hinged self-revealing shelves, containing equipment necessary for emergency resuscitation of children of all ages. Basic equipment for respiratory resuscitation and drugs useful for cardiac resuscitation are included.

An emergency oxygen supply and a suction machine should be available in the emergency department so that they can be brought to the site of resuscitation.

The endotracheal tubes should be individually sterilized so that the entire package is not contaminated when opened. This provides for easy replacement of the tubes that are used.

Medical Emergencies

The most common medical emergency seen in the emergency department is infection, and the most frequent sign is hyperthermia. This feature may be accompanied by vomiting, irritability, diarrhea, lethargy, and refusal to eat. A thorough history and physical examination, along with appropriate laboratory and radiologic investigations, are necessary. Depending on the condition of the patient, the emergency department procedures should be limited and the patient immediately transferred to the appropriate in-patient facility.

It is helpful to classify diseases according to the age of the patient. In neonates, specific signs and symptoms are often absent. Every neonate should be investigated for sepsis, meningitis, and urinary tract infections. Lumbar puncture, blood culture, chest x-rays, urinalysis, and blood count should be done on an in-patient basis.

Children less than 3 years of age are unable to communicate their symptoms. They should be managed in the same manner as the neonate. While the child is being investigated, the hyperthermia should be limited to 103° F by sponging him with alcohol and administering acetylsalicylic acid (65 mg. per year of age). Convulsions are common. Until the temperature is reduced, maintain the airway, administer oxygen, and stop the convulsions with sodium pentobarbital (5 mg. per kilogram of body weight). Be prepared to undertake manual mechanical ventilation.

Most older children relate a specific complaint. It is easier to elicit a good history and accomplish a satisfactory physical examination in these patients. Additional diagnostic measures should include a tuberculin test and urinalysis.

Convulsions in an Afebrile Child

The etiology of convulsions in an afebrile child include metabolic disorders (hypoglycemia, hypocalcemia, water intoxication, and electrolyte disturbances), intoxication (lead and phenothiazine), intracranial hemorrhage (vascular accidents and coagulation disturbances), brain tumors, defects or degenerative diseases, hypertensive encephalopathy (acute glomerular nephritis), and idiopathic epilepsy.

Immediate treatment includes administration of oxygen and establishment of the airway. Diazepam may be preferred to sodium pentothal. The dose is 0.2 to 0.4 mg. per kilogram of body weight with incremental increases to 1 mg. per kilogram for status epilepticus.

Dehydration

Information on sudden body weight changes is helpful in assessing the state of hydration. In infants the percentage of dehydration is estimated on the basis of the physical signs: poor tissue turgor (5% dehydration); sunken fontanella (10% dehydration); sunken eyes (10 to 20% dehydration); and sudden weight loss (percentage of dehydration equals the weight loss as a percentage of the weight before illness) (Levin, 1973).

Replacement fluids should consist of balanced electrolyte solutions (Ringer's lactate) in most states of dehydration. Plasmanate (10 ml. per kilogram of body weight) is an excellent volume expander and should be considered as a partial substitute for the electrolyte replacement solution, especially in the presence of shock. The replacement volume should be 10 ml. per kilogram per percent dehydration. Potassium deficits should be considered in the dehydrated patient, but adequate urine output must be present before potassium replacement begins. The acid-base imbalance is also a consideration, for which Anderson's formula is a good guideline:

$$\text{ml. NaHCO}_3 = (0.3 \times \text{body weight in kilograms}) \times \text{base deficit}$$

14

Comparison between the isomolarity of the plasma and the urine is also helpful.

Laryngitis

Laryngitis (croup) is usually viral in origin. Treatment with ultrasonic mists has radically reduced the need for tracheostomy.

Laryngeal stridor can also result from trauma, allergy, or foreign bodies.

Epiglottitis

Before examining a patient suspected of having epiglottitis, an expert in endotracheal intubation and bronchoscopy should be instantly available. The usual cause of epiglottitis is *Haemophilus influenzae,* which is controlled by antimicrobial therapy, ultrasonic mist therapy, and intermittent positive pressure breathing with racemic epinephrine. Epiglottitis should be treated in a special care unit. The *H. influenzae* may also cause laryngotracheobronchitis. In addition to the aforementioned therapy, respiratory physical therapy aids in the removal of secretions.

Bronchiolitis

Bronchiolitis is frequently caused by a virus, but *H. influenzae* has been implicated for which ampicillin (30 to 50 mg. every 6 hours) is indicated. The general therapy for any acute infective airway disease is adequate hydration, mist therapy, and respiratory physical therapy.

Asthma

Adequate hydration is essential in this disease. For moderate to mild attacks, intermittent positive pressure breathing with isoproterenol hydrochloride or racemic epinephrine usually suffices. If this fails, aqueous epinephrine (1:1,000) is administered subcutaneously in a dose of 0.01 ml. per kilogram of body weight (not to exceed 0.5 ml.). An alternative is aminophylline; 3.5 mg. per kilogram is diluted with 200 ml. of 5% dextrose in water and administered intravenously.

Status asthmaticus is best treated with intravenous isoproterenol hydrochloride at the rate of 0.1 μg. per kilogram of body weight per minute. The electrocardiogram must be monitored because overdosage causes ventricular fibrillation.

Pneumonia

The diagnosis of pneumonia can be suggested by flaring of the alae nasi, tachypnea, or costal retractions. Auscultation may be misleading and a chest x-ray is mandatory. Hospitalization is advisable. Besides antimicrobial therapy, the airway is kept clear with mist therapy and respiratory physical therapy in the drainage positions. In the severe viral forms, oxygen therapy may be necessary for hypoxemia, and mechanical ventilator for hypoventilation. The status of respiratory insufficiency is diagnosed and monitored by blood gas analysis.

Angioedema and Anaphylaxis

In these entities, the airway can be rapidly compromised. Aqueous epinephrine 1:1,000 administered subcutaneously in a dose of 0.01 ml. per kilogram of body weight, is the treatment of choice.

Diabetic Coma

Diabetes mellitus in the young can be very difficult to manage. Coma is not infrequent and may result from both hypoglycemic and diabetic ketoacidosis. The glucose, carbon dioxide, sodium, chloride, potassium, blood urea nitrogen, pH, and serum acetone levels should be monitored. The immediate treatment for hypoglycemic coma is the administration of glucagon (0.1 mg. per kilogram, not to exceed 1.0 mg.), followed by 50% glucose solution at the rate of 2 ml. per kilogram, and then 10% glucose, all intravenously.

Diabetic coma is managed by the intravenous administration of crystalline insulin at the rate of 2.0 units per kilogram. Fluids and electrolytes are then balanced along with glucose levels.

Acute Adrenocortical Insufficiency

This may occur in a child with chronic adrenal insufficiency who undergoes stress from a concomitant disease. Treatment consists of intravenous administration of 50 to 150 mg. of hydrocortisone sodium succinate. Fluids and electrolytes are then corrected.

Meningococcemia

This is a serious medical emergency. A blood sample not only has to be cultured and analyzed (complete blood count), but coagulation studies are also necessary. Large doses of penicillin (1,000,000 units intravenously every 2 hours) are mandatory. If intravascular coagulation is diagnosed, heparinization is indicated. Shock may be treated with plasma or plasmanate, and corticosteroids may be helpful.

Meningitis

Acute purulent meningitis requires immediate aggressive management. Before bacteriologic identification is undertaken, the following therapy is initiated: up to three months of age, ampicillin in a dose of 50 mg. per kilogram of body weight intravenously every 8 hours and kanamycin in an initial dose of 15 mg. per kilogram followed by 7.5 mg. per kilogram intramuscularly every 12 hours; after three months of age, ampicillin is given in a dose of 50 mg. per kilogram intravenously every 6 hours.

Measles

Any child with measles who has a complication such as encephalopathy or chest infection should be hospitalized and vigorously treated. The younger the child, the higher the morbidity and mortality rates.

Conclusion

In this brief overview of pediatric emergencies, it is obvious that all the components of an emergency medical health delivery service are necessary. A Class I comprehensive emergency department can accomplish the immediate care, but a secondary transport system to provide mobile intensive care is necessary so that the same standard of intensive care can be maintained during transport to a suitable special care unit. The mobile intensive care units of the Illinois system are designed to handle patients of all ages and with all types of diseases. They have the same capability as a first class pediatric or adult special care unit.

This overview has been directed to pediatric emergencies in a developed country. In underdeveloped or developing countries, the emphasis is dramatically changed. Gram negative shock is by far the most common pediatric emergency. In addition, vast epidemics of communicable diseases occur with severe complications leading to high morbidity and mortality rates. Malnutrition plays a large part in the morbidity and mortality statistics.

References

1. Swenson, O. (ed.). 1969. *Pediatric Surgery*. 3rd ed. New York, Appleton-Century-Crofts, Inc.
2. Beal, J. M., and Eckenhoff, J. E. 1969. *Intensive and Recovery Room Care*. New York, Macmillan Publishing Co.
3. Gellis, S. S., and Kagan, B. M. (eds.). 1972. *Current Pediatric Therapy*, Philadelphia, W. B. Saunders Co.
4. Norlander, O. (ed.). 1971. *Anesthesia in Thoracic Surgery*. Boston, Little, Brown and Co.
5. Allan, D. 1973. Trauma as a component of critical care system. *J. Trauma*, 13:314.
6. Levin, R. (ed.). 1973. *Pediatric Anesthesia Handbook*. Flushing, N.Y., Medical Examination Publishing Co.

24

"Expressway Syndrome"

Herbert Kaufer

Traumatologists have defined an easily recognized "expressway syndrome" characterized by multiple injuries distributed over a large area and involving multiple organ systems. A recent patient had a fractured larynx, rib fractures with a pneumothorax, a ruptured spleen and liver, tears of the mesentery, and fractures of the mandible, the second cervical vertebra, both femurs, the left patella, and the right ankle (Fig. 24-1). This patient's area of injury extended from the head and neck region down to the ankle. Injured organ systems included the respiratory system, the gastrointestinal tract, and the musculoskeletal system. There is nothing unique about each component of the syndrome. For example, an identical laryngeal fracture could have been sustained in a fist fight, and an identical femoral fracture might have been sustained in a fall from a ladder. When one sees the pattern of injury spread over so wide an area and involving three or more organ systems, however, it is almost certainly the result of an automobile collision.

This patient's laryngeal, thoracic, and abdominal injuries are potentially life threatening and have the highest treatment priority. Unless associated with major nerve or vascular disruption, musculoskeletal injuries, no matter how numerous or severe, are seldom life threatening and therefore have a low immediate treatment priority. Fortunately, it is usually possible to delay definitive treatment of musculoskeletal injuries for several days without compromising ultimate restoration of function. During this period of grace, one can devote maximal energy to the components of the "expressway syndrome" that threaten survival. It is essential, however, that one does not develop a casual or cavalier attitude toward the musculoskeletal component of the syndrome. Once the question of survival has been resolved, energetic and expert management of the musculoskeletal injuries is essential to minimize the degree

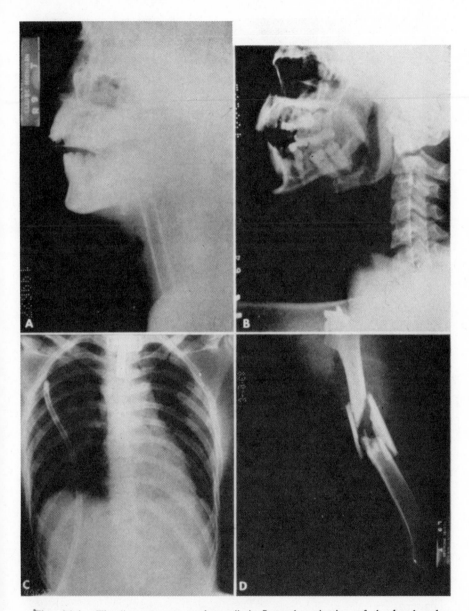

Fig. 24-1. The "expressway syndrome." A, Lateral projection of the head and neck with intratracheal tube in place shows free gas in the anterior soft tissues of the neck, indicating a fracture of the larynx. B, Lateral projection of the neck with greater x-ray penetration shows a slightly displaced transverse fracture of the second cervical vertebra. C, Posteroanterior projection of the chest shows the tracheostomy tube in place as well as a thoracotomy tube in the right side of the chest. The mediastinum is shifted to the left, indicating a tension pneumothorax on the right. Rib fractures are not apparent in this reproduction. D, An obvious, markedly comminuted fracture of the left femoral shaft. (*Continued on p. 410.*)

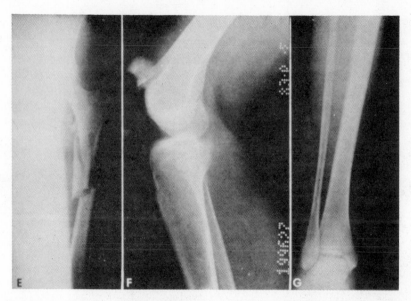

Fig. 24-1. (Contd) E, A similar fracture of the opposite (left) lower extremity. F, A comminuted fracture of the right patella with marked separation of fragments and complete disruption of knee extension mechanism. G, A fracture of the left distal tibia entering into the ankle joint. If badly managed, even this comparatively trivial injury can be a source of significant disability.

of crippling and disability. It is the end result obtained in treatment of the musculoskeletal injury that, more than any other, determines the patient's degree of permanent disability.

As in most other medical situations, accurate and complete diagnosis is the key to effective treatment. Diagnosis of fractures, dislocations, and other major musculoskeletal injuries is usually obvious. In dealing with the expressway syndrome, however, a significant injury may be missed because attention is diverted by a life-threatening or extremely obvious associated injury. These undiagnosed and therefore untreated musculoskeletal injuries are most likely to result in unnecessary disability. In order to avoid such an error of omission, it is useful to be aware of, and to understand, frequently repeated patterns of musculoskeletal injury so that a search can be made for each component of the pattern.

One such pattern is usually seen in unrestrained occupants of rapidly decelerated vehicles. As he is thrown forward, his flexed knee strikes the dashboard or other solid objects and a patellar fracture occurs (Fig. 24-2). Occasionally the major knee ligaments are also torn. Energy absorbed in the collision of the knee and dashboard is almost instantaneously transmitted along the shaft of the femur, sometimes causing

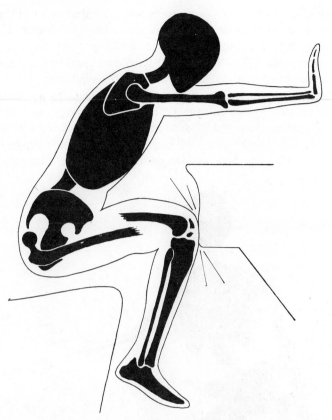

Fig. 24-2. During rapid deceleration an unrestrained automobile passenger is thrown forward and his knee strikes the dashboard. An enormous amount of energy is absorbed by the limb and causes patellar and femoral fractures as well as hip dislocation and occasionally disruption of knee ligaments.

it to fracture. A large amount of the absorbed energy is dissipated when this femoral shaft fracture occurs and the thigh deforms. If the initial energy absorption is sufficiently large, however, there may be enough residual energy to force the head of the femur through the posterior acetabulum and hip joint capsule and produce a hip dislocation. The patellar and femoral shaft fractures are usually obvious, but the hip dislocation and torn knee ligaments tend to be missed. Torn knee ligaments, patellar and femoral fractures, and hip dislocation in the same limb are becoming increasingly common.

Twenty years ago, femoral fracture and hip dislocation in the same limb were rare. If the femur broke, so much energy was dissipated at the fracture site that the hip was protected from dislocation. Today, however, collision deceleration at expressway speeds produces such enormous loads and peaks of energy transference that even after energy loss at the femoral fracture, there is ample residual energy to cause hip dislocation. This superabundance of traumatizing energy is a predominant characteristic of the "expressway syndrome" and explains the wide area and multiple organ systems involved in the syndrome.

Another pattern is frequently seen in pedestrians. In an attempt to avoid the on-coming vehicle, the pedestrian turns away, in which case the car strikes his side, and he sustains femoral and tibial fractures on that side as well as disruption of knee ligaments on the opposite side (Fig. 24-3). The fractures are frequently compound, attesting to the

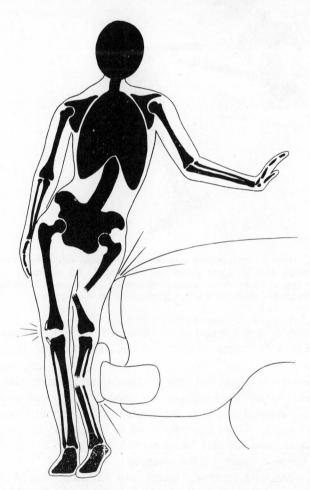

Fig. 24-3. A pedestrian struck from the side may sustain open fractures of the femur and tibia on the side that contacts the vehicle. The knee on the opposite side is subjected to enormous valgus stress, and disruption of collateral and cruciate ligaments is likely.

magnitude of the traumatizing force. The dramatic and obvious fractures frequently divert attention from the injured opposite knee, which, without treatment, is likely to progress to chronic instability and may be the patient's major permanent disability.

A typical upper extremity pattern is the so-called "side swipe" injury produced by collision forces acting on the elbow, as shown in Figure 24-4. This mechanism characteristically produces a fracture of the humerus, fracture-dislocation of the elbow, and fractures of the shaft of the radius and ulna. There are often associated peripheral nerve palsies. The skeletal destruction in this injury is so dramatic that attention may be diverted from the peripheral nerve injuries, which have great potential for causing functional loss.

The "expressway syndrome" is a highly lethal disease. During 1973, approximately 55,000 Americans died as a result of vehicular trauma. Many lives were saved by expert and prompt medical care; otherwise the toll would have been greater. Under the best conditions, we do very

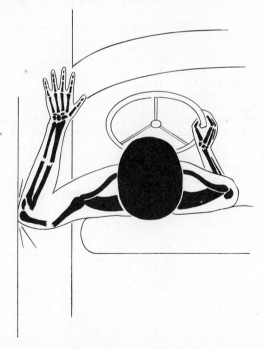

Fig. 24-4. The "side swipe" injury is a particularly devastating injury of the upper extremity, characterized by fractures of the radius and ulna, open fractures of the humerus and olecranon, and dislocation of the elbow. Major peripheral nerve loss is common. The pathogenesis of this injury is depicted in a Burma-Shave slogan, which reads: "Don't ride with your elbow out too far, it may go home in another car."

well, indeed, in terms of survival. When one considers crippling and disability, however, the record is not as good. Unnecessarily often, an accident victim is condemned to permanent and severe disability because nonlethal components of his injury were either overlooked or ignored.

As we have tried to show, if one is aware of the direction and magnitude of forces involved in a specific accident situation, it is often possible to anticipate these otherwise occult components of an injury. Although these additional components may have little effect on survival, they can exert a strong influence on disability. Complete care for the accident victim must go beyond mere survival and include all available measures to insure maximal functional capacity as the end result.

References

1. Committee on Injuries. 1971. *Emergency Care and Transportation of the Sick and Injured.* American Academy of Orthopedic Surgeons.
2. Pedersen, H. E., and Serra, J. B. 1968. Injury to the collateral ligaments of the knee associated with femoral shaft fractures. *Clin. Orthop. Rel. Res.,* 60:119–121.
3. Watson-Jones, R. 1952-1955. *Fractures and Joint Injuries,* 4th ed., vol. II. Baltimore, Williams and Wilkins, p. 552.
4. Horwitz, T. 1972. Ipsilateral fractures of the femoral shaft and neck associated with patellar fracture and complicated by entrapment of a major fragment within the quadriceps muscle. A report of two cases. *Clin. Orthop. Rel. Res.,* 83:190–193.
5. Kulowski, J. 1964. Fractures of the shaft of the femur resulting from automobile accidents. *J. Int. Coll. Surg.,* 42:412–420.
6. Lyddon, D. W., and Hartman, J. T. 1971. Traumatic dislocation of the hip with ipsilateral femoral fracture. A case report. *J. Bone Joint Surg.,* 53A: 1012–1016.
7. Shelton, M. L., Neer, C. S., II, and Grantham, S.A. 1971. Occult knee ligament ruptures associated with fractures. *J. Trauma,* 11:853.
8. Bernstein, S. M., and Meyers, M. H. 1975. Fractures of the femoral shaft and associated ipsilateral fractures of the hip and/or patella. *J. Bone Joint Surg.,* 57A:1029.

25

Initial Management of Bone and Joint Injuries of the Extremities

Waldomar Roeser

Injuries of the extremities occur with great regularity in trauma patients, partly because they represent a large portion of the total body area, and partly because of their flagelliform attitude, which places them in jeopardy. This chapter presents a brief, superficial view of extremity trauma, emphasizing initial management on the scene and in the emergency department. The orthopedic and surgical literature is replete with books[1-4] and journals that deal in depth with the specific management of fractures, and new work is being published every month. In lieu of detailed coverage of the topic, a short bibliography is included for those interested in pursuing a specific problem further.

Evaluation of any patient begins with a careful history of the problem. This is as true for patients with extremity injuries as for those with any other medical problems. The history should include details of time and place of injury and, most important, as detailed an account of the mechanism of injury as can be obtained. Symptoms produced by the injury and disability accompanying the injury should be noted. In this way, the amount of force and direction of application can be estimated, and the type of injury can be predicted.

Physical examination of the injured patient is necessary to ascertain areas of injury. Fractures, dislocations, and sprains cause pain in the area of injury. A cardinal sign of a fracture is point tenderness at the site; local swelling also is usually present. Deformity may be noted, but its absence does not rule out a fracture. Each extremity should be palpated to reveal tenderness at the sites of injury. Complete evaluation must also include assessment of the neurovascular status of the extremity. This examination should be performed on all injured patients and the results recorded before x-rays are obtained.

Proper x-rays are necessary because they are the basis of accurate diagnosis in bone and joint injuries.[5] Whenever substandard or inadequate x-ray examination is accepted by the physician, he is courting disaster and may very well miss an important injury. The *entire* injured bone must be visualized in at least two planes (anteroposterior, lateral, and possibly oblique views), and the joints proximal and distal to the injury *must* be seen. It is not unusual for a dislocation to be overlooked when it is associated with a fracture of the same bone. If the x-rays are equivocal or inadequate, the physician should not hesitate to obtain other views, or even comparison views of the opposite, uninjured extremity. (This is particularly helpful in children.)

It must also be kept in mind that bone and joint injuries are rarely life threatening.[6] In the patient with multiple injuries, initial attention must be directed to the treatment of life-threatening problems, such as airway compromise, major hemorrhage, and shock. Reduction of dislocations and splinting of fractures can be undertaken at the same time if they do not interfere; otherwise, they can be postponed until the lifesaving measures are complete. Definitive fracture management can often be delayed for a number of days or even weeks until the patient is stable.

Terminology. The use of specific orthopedic terminology is important to the understanding and description of musculoskeletal injuries. Initially, any disruption of a bone's structural integrity, from a simple compression or buckle of the cortex to the most severely crushed and displaced break, is termed a *fracture*. There is no difference between a break and a fracture, as many laymen believe.

The foremost consideration in diagnosis is to differentiate between *open* and *closed* fractures. An open fracture is any fracture in which the bone ends have come in contact with the external environment, either from protrusion through the skin or from a foreign object penetrating the skin to the fracture site. A clean sterile dressing should be applied at the earliest opportunity to prevent further contamination. A closed fracture is not associated with a break in the skin.

Another basis of classification is the x-ray appearance of the fragments. The fracture may be *transverse, oblique,* or *spiral*. It may be *comminuted* (have a number of fragments), *impacted* (the bone ends driven together rather than apart), *greenstick* (an incomplete fracture in children), or *segmental* (a second major fracture in the same bone, isolating a middle segment). Fractures are also classified according to the amount of *displacement* or separation of the ends, and to the *angulation* or angle formed between the two fragments. A fracture may therefore be undisplaced, minimally displaced, or completely displaced when there is no contact between the ends. By convention, angulation is measured in degrees and described by the direction of the distal frag-

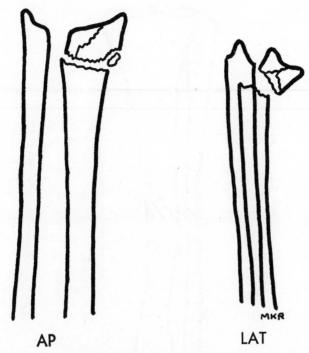

AP **LAT**

Fig. 25-1. A closed, comminuted fracture of the distal left radius with 50% displacement and 30 degrees of dorsal angulation.

ment in relation to the proximal fragment. Apposition refers to the percentage of bone end contact. Examples are a closed, comminuted fracture of the distal left radius with 50% displacement and 30 degrees of dorsal angulation (Fig. 25-1), and an open spiral fracture of the middle third of the right tibia with minimal displacement and 15 degrees of varus angulation (Fig. 25-2). By using proper terminology, a word picture is painted whereby the injury is visualized without confusion.

Principles of Management. Principles of fracture management are directed to restoring painless function to the injured extremity in the least restricting manner to the patient and in the shortest possible time. The goals of initial management are to avoid and prevent further injury to the extremity, to make an accurate and complete diagnosis of the injury, and to keep the patient as comfortable as possible during transportation and while awaiting definitive management. The four Rs of definitive fracture management are recognition, reduction, retention of reduction, and rehabilitation.

A splint is used to immobilize the extremity and prevent further soft tissue damage by motion of the sharp fracture fragments. It also re-

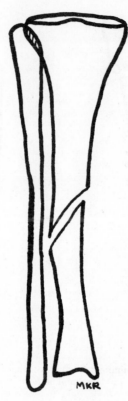

Fig. 25-2. An open spiral fracture of the middle third of the right tibia with minimal displacement and 15 degrees of varus angulation.

lieves pain, thereby making the patient more comfortable. There are many methods of splinting. Each type of fracture is best splinted in a distinct manner and will be discussed under the individual fractures.

The injured extremity should be splinted at the scene of the accident and maintained in this manner until definitive treatment is instituted. Swelling accompanies almost all injuries and increases pain as well as tissue damage. It can be controlled by ice, elevation, and compression and should be used, along with the splints, in the emergency department. Again these procedures should be continued until definitive treatment is begun. The importance of proper early management can be understood in the context that it sets the stage for all further treatment. If it is not done correctly, the end result will be compromised or at least delayed.

Fractures in Children. There is a significant distinction between fractures in children and those in adults.[7] By convention, until epiphyseal closure occurs, the patient is considered to be a child. The anatomy of the growth area and the thickness of the periosteal tube account for the major differences between fractures in adults and children. Definitive treatment varies also because of the potential of the child's bone to remodel and because of the more rapid healing in the smaller, more metabolically active bone in the child. The initial principles—splinting, ice, elevation, and compression—are still important in these patients.

The thick periosteal tube is the major factor resulting in the greenstick fracture. The bone bends like a green twig but does not break completely, leaving the concave cortex bent and supported by the thick periosteum. Clinically this fracture appears to be serious, but it actually is relatively minor. There usually is little other soft tissue damage, and reduction is accomplished simply by completing the fracture through the intact cortex and then realigning the two ends.

The epiphyseal growth plates are the major concern in fractures in children. The epiphyses are relatively weaker areas in the long bone. Also, these plates are located at the ends of the bone where the stress of trauma is usually concentrated. For these reasons, fractures in children frequently involve the epiphyses. These injuries are important because if they are severe, growth disturbances may result. The disturbances may be complete, resulting in total growth arrest and shortening of the bone by the amount of growth potential left. The damage may involve only a portion of the epiphysis, leaving the rest of the bone undisturbed, and this results in progressive angular deformity.

In order to afford some degree of predictability in epiphyseal fractures, classifications have been developed to describe them. One of the most convenient classifications, that described by Salter and Harris, is based on the course of the fracture line through the epiphysis and given a rating of I through V (Fig. 25-3).[8] In the type I epiphyseal fracture

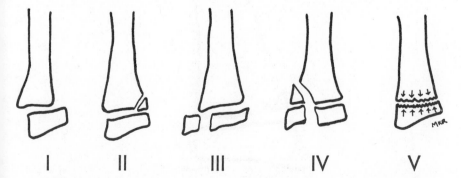

I   II   III   IV   V

Fig. 25-3. Salter-Harris classification of epiphyseal fractures, which is based on the course of the fracture line through the epiphysis.

(a fracture extending only through the growth plate without involvement of the bone on either side), the growth potential is rarely disrupted. The incidence of growth disturbance increases with the subsequent types. In a type V fracture (a vertical crushing type injury), growth arrest almost always results. By use of proper terminology in the description of the injury, communication is facilitated and understanding is increased.

The Salter-Harris type II fracture that has undergone spontaneous reduction is a special type that is often misdiagnosed. In this injury, the only abnormality seen on x-ray is a small fragment of bone at the epiphyseal-metaphyseal junction. This is known as the Thurston-Holland sign and indicates a significant epiphyseal fracture (Fig. 25-4).

Children's injuries present another difficulty in exact diagnosis. Epiphyses appear and then close with regularity, and the timing is relatively predictable. For those unfamiliar with the appearance and timing of these events, however, they may appear as fractures. Aside from familiarity with the normal appearance (which admittedly is difficult), careful examination of the area should reveal the presence or absence of a fracture. Fractures demonstrate exquisite point tenderness at the site of injury; an extremity with a normal growth area may be generally tender from injury, but localized tenderness is usually absent. A com-

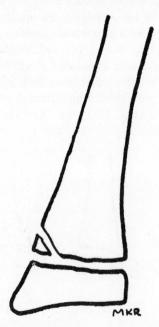

Fig. 25-4. The Thurston-Holland sign: a small bone fragment seen at the epiphyseal-metaphyseal junction on x-ray.

parison x-ray of the opposite, uninjured part is often of value in making an accurate diagnosis.

Injuries not Involving Bones. Extremity injuries not involving bones are also common, and proper diagnosis is essential. Again, recognition and terminology are important in differentiating serious from nonserious problems. A *strain* is a stress injury, and the term is usually applied to muscles and tendons, indicating overuse or overstretching but not complete traumatic disruption. The term is sometimes applied to joint injuries (probably incorrectly) but should be applied to minor problems resulting from excessive or abnormal use. Strains, in general, are best treated by resting the injured part. Other conservative measures, such as ice, heat, strapping, and mild analgesics, may also be used.

The word *sprain* indicates traumatic disruption or tearing of the ligaments and supporting structures of a joint. Some sprains are relatively minor, but because of the potential seriousness of these injuries, a high degree of suspicion is necessary. If the sprain is severe enough to cause joint instability, more extensive treatment is indicated, *i.e.,* plaster immobilization or, in special instances, surgical repair of the torn ligaments. These patients should be completely evaluated, including the use of stress x-rays if necessary, before they are dismissed with a simple elastic wrap.

A *subluxation* is a partial dislocation of a joint. By description, it must be accompanied by tearing of at least some of the supporting ligaments (a severe sprain). It is a significant injury and requires definitive treatment.

A *dislocation* is a complete separation of the joint surfaces. It indicates major trauma to the area, results in major disruption of the supporting structures of the joint, and is one of the true orthopedic emergencies. In general, a dislocation should be reduced at the earliest possible time after confirmatory x-rays have been obtained.

Scapula

Fractures of the scapula are relatively rare. Fractures of the *body of the scapula* are, in general, the result of a direct blow. The bone is encased in muscles and displacement is minimal. Healing takes place without difficulty and only symptomatic treatment is required. A sling to rest the arm is usually adequate. Of more importance is the possibility of associated injury. One must be certain that underlying rib fractures and pulmonary injuries are not present.

Fracture of the *acromion process* is also a rare injury and results from a direct blow. It also heals readily with only symptomatic treatment. In children, one must be aware of the timing of epiphyseal appearance and closure in order to recognize this fracture.

Fracture of the *scapular neck* is a more common injury that usually consists of an impacted fracture with little or no displacement. It usually responds to treatment involving a sling and rest, but it occasionally requires more sophisticated management.

Clavicle

A fracture of the *body of the clavicle* is one of the most common fractures seen in children and adults. It is painful, and clinically and radiographically may appear as a severe deformity, but it rarely requires more than simple measures of treatment. Initial treatment is directed to making the patient comfortable by use of a sling, ice bags to decrease swelling, and analgesics. A figure-of-eight dressing is applied to hold the shoulder in abduction. As it is gradually tightened, traction is placed on the fracture, which satisfactorily aligns the fragments even when comminuted, and healing occurs. It is extremely rare that surgical intervention is indicated, and it can result in nonunion. This is rarely, if ever, seen in fractures treated by closed methods.

Sternoclavicular dislocation is also a relatively rare injury. Treatment is usually conservative and consists of protecting the arm in a sling and allowing motion when comfortable. One must be aware of the possibility of an associated chest injury.

Dislocation of the outer end of the clavicle, *acromioclavicular dislocation* (or shoulder separation), is more common. The injury can be a painful strain, a partial separation showing only mild asymmetry, or a complete dislocation.[9] In a *simple strain,* the area is acutely painful and swelling is present, but gross deformity is absent. A shoulder x-ray taken with the patient holding weights may be normal or show only mild asymmetry. In a *complete dislocation,* the gross deformity is obvious clinically with the end of the clavicle protruding above and behind the acromion process. In this injury the x-ray merely confirms the clinical findings. A *partial separation* is manifested by a palpable deformity without complete dislocation.

The initial treatment of all these injuries is essentially the same. The arm is protected by a snug sling and the patient is made more comfortable with ice and analgesics. For cases involving strains or partial acromioclavicular separation, this treatment is entirely sufficient. For complete dislocation, surgical repair, particularly in the young athletic patient, is usually the treatment of choice. Various casts and braces are also used in certain patients, and occasionally only a sling is used.

Humerus

Dislocation of the *glenohumeral joint* (true shoulder dislocation) is also a common injury. Most are anterior and have a characteristic clinical picture. There is extreme pain about the shoulder, and the arm is held apprehensively by the patient in a neutral or externally rotated position. There is characteristic flatness or indentation lateral to the acromion process. The x-rays must be obtained as soon as possible and include an anteroposterior and a lateral view, either cross chest or preferably an axillary lateral view. The axillary lateral view can be obtained with the patient supine, the film above the shoulder, and the x-ray beam directed into the axilla. Only 15 to 20 degrees of abduction is necessary to obtain this view. These films document the position of the humeral head and confirm its usual anteroinferior position. They also provide assurance that a concomitant fracture does not exist.

The dislocation should be reduced as soon as possible. Muscle relaxation is mandatory to effect reduction, because spasm of the large shoulder muscles maintains the dislocation. This can be done with anesthesia, analgesics, and muscle relaxants (meperidine and diazepam, preferably intravenously), or continuous traction to fatigue and relax the muscle spasm. Traction is often preferred because it is simple and atraumatic. It is accomplished by placing the patient prone on a high stretcher with the arm hanging over the side. Weights are attached to the hand or wrist, analgesics are given, and after 10 or 20 minutes, the dislocation is reduced spontaneously. If not, gentle rotation of the arm effects the reduction. Once reduction is obtained, it should be confirmed by follow-up x-rays. The patient should be maintained in internal rotation and adduction by use of a Velpeau dressing, or sling and swathe. The period of immobilization is controversial, but the incidence of recurrent dislocation is less in persons immobilized for four or six weeks than in those held only until symptoms have subsided. Recurrent dislocations require surgical repair to prevent the repetition.

Fracture of the proximal end of the humerus, or *humeral head fractures,* are common in children and the elderly.[10] The most common is a fracture of the surgical neck, basically a transverse fracture at the lower end of the humeral head. In children, it frequently involves the epiphyseal plate. Despite the fact that the x-ray may show severe displacement, the treatment is relatively simple. Initially, a simple arm sling, ice, and analgesics are adequate for comfort. The patient is most comfortable in the sitting or upright position because the weight of the arm affords traction to effect reduction and immobilization of the fracture. If greater traction is needed, a short arm plaster cast can be used as weight, but a collar and cuff device usually suffices. Again, the upright position, including sleeping in the sitting position, is necessary. In the elderly, the major concern is preventing shoulder stiffness. For this reason, rotation type exercises are begun early, and more attention is paid to joint motion than to the x-ray appearance of the fracture.

Fractures of the anatomic neck are less common, but the treatment is essentially the same. The fractures may be comminuted, having more than one associated fracture, including the so-called "four part" fracture. There is some controversy concerning the best definitive treatment for these fractures, and factors such as age, displacement, and personal needs enter into the decisions. At any rate, the initial treatment is as previously discussed, including the use of a sling, ice, and analgesics.

The major problem in this area is an associated dislocation of the fractured humeral head. The initial problem is to recognize the dislocation, and proper x-rays must be obtained to confirm it. It must be ruled out in *all* fractures of the proximal humerus, and again an axillary lateral x-ray is helpful. If this combination is present, generally the dislocated head must be reduced. If closed reduction can be accomplished, it is fortunate and subsequently the fracture can be treated as previously mentioned. If closed reduction is unsuccessful, the decision regarding open reduction must be made. In young people, it probably is indicated. In the elderly, a satisfactory functional result may be obtained even with the head remaining dislocated if attention is paid to encouraging early motion as soon as symptoms allow it.

Fractures of the *shaft of the humerus* are common at all ages, from the newborn to the elderly. Initial evaluation must include the neurovascular status of the forearm and hand. The radial nerve (to the wrist and hand extensors) spirals around the humerus and is particularly susceptible to injury. Initial treatment is directed to making the patient comfortable and protecting the injury. A Velpeau sling, or sling and swathe, will immobilize the arm against the body. Alignment of the fracture need not be anatomic and again is best achieved by traction. This can usually be readily accomplished in a collar and cuff or hanging arm cast if more weight is needed. The patient must remain in the upright position at all times, even when sleeping. In general, these fractures heal well, but some situations make control difficult and open reduction and internal fixation may be necessary.

Fractures about the *distal end of the humerus* are of particular concern. In children, these injuries nearly always involve the growth areas, making recognition more difficult and treatment more complicated. Adequate x-rays are mandatory, and if the observer is not familiar with the normal appearance of the epiphyseal centers, comparison views of the normal side must be obtained. Neurovascular complications are frequently seen in both adults and children. A very careful assessment of these functions must be made and recorded. The supracondylar fracture is the notorious fracture that may be associated with a Volkmann's ischemic contracture, a medical tragedy.

Supracondylar fractures are often best treated by skeletal traction unless they are absolutely undisplaced. Even then, one must be concerned about neurovascular problems. Plaster splints rather than circular casts are usually used for initial immobilization so that one can follow this problem closely. In displaced fractures, traction may be the treatment of choice. A Kirschner wire is placed in the proximal part of the ulna, and side-arm or preferably overhead traction is applied. This allows accurate control of the fracture and close observation of the neurovascular status. It should also allow the treating physician to avoid a cubitus varus deformity.

Medial and lateral condylar fractures are frequently seen in children. They are epiphyseal fractures, and reduction must be accurate for proper healing. They are usually avulsion fractures with the fragment pulled off by the attached muscles when the elbow is subjected to the opposite stress. The elbow is usually dislocated at the time of injury, and with fracture, it may be quite unstable. Initial treatment, after accurate diagnosis is made, involves reduction of the dislocation if present, splinting of the elbow in neutral flexion, and use of ice to help control swelling. Many of the fractures are best treated by effecting open reduction, anatomically positioning the fragment, and pinning it with two small Kirschner wires.

An *elbow dislocation* is a common injury in sports. The x-rays show dissociation of the ulnar olecranon fossa and the trochlea of the humerus. Also, the radial head does not point at the capitulum in all views. As in any dislocation, after recognition, reduction of the dislocation is an urgent matter. The sooner it is accomplished, the easier it is done and the less permanent damage expected. Once reduced, the elbow should be splinted at approximately a right angle, because in this position the elbow should be stable. Considerable swelling may accompany this injury. Accurate initial assessment of neurovascular status and close follow-up are essential. Frequently, these patients are hospitalized for a day or so for this observation.

Forearm Bones

A fracture of the *head of the radius* may result from a fall on an outstretched hand. There is pain at the elbow with point tenderness laterally over the radial head. Many of these fractures are obvious with deformity and displacement evident on x-ray. Relatively undisplaced fractures, however, may not be seen unless multiple x-rays at various degrees of rotation are obtained. Initially, a sling and ice for comfort are adequate for all fractures. Those with minimal displacement are treated by splints and sling for comfort, followed by protected range-of-motion movements as soon as symptoms allow, progressing to more extensive use at six to eight weeks. Fractures with significant displacement or articular surface disruption are best treated surgically by radial head excision.

A unique injury of the first three years of life is *subluxation of the radial head* or "nursemaid's elbow." This usually results from longitudinal traction on the child's arm, such as when he falls while holding his mother's hand or when he is lifted suddenly by the hands. The child frequently does not localize the pain to the elbow but refuses to move the extremity, demonstrating a pseudopalsy. The x-rays of the extremity show no obvious abnormalities. When a fracture is ruled out, the subluxation is easily reduced by supination of the forearm, which is frequently accompanied by a small audible click at the radial head. The actual reduction may have already been accomplished in the initial examination or by the x-ray technician while obtaining the films. At any rate, use of an arm sling for a few days is all that is required.

The *olecranon process* of the ulna is exposed and subject to fracture from a direct blow, or the avulsing stress of the powerful triceps muscle attachment, or both. The fragments are usually displaced, with the proximal fragment being pulled up by the triceps. These displaced fractures require surgical repair by one of a number of methods. The occasional nondisplaced fracture may be treated by casting or splinting in extension until healing occurs.

A *Monteggia fracture* is a specific injury in which there is an ulnar fracture with concomitant dislocation of the radial head. The radius and ulna form a two-bone complex giving stability while allowing 150 degrees of free rotation to the forearm. If only one bone fractures, it may angulate, but it *cannot* show overriding of bone ends unless the other bone dislocates at one end or the other. In the Monteggia fracture, the ulna is fractured and demonstrates overriding, and the radial head is dislocated by the force that broke the ulna. It must be looked for to be recognized because it may be subtle on a routine x-ray. Again, a line drawn through the radial shaft and head should point toward the capitellum of the humerus on all views. This injury requires reduction and immobilization as early as practical. In children, this can usually be accomplished by closed means, but nearly all adults require open reduction and internal fixation of the ulnar fracture and sometimes of the radial head dislocation.

Fractures of the *shafts of the radius and ulna,* both forearm bones, are more common than the Monteggia fracture. In children, these frequently are greenstick fractures with considerable angulation and grotesque deformity. These fractures are not serious, however, because neither the trauma causing them nor the accompanying soft tissue damage is great. After initial x-rays of the entire bones are obtained, reduction is easily accomplished by increasing the deformity to complete the fracture and then realigning the arm and applying a long arm cast. Healing is usually rapid, and deformity and disability negligible. Even displaced fractures in children are usually easily reduced with traction, but anesthesia by intravenous lidocaine, axillary block, supraclavicular brachial plexus block, or general anesthesia is usually preferred. Immobilization in a long arm plaster cast allows healing, and in children, bone remodeling allows healing in somewhat less than anatomic position and alignment to result in an excellent functional and cosmetic result. Rotatory malalignment cannot be accepted, however, because remodeling will never occur.

In the adult, the approach to both bone fractures, or isolated radius and ulna fractures, is different. Near anatomic position and alignment are mandatory to allow synchronous forearm motion and normal rotation. Because of the muscle attachments and pull, adequate fracture position can almost never be maintained by closed means. Open reduction and internal fixation, therefore, are advised in nearly all of these fractures in the adult.

The *Galeazzi fracture* is an injury related to the Monteggia fracture in which the radial shaft is fractured with a concomitant dislocation of the distal part of the ulna. Again, it must be looked for to be recognized. Treatment is usually closed reduction in children, and open reduction and plate fixation of the radius in adults.

Fractures of the distal end of the forearm bones can basically be divided into four groups. The *Colles fracture* is the most common. This term is often applied to all fractures of forearm bones in the region of the wrist. The term is classically used to describe fractures of the distal radius with dorsal angulation and deformity, producing the so-called "silver fork" clinical deformity. Initial treatment involves splinting; an air splint is excellent for this injury. Ice helps to control swelling while the patient waits in the emergency department. In both children and adults, if the fracture is displaced, it should be reduced, and immobilization in a long arm cast is mandatory. Anesthesia is helpful, and reduction can be obtained by manipulation or by traction, which does not increase the soft tissue trauma. Because of the remodeling potential of children's bones, some deformity can be accepted, but in the adult, wrist dysfunction will result if residual deformity exists. This deformity may be acceptable, and in some situations it is preferable to applying a cast in an awkward position, pinning the fragments, or maintaining traction with metacarpal and proximal ulnar pins. In this fracture, one must keep in mind that the median nerve can be stretched across the proximal fragment and compressed at the point at which it then passes under the volar carpal ligament. Clinical assessment of median nerve function is mandatory.

A *Smith fracture* is also a distal radial fracture, but the distal fragment is angulated and displaced in the volar direction. It is a reverse Colles fracture. Treatment consists of reduction, and a long arm cast is applied with the forearm in full supination.

A *Barton fracture* is an articular fracture of the distal radius, involving the anterior articular margin. It may be associated with volar dislocation of the carpus on the radius, and this must be looked for on the x-rays. The dislocation must be reduced and then maintained in plaster until stability is obtained by healing.

The *comminuted articular fracture of the distal radius* is a severe and potentially disabling injury. Whenever a fracture involves a joint, function is disturbed if the joint surface is not reapproximated anatomically and sometimes even when it is. In this fracture, the hand and the carpal bones are forced into the distal radius, shattering the articular surface. There is usually considerable compression of the distal radius and loss of the radioulnar and dorsovolar angles. The best means of treating this fracture is by traction. A Kirschner wire in the proximal ulna and another in the metacarpus allow traction to be applied. This reduces the fracture and allows close monitoring of swelling and the neurovascular status of the hand, which are important because there is usually considerable soft tissue trauma, swelling can be massive, and neurovascular compromise is not unusual. When the danger period is over, the cast can be applied, incorporating the two pins.

Another special fracture seen in children is the *torus or buckle fracture* of the distal radius. This is a compression type fracture in which one cortex buckles on itself. This is different from the greenstick fracture, which breaks apart. It is a stable fracture and reduction is rarely indicated or necessary. A short arm cast protects the injury, and healing is rapid.

Carpal Bones

The *carpal-scaphoid fracture* is the most common type of carpal fracture. The most important step in the treatment of this injury is recognizing the fracture. One must have a high index of suspicion when a patient is seen after a fall on the hand and is experiencing pain, particularly on the dorsoradial aspect of the wrist. Tenderness is a classic sign, but it may be diffuse. Again, x-rays are mandatory in the diagnosis and they must be adeqate.[11] The routine anteroposterior, lateral, and oblique views may not show the scaphoid in profile, and, therefore, the fracture may be missed. One should order a "scaphoid series" that will show the scaphoid bone in a number of planes and will demonstrate most fractures, even the small linear undisplaced fractures. If the x-rays appear to be normal, but clinical suspicion is high, the injury should be treated as a fracture. The cast can be removed in two or three weeks and another x-ray series obtained. If a fracture still is not seen and the patient is no longer in pain, immobilization can be discontinued. There is a large volume of literature concerning scaphoid fractures, dwelling on the incidence of nonunion in this fracture and its treatment.[12] Certainly, nonunions are encountered, and other problems develop, but if the fracture and extent of injury are recognized early and proper treatment initiated, these problems will be minimal.

Lunate dislocation is another wrist injury that may easily be missed if it is not carefully sought. Again, adequate x-rays are mandatory. On the lateral view, one must look for the crescent-shaped lunate bone. It should be directly in line with the radial shaft and its concave surface should accept the large carpal capitatum. This dislocation should be reduced as soon as possible, and adequate anesthesia is required. Often open reduction is necessary. When the lunate dislocates volarward, it is located in the carpal canal and can cause compression of the median nerve.

The *perilunate dislocation* involves dislocation of all the carpal bones except the lunate, which remains in contact with the distal radius in essentially a normal position. The clinical deformity is usually striking and resembles a Colles fracture, whereas the clinical deformity in a lunate dislocation may be minimal. This injury is often accompanied by a scaphoid fracture resulting in a *transscaphoid perilunate dislocation*. This is an unstable condition, and nonunion of the scaphoid fracture is to be expected. Often the best treatment is open reduction and internal fixation.

Other carpal bones can be fractured but this is relatively rare. They must be carefully sought, and the suspected x-ray abnormality should correlate with the clinical findings of localized tenderness and swelling. Many of these are avulsion fractures with only small fragments of bone in the region of the tendon attachments. These injuries usually respond well to a limited period of immobilization followed by rehabilitation.

Hand

Fractures occur more frequently in the hand than in any other area. Crush fractures of the distal phalanges are probably the most common of all fractures, and the boxer's, or impacted, fracture of the neck of the metacarpal bone of the little finger is the second most common.

The initial treatment of all fractures of the hand is basically the same. Open fractures, or associated soft tissue lacerations, should be covered with clean dressings to prevent further contamination. If any delay is expected, the hand should be placed in the position of comfort and function with the wrist at neutral or slight extension, the thumb abducted and in palmar opposition, and the fingers in partial flexion (as when grasping a glass). A soft, fluffy, bulky dressing can be applied and the hand elevated. This splints the injuries, decreases pain, controls swelling, and makes future treatment easier.

The volume of literature concerning fractures and other injuries of the hand would fill libraries. This section will touch on certain problems in hand injuries, emphasizing injuries that pose problems in diagnosis as well as treatment. The section on soft tissue injuries of the hand should also be consulted because fractures are frequently accompanied by injuries to the soft parts (see Chapter 27).

Injuries to the basal joint of the thumb must be carefully evaluated with x-rays. The carpometacarpal joint may be dislocated, there may be a fracture-dislocation (Bennett's fracture), or there may be a fracture of the base of the metacarpal bone. These must be differentiated because each portends a different problem in treatment and expected results. Proper x-rays in multiple planes must be available for careful evaluation.

The major injury of concern at the metacarpophalangeal joint of the thumb is rupture of the ulnar collateral ligament.[13] This results from forced abduction of the thumb, such as in a fall, and is frequently called "gamekeeper's thumb." Clinically, there is tenderness on the ulnar side. Routine x-rays may be normal. The thumb must be examined clinically and the ulnar collateral ligament stressed, or an x-ray, while stressing the injured thumb, can be taken and compared with the normal one. Complete rupture requires surgical repair for best results.

Fractures of the metacarpal bones of the other digits are common and seldom missed. The major problem that must be looked for is the rotational alignment of the fragments. The fracture is frequently oblique or spiral and tends to rotate because of the intrinsic muscle attachments. Slight malrotation is translated to the fingertip, which then overlaps an adjacent digit when the patient attempts to grip something. This is a disabling deformity, and open reduction and pinning may be necessary if it cannot be controlled by closed means. It must be looked for by observing finger alignment during flexion, as in making a fist.

A related injury that is often missed is a fracture-dislocation of the base of the metacarpal bone of the little finger; this is a carpometacarpal dislocation.[14] Again, this injury must be suspected in injuries to the ulnar side of the hand with pain and swelling in the area of the base of the metacarpal. Oblique x-rays must be closely evaluated to see the metacarpal base sitting dorsal to the hamate bone. A metacarpal fracture may also be present, but the dislocation is the important injury and may require open reduction for stabilization.

Fracture of the neck of the metacarpal bone of the little finger usually is the result of striking an object with the fist (the boxer's fracture). There is volar angulation of the metacarpal head with impaction and comminution of the volar cortex. Most of these fractures heal readily and cause no functional disability even when there is considerable angulation. Bony prominence and shortening of the metacarpal bone are seen clinically. Severely displaced fractures may require reduction as does a rotated fracture that allows the little finger to underlap the ring finger.

Dislocation of the metacarpophalangeal joint of the index finger is a rare but interesting injury. The phalanx is forced dorsally and the metacarpal head is pushed into the palm. Because of the anatomy of the ligaments and tendons in this area, closed reduction is seldom possible, and open reduction through a palmar incision is necessary.

Fractures of the proximal and middle phalanges of the digits are seldom missed on x-ray but may be particularly troublesome if treatment is not timely and proper. Because of tendon pull, transverse fractures tend to buckle and progressively collapse; oblique fractures tend to rotate, again resulting in overlapping of the fingers during grasp. Many of these fractures may be treated by closed means, but open reduction and pinning may be necessary. While definitive treatment is being awaited, these fractures are again splinted, but use of the straight tongue blade splint is to be condemned; this is a nonfunctional and uncomfortable position for the finger. These injuries are best splinted in the position of comfort and function, which is partial flexion, using a malleable aluminum splint or a commercial "frog" splint.

Distal phalanx fractures are usually the result of crushing injuries to the distal segment of the finger. These are frequently open injuries, and if the nail bed is damaged, they are considered to be open by definition. As with any open fracture, the treatment includes cleaning and dressing of the wound, consideration of antibiotics, close observation of the soft tissues, and splinting of the distal joint during healing.

Dislocations of the interphalangeal joints are common.[15] Reduction is usually readily obtained with traction. The dislocation of the middle joint may be accompanied by an avulsion fracture of the volar base of the middle phalanx. This may result in instability even after reduction if extension is permitted. Open reduction and fixation of the fragment may be recommended, or splinting in flexion may be adequate. Motion in flexion can often be allowed as long as extension to the point of instability is blocked.

Pelvis

The pelvis forms a strong ring, or girdle, with the sacrum to support the trunk. To perform its function, it must be exceedingly strong and can withstand considerable stress. When stress is great enough, however, it will fracture. The major concern with any pelvic girdle fracture is accompanying soft tissue injuries, which can be not only severe but also fatal.[16] They therefore are of more medical importance than the x-ray evidence of fracture indicates. Most of these patients are seen after major trauma, such as motor vehicular accidents, falls from significant heights, and cave-ins. In most cases, routine supportive care should be instituted even before x-rays are ordered. Intravenous fluids should be begun, blood should be drawn for routine studies and typing and crossmatching ordered, urinalysis should be obtained, and if this is not possible, a catheter should be inserted. If hematuria is present, an intravenous pyelogram or further urologic studies should be obtained. These patients may die immediately from blood loss (which can be massive intrapelvically and never seen externally) or later from rupture of the bladder, intestines, or even the uterus.

Pelvic fractures of a significant degree are seldom missed on x-ray, but the accompanying injuries are frequently overlooked in the emergency department. Also, most pelvic fractures heal satisfactorily with just bed rest and symptomatic treatment. These fractures can basically be considered as stable, unstable, and avulsion fractures. The avulsion fracture results from a sudden muscle pull that tears off its bony attachment, such as the anterior superior iliac spine, or the ischial tuberosity. Most of these injuries seem to do well with bed rest followed by progressive mobilization.

Most pelvic fractures are stable and involve the pubic or ischial rami, the body of the sacrum, or an iliac wing. In these injuries, the only real medical concern is relief of pain and care of the associated major intrapelvic injuries, which are seen in more than 25% of patients.

The unstable fractures are those involving the weight-bearing portion of the pelvis. These are the result of more severe trauma, and nearly 75% of patients have associated major injuries, with as many as 10% dying from their injuries. These fractures require active treatment, such as reduction, traction, and prolonged recumbency, but the major initial concern is the associated problems.

Central fractures of the acetabulum are frequently discussed with hip dislocations, because the femoral head dislocates centrally through the acetabulum. The fracture seen, however, is of the pelvic acetabulum. Again, close attention must be given to associated injuries, particularly the urinary tract. Hospitalization with traction is usually necessary.

Femur

Hip dislocation is seen fairly frequently in trauma and is usually posterior (the femoral head lying posterior to the acetabulum).[17] The clinical picture is usually diagnostic, with the patient in considerable pain and the thigh flexed, adducted, and internally rotated. There is extreme irritability with any attempt to test range of motion. The sciatic nerve may be trapped or compressed by the femoral head; the neurovascular status of the leg therefore must be checked. This injury is one of the few true orthopedic emergencies. Reduction must be achieved as soon as possible. Studies indicate that the longer the hip is left dislocated, the greater the chance of developing avascular necrosis of the femoral head and obtaining a poorer functional result. The posterior dislocation may be accompanied by a fracture of the posterior part of the acetabulum that renders the dislocation unstable and requires surgical correction. The dislocation can be anterior or at the obturator, but expeditious reduction is still mandatory.

Hip fractures are commonly seen in the elderly following relatively minimal trauma and in younger people following severe trauma. They are rarely seen in children, but when they do occur they are serious and potentially disabling problems. The fractures are named according to where they occur: *subcapital*—at the junction of the femoral head and neck; *transcervical*—across the femoral neck; *basilar neck*—at the base of the neck; *intertrochanteric*—through the region of the greater and lesser trochanters; and *subtrochanteric*—across the femoral shaft but less than 3 inches below the lesser trochanter. Most of these fractures require surgical repair or replacement of the femoral head. The elderly person with a hip fracture usually requires close medical management before, during, and after surgery; this is perhaps the most important part of the treatment of this injury.

Fractures of the *femoral shaft* occur at all ages but perhaps most commonly in young adults, who are subject to athletic and motor vehicular trauma. These fractures are usually due to significant trauma, and other injuries must be suspected and looked for carefully. The neurovascular status of the rest of the extremity must be evaluated. (See chapter on vascular injuries.) Blood loss must also be considered, even in closed fractures, because 1 or 2 liters may be lost in the tissues of the thigh after a femoral fracture. (See chapter on shock.) These fractures can be well splinted in a Thomas leg splint with elastic bandages or triangle bandage support, and traction can be applied to the foot. This allows control of the fracture in the emergency department, during transportation, and even while other medical problems are being handled in the hospital. Initial treatment of most of these fractures is traction, preferably skeletal traction with a pin in the distal femur or proximal tibia. In this manner, the powerful thigh muscles, which are in spasm, can be overpowered. This reduces pain and regains length of the femur. With adjustment of the traction, proper alignment and position of the fracture can be maintained during healing. This, of course, is done in the hospital where subsequent treatment such as internal fixation can be considered at the proper time. In some young children, femoral fractures can be treated by immediate application of a hip spica plaster cast, but most also require traction in the hospital.

Patella

Patellar fractures are usually the result of direct blows and therefore are often seen in automobile accidents when the knees strike the dashboard. Clinically, there is pain, considerable swelling, and usually loss of the ability to lift the leg off the stretcher with the knee extended. Ice should be used to help control swelling, and the extremity should be splinted with the knee extended. Fractures that do not show significant displacement or disturbance of the articular surface may be treated with a cast in extension. In most cases, however, the fractures are either badly comminuted or transverse with significant separation, indicating a disruption of the quadriceps mechanism. These fractures require surgical repair by performing a patellectomy or reconstituting a smooth, anatomically accurate articular surface.

Patellar dislocations are commonly seen in teenage girls. The dislocations are always lateral, and patients with valgus knee with lateral insertion of the patellar tendon and a weak or high inserting vastus medialis portion of the quadriceps are predisposed to these dislocations. These and other structural variations allow the patella to be forced around the lateral side of the lateral femoral condyle where it becomes lodged. There is pain and the knee is locked in the semiflexed position. This dislocation is usually easily reduced by extending the knee while lifting the patella anteriorly. It should be done gently to prevent excessive trauma to the articular surface of the patella. In recurrent patellar dislocations, surgical reconstruction of the quadriceps mechanism may be necessary.

Knee

Knee injuries are very frequent in athletics and other trauma-inducing situations and are perhaps more often overlooked in the emergency department than is any other significant orthopedic problem.[18] Perhaps the reason is that the x-rays are usually normal because the injury is to the soft tissues. The knee must be adequately and carefully examined clinically or these injuries will certainly be missed.

The *meniscus cartilages* in the knee may be torn by twisting injuries to the knee when it is in semiflexion while bearing weight. This is a frequent result of a clipping type injury in football and is also seen in activities such as rising from a full squatting position.[19] The medial meniscus is more susceptible to tear than is the lateral meniscus. The patient experiences acute tearing pain along the joint line and is unable to bear weight on the knee. Also, the knee is often locked in semiflexion if the torn cartilage has shifted into the knee. An effusion develops but may not be present immediately unless the tear involves the peripheral attachment or the synovium where a hemarthrosis will result. If this lesion is suspected, the most critical part of the examination is to be certain that the collateral and cruciate ligaments were not torn at the time of injury. Their integrity must be ascertained by examination before further disposition is made. Once ligament integrity is proven, initial management of the injury may include crutch ambulation (without weight bearing), ice packs, and possibly splinting. If the meniscus cartilage is truly torn, it will almost certainly require surgical excision but not necessarily as an emergency procedure.

Tears of the collateral ligaments are serious knee injuries that are too often missed. The medial or lateral ligaments as well as the cruciate ligaments may be torn. The injury usually is the result of a significant force applied to the side of the knee, forcing it into varus or valgus position and often with rotation. The classic mechanism is the clipping injury in football in which the valgus stress results in tearing of the medial collateral and the anterior cruciate ligament, and disruption of the posterior medial corner of the joint capsule, producing an unstable knee. The medial meniscus cartilage is usually also torn. Pain is usually diffuse along the medial (or lateral) side of the knee along the femoral condyle and the proximal tibia. Stressing the ligament reveals the lack of stability of the knee by its opening abnormally when compared with the opposite normal knee. In a complete tear, there very well may be no effusion or hemarthrosis because the accompanying synovial and capsular tears may allow the effusion to escape into the soft tissues. This lack of effusion in an obviously significantly injured knee must be a point of concern to the examiner. Further evaluation may include obtaining "stress x-rays" while attempting to open the knee, or even examination under anesthesia to determine the extent of damage. These injuries are to be considered urgent orthopedic problems; most require surgical repair to restore ligament stability.

True *knee dislocation,* or tibiofemoral dislocation, is a relatively rare but extremely serious injury. In this injury, there is complete disruption of all supporting ligamentous structures of the knee. With this much disruption, the x-ray usually shows the tibiofemoral dissociation. Perhaps the most serious accompanying problem is disruption of the popliteal artery, which may be seen in 50% of these cases. This must be suspected, and if there is any question, an arteriogram should be obtained to confirm its integrity. (See chapter on vascular injuries.) Even when an intact vascular system is demonstrated, there very well may be intimal damage that can result in delayed thrombosis and loss of circulation to the leg. The peroneal nerve winding around the lateral side of the knee and fibular neck also is susceptible to damage and its function in the leg must be evaluated. This injury requires surgical repair of the knee and often surgical reconstruction of vascular integrity.

Another knee injury that is too frequently missed is disruption of the quadriceps mechanism, either by rupture of the quadriceps attachment to the superior aspect of the patella or by rupture of the patellar tendon distally. This may be seen after direct trauma to the tensed mechanism, or the tendon may separate with sudden, severe muscular contraction. There is pain and localized tenderness, and the gap may be palpable. So much swelling may be present that the gap is not appreciated. The patient is unable to lift the leg with the knee extended, and for this reason the injury may be clinically mistaken for a patellar fracture except that the x-rays may be normal. Treatment is usually surgical repair.

Tibia

The *anterior tibial spine* may be avulsed as an intraarticular fragment in the knee joint. There is pain and a large hemarthrosis. Treatment involves controlling the swelling and obtaining full knee extension and immobilization by applying a long leg cast. In general, this fracture is reduced when in extension, and immobilization is all that is required. If it is not reduced in this way, open reduction may be necessary.

Tibial plateau fractures are the result of direct trauma, often by a fall from a height. The medial or lateral plateau may fracture, or both may fracture. Small, linear, minimally or nondisplaced fractures may be missed unless adequate oblique x-rays are also obtained. If the fractures are significantly depressed or displaced, open reduction may be required. Others may be treated with traction and motion exercises or with a plaster-of-paris cast.

Injuries to the *tibial tubercle* may occur, but rarely is an acute fracture seen here. It is not unusual, however, to see an accessory bony ossicle on the lateral x-ray, a condition known as Osgood-Schlatter's disease. There certainly can be considerable pain associated with a direct blow, but if the quadriceps mechanism is intact, this can be treated with ice, use of crutches, and rest until the contusion and irritation subside.

Fracture of the tibial shaft is one of the more common injuries seen in an emergency department. The motorcyclist is a frequent patient with this injury as an open fracture, and the skier is frequently seen with a spiral fracture just above his boot due to the severe torsional stress of the ski and boot during a fall. Splinting of this injury is relatively easy; a commercial air splint is preferred, but one of the other leg splints from the groin to the toes can be used. This allows the patient to move and undergo further evaluation with minimal discomfort and excellent immobilization. Any open wound can be covered with a clean or sterile dressing before application of the splint to prevent further contamination. The neurovascular status of the foot should be evaluated and recorded. The tibia alone may be fractured, in which case the intact fibula affords an excellent internal splint. It is more common, however, for both tibia and fibula to fracture together, leaving a severely unstable situation. Tibial fractures require careful, knowledgeable management, and there is a considerable volume of literature concerning the preferred method. The goal, again, is to obtain a functional extremity for weight bearing in the shortest time period possible. This may require open reduction and internal fixation, or treatment in a plaster-of-paris cast.

Fibula

The *proximal tibiofibular joint may dislocate* with torsional injuries that force the fibula anterior to the tibia. This is a rare injury, and when it is seen, the integrity of the peroneal nerve must be carefully evaluated because it is vulnerable as it winds around the proximal part of the fibula.

Fractures of the fibular shaft usually accompany tibial fractures. They can occur, however, as isolated fractures or even as stress fractures with the crack appearing slowly over a period of time from excessive demands placed on the leg. These fractures are relatively inconsequential except for the symptoms they cause. Treatment is therefore symptomatic. A cast may be applied as necessary to relieve pain. When the fracture is proximal, one must again be conscious of the vulnerable peroneal nerve in this area.

Ankle

The ankle is very frequently injured, and careful evaluation is necessary to determine the extent of damage. This requires assessment of the method of injury, clinical examination of the ankle, and careful evaluation of the x-rays.[20] Some injuries require surgical repair, whereas others require only a cast or even no active treatment. The x-rays must include anteroposterior, lateral, and mortice views. The mortice film is the most important because only on it can an accurate assessment of the tibiotalar relationship be made. It must be insisted upon in all ankle injuries. Perhaps the most common injury is a strain or sprain of the lateral or fibular collateral ligaments and usually the anterior capsule. There is pain and usually significant swelling in the region of the injury. The x-rays confirm the soft tissue swelling but show no fracture, and the mortice is intact with a normal tibiotalar relationship. Initial treatment usually involves controlling swelling and pain by ice, compression dressings, elevation, and use of crutches. If the damage is thought to be significant, a short leg walking cast may be used, and in some areas surgical repair of the ligaments is recommended.

Isolated *fracture of the lateral malleolus* is also a common injury. There may be a small avulsion fracture of the tip, which dynamically is the same as the ligamentous sprain previously described. The typical injury is the spiral fracture of the lateral malleolus resulting from external rotation stress that twists the ankle. Again, the ankle mortice must be carefully evaluated on the x-rays. One must be certain that the distance between the medial malleolus and the talus is no greater than the distance between the tibial plafond (or ceiling) and the dome of the talus. If such is the case, the deltoid ligament must be torn and the ankle subluxed. If this is not the case, initial treatment frequently involves control of the swelling with ice, compression dressings, elevation, and use of crutches. Definitive management is controversial, with recommendations varying from ambulation in a tightly laced boot to surgical repair. Perhaps most authorities recommend a plaster-of-paris cast with or without a walking heel.

Fractures of the medial malleolus may be particularly troublesome and are usually considered as surgical and nonsurgical fractures. Those that are well below the tibial plafond (or ceiling), such as avulsion fractures of the tip of the medial malleolus, do well with a plaster-of-paris cast after swelling is controlled. Fractures at the level of the plafond interfere with ankle joint stability and integrity and heal poorly. Almost all of these require open reduction and internal fixation for best results.[21]

Other more serious fractures include the *bimalleolar fracture,* in which both medial and lateral malleoli are fractured, and the *trimalleolar fracture,* in which the medial and lateral malleoli and the posterolateral malleolus of the tibia are fractured. These are serious injuries and essentially are fracture-dislocations because the tibiotalar relationships are disrupted. Essentially all these fractures require surgical repair, and even then the results are less than ideal. Initial treatment of these injuries must include aligning the foot on the leg, applying a compression dressing and splint, using ice, and elevating the foot. Surgical repair is usually carried out early before fracture blisters develop.

Injuries in which one malleolus is fractured and the ligaments to the opposite malleolus are torn also represent fracture-dislocations and are dynamically the same as the bimalleolar fracture. Again, the clue is in the mortice x-ray in which the tibiotalar relationships are disturbed. These injuries, like the bimalleolar fractures, in general require surgical repair, but they must be diagnosed correctly. A related injury that also requires accurate evaluation is a tear of the distal tibiofibular syndemosis, which is usually associated with a high fibular fracture and deltoid ligament tear or medial malleolar fracture. This is also a fracture-dislocation, and the disruption of the tibiotalar relationship must be recognized and carefully evaluated.

True *ankle dislocation,* with no accompanying fracture, is rare. Because the clinical deformity is severe, it is often open. Reduction should be accomplished as soon as possible, and surgical repair is usually necessary. The soft tissue trauma can be severe and vascular damage can be enough to cause loss of the foot. This is a serious injury.

Foot

An injury that bridges the leg-foot axis is rupture of the heel cord. *Tendo-Achilles rupture* frequently occurs in the middle-aged athlete during push-off while running and jumping. He feels sudden pain behind his ankle as if someone has kicked him in this region. Subsequently, he finds he is unable to walk normally because he cannot push off. Clinically, the gap in the Achilles tendon is usually palpable, and squeezing of the calf muscles above the injury does not produce the normal plantar flexion. The x-rays may be interpreted as normal, but close inspection of the lateral view indicates a soft tissue defect in the tendon. Treatment may involve surgical repair; recently, placing a cast on the foot in the equinus position has been recommended.

Fractures of the foot are frequently misdiagnosed because of lack of familiarity with the normal tarsal and metatarsal appearance and with the multitude of accessory ossicles in the foot. A careful physical examination discloses the point of maximal pain and swelling and any obvious deformity. When this information is correlated with the x-rays, a more accurate appraisal should be possible. If one sees on the x-ray a suspicious ossicle or unfamiliar appearance of a bone, but the pain is localized in another area, one can be relatively confident that there is no clinical significance to the x-ray finding. Acute fractures are painful. Initial management first involves making the correct diagnosis. The extremity then should be elevated above the heart, with the use of ice and a bulky compression dressing to control swelling and make the patient comfortable. Definitive management depends on the specific injury.

Fractures of the *tarsal talus* are potentially disabling. In its protected position in the ankle mortice, the body of the talus is seldom fractured. The neck is frequently fractured, however, in injuries causing sudden forced dorsiflexion of the foot, such as in a fall on the ball of the foot. This is particularly serious because the major blood supply to the body of the talus is across the neck, and avascular necrosis is a common result. The displaced fractures are usually easily seen on lateral and oblique x-rays of the foot. Accurate reduction is mandatory, and internal fixation may be advised. With nondisplaced or minimally displaced fractures, the major concern is to recognize the fracture. Again, careful evaluation of the mechanism of injury, location of the site of tenderness and swelling, and correlation with close inspection of the x-ray lead to the correct diagnosis. In these injuries, treatment is usually a plaster-of-paris cast with non-weight bearing until healing occurs.

Fractures of the *tarsal calcaneus* are almost always the result of a fall from a height and landing on the heels. They are frequently bilateral. Because of the mechanism of injury, other fractures, including tibial plateau fractures, hip fractures, and compression fractures of the spine, are also frequently seen and the patient must be carefully evaluated for these. Calcaneal fractures are seldom missed because pain is usually severe and localized to this area. If clinical suspicion is high and routine anteroposterior, lateral, and oblique x-rays are equivocal, multiple oblique x-rays (Broden's views) can be obtained. These usually show minimal fractures and accurately demonstrate the extent of deformity in more severe fractures. Calcaneal fractures are usually accompanied by considerable swelling. Initial treatment usually requires continuous elevation of the extremity above the heart for a number of days. Ice and bulky compression dressings help to control the swelling and the pain. When the swelling is controlled, plaster-of-paris immobilization is used. Some orthopedic surgeons recommend surgical treatment for some of these fractures.

Perhaps the most serious injury to the foot is a dislocation through the midtarsal region (a *Chopart dislocation*). This results from severe torsional stress on the foot. Deformity may be significant and the injury is frequently open. Pain and tenderness are severe and diffuse across the midfoot region, and swelling is usually massive. This dislocation should be reduced as soon as practicable after x-rays are obtained. It is frequently unstable and often requires open reduction and pin fixation to afford stability during healing. Circulatory compromise is a frequent sequela to this injury and 30% of patients may develop necrosis, resulting in partial foot amputation. Occasionally this dislocation may be spontaneously reduced or at least be only minimally displaced at the time x-rays are obtained. The x-rays must be carefully scrutinized and multiple oblique films may be needed. Small avulsion fractures at the calcaneocuboid joint laterally, or about the tarsal navicular dorsally and medially, may be clues that the joints were dislocated at the time of injury. When this injury is suspected or confirmed, it should not be neglected.

Isolated fractures of the *individual tarsal bones* are usually due to direct blows or tendon or ligament avulsion. The history or mechanism of injury and the site of tenderness and swelling indicate the area of concern on x-ray. Stress on the posterior tibial tendon insertion on the tarsal navicular bone may result in an avulsion fracture. It is much more likely, however, that the ossicle seen in this region on the x-ray represents a developmental accessory navicular bone and the actual injury is just a strain of the tendon. Fractures of the distal tarsal row can result from direct trauma, but one must be certain that they are not part of a more serious injury, such as a midtarsal fracture-dislocation (Chopart's fracture-dislocation). The isolated fractures usually require only elevation, a bulky compression dressing, ice bags, and use of crutches, but if symptoms warrant, a short leg walking cast may be used.

Tarsal-metatarsal dislocation is also a potentially disabling injury and may be misdiagnosed. It also is the result of a torsional injury to the foot and usually involves lateral displacement of the second, third, fourth, and fifth metatarsals with the first metatarsal remaining intact. Considerable pain and swelling are present, and the swelling may mask any deformity. The key to recognizing this injury on x-ray is to assess carefully the relationship of the tarsals to the metatarsals, comparing them with x-rays of the uninjured foot if necessary. Of most importance is the relationship of the first to the second metatarsal. Usually the space between the two is widened and there may be small avulsion fractures in the vicinity. This is a serious injury and surgical repair is usually recommended.

Metatarsal fractures are usually the result of direct blow trauma, except for the avulsion fracture of the base of the fifth metatarsal. Fracture of the *base of the fifth metatarsal* (the Jones fracture) results from inversion stress on the foot, causing avulsion of the attachment of the peroneus brevis tendon to the base of the fifth metatarsal. There is very localized tenderness and swelling in the area. It is often difficult to confirm the diagnosis unequivocally, because this area is often the site of a developmental accessory bone. Regardless of whether the injury is a true fracture or a tendon strain with an associated accessory bone, treatment is symptomatic with use of a compression dressing, ice bags, crutch ambulation, and a plaster-of-paris cast as necessary.

Fractures of the metatarsals from direct trauma are painful injuries but usually of little permanent significance. Displacement is usually minimal because of the connecting intermetatarsal ligament system. Treatment, in general, is symptomatic with the use of compression dressings, ice bags, and crutches initially, followed by strapping with tape or a plaster-of-paris cast as needed. Open fractures, such as those seen in rotary lawnmower injuries, require surgical debridement and must be repaired. A special situation is the *stress fracture,* usually of the third or fourth metatarsal shaft which is called the *march fracture* because of the frequency with which it is seen in military recruits who do considerable marching during basic training. In this injury, pain develops over a period of time related to the increased foot stress, and swelling appears. The x-rays show the fracture developing at the same time as healing callus is seen. Treatment is symptomatic and involves decreasing the stress and immobilization while healing occurs.

Fractures and dislocations of the phalanges of the toes occur frequently. They are often due to stubbing the bare toes on a hard object, such as a chair or table leg. The dislocation is easily reduced by direct traction, using digital block anesthesia as required. Fractures are well treated by grossly aligning the toes and then taping adjacent toes together for immobilization. Additional treatment usually is not required.

References

1. Conwell, H. E., and Reynolds, F. C. 1961. *Management of Fractures, Dislocations, and Sprains,* 7th ed. St. Louis, C. V. Mosby Co.
2. Crenshaw, A. H. 1971. *Campbell's Operative Orthopaedics.* St. Louis, C. V. Mosby Co., pp. 477–691.
3. Rockwood, C. A., and Green, D. P. (in press). *Fractures.* Philadelphia, J. B. Lippincott Co.
4. Watson-Jones, R. 1955. *Fractures and Joint Injuries,* 4th ed., Baltimore, Williams & Wilkins Co.
5. Kohler, A., and Zimmer, E. A. 1968. *Borderlines of the Normal and Early Pathologic in Skeletal Roentgenology,* S. P. Wilk (ed.). New York, Grune & Stratton.
6. Hampton, O. P. 1951. *Wounds of the Extremities in Military Surgery.* St. Louis, C. V. Mosby Co.
7. Blout, W. P. 1955. *Fractures in Children.* Baltimore, Williams & Wilkins Co.

8. Salter, R. B., and Harris, W. R. 1963. Injuries involving the epiphyseal plate. *J. Bone Joint Surg.,* 45A:587.
9. Behling, F. 1973. Treatment of acromio-clavicular separations. *Ortho. Clin. N. Amer.,* 4:747.
10. Neer, C. S. 1970. Displaced proximal humeral fractures. Part I: Classification and evaluation. *J. Bone Joint Surg.,* 52A:1077.
11. O'Rahilly, R. O. 1953. A survey of carpal and tarsal anomalies. *J. Bone Joint Surg.,* 35A:626
12. Russe, O. 1960. Fracture of the carpal navicular. Diagnosis, non-operative treatment and operative treatment. *J. Bone Joint Surg.,* 42A:759.
13. Moberg, E. 1960. Fractures and ligamentous injuries of the thumb and finger. *Surg. Clin. N. Amer.,* 40:297.
14. Stark, H. H. 1970. Troublesome fractures and dislocations of the hand. *A.A.O.S. Instruct. Course Lectures,* 19:130.
15. Eaton, R. G. 1971. *Joint Injuries of the Hand.* Springfield, Charles C Thomas.
16. Dunn, A. W., and Morris, H. D. 1968. Fractures and dislocations of the pelvis. *J. Bone Joint Surg.,* 50A:1639.
17. Gregory, C. F., Epstein, H. C., and Lowell, J. D. 1973. Fractures and dislocations of the hip and fractures of the acetabulum. *A.A.O.S. Instruct. Course Lectures,* 22:105.
18. O'Donoghue, D. H. 1962. *Treatment of Injuries to Athletes.* Philadelphia, W. B. Saunders Co.
19. Helfet, A. J. 1970. Diagnosis and management of internal derangements of the kneejoint. *A.A.O.S. Instruct. Course Lectures,* 19:63.
20. Lauge-Hansen, N. 1946. Fractures of the ankle. *Arch. Surg.,* 56:259.
21. Malka, J. S., and Taillard, W. 1969. Results of non-operative and operative treatment of fractures of the ankle. *Clin. Ortho. Rel. Res.,* 67:159.

26

Initial Evaluation and Management of Spinal Injuries

Louis W. Meeks

All patients seen in the emergency department who have a history of significant trauma must be carefully evaluated and prophylactically managed for a spinal injury, particularly if the trauma is associated with a motor vehicular accident, diving mishap, contact sports injury, or a fall from a height. Fractures, dislocations, and soft tissue injuries of the spine are becoming increasingly common. The physician must be continually aware that additional spinal cord damage can be caused by injudicious manipulation of the patient with a skeletal injury.

Initial Examination and Immobilization

Patients with spinal injuries often relate a fear of a broken back or neck. The cardinal symptom of a fractured spine is acute local pain, which may radiate into the arms, shoulders, chest, abdomen, or lower extremities. These patients may also be comatose, have head injuries, or have evidence of multiple trauma. At this point, further evaluation should be carried out without moving the patient's spine.

Initial examination consists of palpation of the entire vertebral column. Local tenderness, prominence of the spinous processes, and muscle spasm are of special diagnostic significance and help to localize the injury.

Immobilization of the spine is imperative prior to further evaluation. The supine patient is gently placed on a rigid surface, such as a "spine board." For cervical injuries, laterally placed sandbags or preferably a headhalter is applied. Eight or ten pounds of longitudinal traction in neutral flexion-extension is helpful. This form of immobilization facilitates the transfer necessary for obtaining x-rays and other procedures.[3]

Neurologic Examination

Following the safe positioning of the patient, documentation of the neurologic defecit is imperative. Motor assessment (corticospinal function) includes voluntary muscle contractions and involuntary response to painful stimuli. Also important is the degree of muscular resistance to passive movements (tone). The ability to contract voluntarily the anal sphincter is tested at the same time that the bulbocavernosus reflex is assessed.

The sensory examination includes the spinothalamic tract, which is assessed by response to pain elicited with a pin. The posterior columns carry the position and vibratory sense, which should be evaluated in both upper and lower extremities.

Finally, the deep tendon reflexes, abdominal and cremasteric reflexes, are assessed. The presence or absence of the Babinski sign is also noted.

The neurologic deficit is usually correlated with the level and severity of the spinal cord lesion.[2] The mildest form of spinal cord injury is concussion; the symptoms are transient and usually disappear within a few hours. In incomplete cord injury, a varying amount of sensation or movement is retained. The most severe and irreversible injury is cord transection, which is characterized by immediate, complete, and permanent motor and sensory loss below the level of the injury. The typical findings of transverse injury of the cord at various levels are as follows:

At the level of the second or third vertebra:

1. Complete flaccid paralysis, respiratory paralysis
2. Complete areflexia
3. Anesthesia up to the level of the mandible
4. Bowel and bladder retention
5. Death unless artificial respiration is maintained

At the level of the fifth or sixth cervical vertebra:

1. Quadriplegia—complete loss of motor power up to the level of the shoulder girdle; possible persistence of some deltoid, pectoral, and biceps function; no intercostal respirations
2. Complete areflexia except possibly for the biceps reflex
3. Anesthesia of the ulnar half of the upper extremities and below the clavicle
4. Priapism as well as bowel and bladder retention

At the level of the first to twelfth thoracic vertebrae:

1. Paraplegia
2. Areflexia of the lower extremities, including the plantar and cremasteric reflexes; upper abdominal reflexes possibly preserved in a low dorsal lesion
3. Anesthesia with a dermatomal distribution depending on level of cord lesion
4. Priapism as well as bowel and bladder retention

At the level of the first to fifth lumbar vertebrae (cauda equina):

1. Partial flaccid paraplegia
2. Abdominal and cremasteric reflexes present; patellar tendon reflex present in injuries below the fourth lumbar vertebra; ankle and plantar reflexes absent
3. Perineal anesthesia; lower extremity anesthesia possibly asymmetrical and spotty
4. Bowel or bladder retention possible

Some of these patients may have pronounced motor and sensory changes in one or more of the extremities immediately after injury. The physician must therefore precisely differentiate between paralysis and paresis when he first examines the patient. The presence of some sensation in the extremities or a flicker of toe motion must be noted. It affords a better prognosis because cord conduction has not been completely interrupted. Following the careful recording of the neurologic findings, a fair assessment of the level and severity of the spinal lesion can be made.

X-Ray Evaluation of the Cervical Spine

After the patient suspected of having a spinal lesion has been examined and immobilized, he can be transported to the x-ray department for the appropriate roentgenographic studies. He should always be accompanied by the examining physician. Neck injuries in particular have extremely serious connotations for major disability. The patient should not be asked to sit or stand under any circumstances.

A cross-table lateral view is obtained with the neck immobilized or supported by the physician in neutral extension or flexion. Roentgenographic visualization of the odontoid process (open mouth view) and the cervicodorsal junction (swimmer's or Twining's view) is imperative. Then an anteroposterior view is obtained. Neck motion should not be allowed or determined until these views have been obtained and evaluated by the physician in charge. If these x-rays are of good quality and reveal no evidence of fracture or dislocation, oblique views of the cervical spine and flexion and extension x-rays may be obtained with the physician in attendance. If there is any question of fracture or instability, a neurosurgeon, orthopedic surgeon, or both, should be consulted before the x-ray evaluation is completed.

The cervical fractures or subluxations that are most commonly missed in the emergency department involve the atlas, axis (including the odontoid process), and cervicodorsal junction. Upon reviewing these cases, the x-rays usually are either of poor quality or do not visualize the entire cervical spine.[1] This is frequently the case in the patient who has a short, thick neck. The special views, therefore, are mandatory.

Complete views of the thoracic, lumbar, and lumbosacral regions may be safely obtained in the lateral position. This requires two persons to turn the patient like a log, using a sheet or blanket so that the spinal alignment is not altered during the maneuver. Spot views of the area of pain and local tenderness are desired in these longer parts of the spine. Occasionally, laminagrams are required to obtain fine detail.

The emergency department physician must be familiar with the proper and systematic approach to spinal x-ray evaluation. The method recommended is the ABC'S of roentgenologic diagnosis: A—alignment, B—bony mineralization, C—cartilage space, and S—soft tissue. The mnemonic ABC'S are easy to remember and allow the physician to isolate unusual findings quickly and in a logical order.[4] The roentgenographic features plus the clinical evaluation, therefore, usually lead to the correct diagnosis.

When multiple bones and joints are included on a single film, an orderly assessment is essential. This is obviously the case in any x-ray of the spine. If localization is a problem, a hypodermic needle may be inserted at the level of localized spinal tenderness, and a coned-down spot view may be obtained.

Alignment is evaluated by observing the contour of an imaginary line drawn along the anterior and posterior margins of the vertebral bodies. A similar line drawn along the anterior margins of the spinous processes is also helpful. These lines should form smooth and continuous arcs. Care is required in comparing the height of the anterior and posterior margins of the vertebral bodies. These are almost equal in adults and older children. If not, the body has a wedge shaped appearance and probably represents a compression fracture. In children less than 10 years of age, however, the ossification of the anterosuperior portion of the cervical vertebrae (especially the third and fourth) is lower than that of the posterior counterpart. This gives a wedge shaped appearance that can be misinterpreted as a compression fracture.

Bony mineralization assessment is important because it may indicate preexisting disease. Osteopenia (decreased osseous density) may represent either osteoporosis or osteomalacia. Further laboratory evaluation is indicated. Rheumatoid arthritis often is also associated with subluxation of the atlas and axis as well as of the other cervical vertebrae. In the atlas, the anterior ring and the odontoid process are separated by more than 2.5 mm. Radiolucent linear or comminuted sharp lines indicate probable fractures of the lamina pedicles or neural arches. Conversely, localized areas of radiodensity may represent compression fractures.

Cartilage space assessment is necessary in evaluating supportive soft tissue disruption with associated subluxation or dislocation. An x-ray of a normal lateral spine demonstrates the alignment of each vertebra and the appearance of the articulating facets. The superior and inferior articulating processes are parallel and there is a well defined, uniform joint space between them. The odontoid process lies in close approximation to the anterior ring of the atlas. It is held firmly in place by a strong transverse ligament that prevents its separation during flexion and hyperextension of the neck. As previously mentioned, disruption exists if this space is greater than 2.5 mm. These areas, as well as the joints of Luschka (the pointed projections at the posterosuperior vertebral margins) are synovial-lined joints. They must be closely scrutinized to rule out traumatic disruption, which may indicate potential instability.

Soft tissues are carefully assessed. Changes in the height of the intervertebral disc spaces are evaluated. The height of the disc space is decreased in degenerative, traumatic, and infectious spondylosis. In the cervical spine, degenerative changes tend to begin at the intervertebral space between the fifth and sixth cervical vertebrae. This is the level at which pivotal motion is greatest. In the lumbar spine, these changes are at the level of greatest mechanical loading, *i.e.,* disc spaces from the fourth lumbar to the first sacral vertebra. Careful observation of the soft tissue space anterior to the cervical spine will aid in detecting fractures. If the retropharyngeal space anterior to the third cervical vertebra is greater than 5 mm., edema or hemorrhage is present in this area.

Roentgenographic examination has a very important place in the diagnosis and management of the patient with a spinal injury. Great consideration must be given to the sequence of obtaining and interpreting the views that are indicated. It is possible for a patient to sustain a serious injury of the cervical spine without radiologic abnormalities. The more frequent flexion injuries, however, are usually visualized. Momentary flexion injuries are rare, but if there is instability, it is recognized on forward flexion films. If the film of the cervical spine is grossly normal in the presence of neurologic deficit, one can practically assume that the injury was one of hyperextension. It is improbable that momentary dislocations would occur in the more stable and less mobile thoracic or lumbar spine. The wedge fracture is by far the most common injury to the thoracolumbar spine.

Transportation

Specific instructions for transporting or transferring the patient with a spinal injury and neurologic deficit are pertinent because specialized medical centers are necessary for these patients. An emergency physician's initial care is directed toward determining if there is shock or embarrassed respiration. Simultaneously, the patient is comforted and neural injury is assessed. If neural deficit exists, one must recognize that only the best medical facilities even approach adequacy. The following outline may serve as a helpful check list when preparing the patient for transfer.[3,11]

1. Immobilize the patient
   A. Fracture board plus sandbags for cervical injuries
   B. Fracture board for thoracic and lumbar injuries
2. Insert a nasogastric tube to decompress a paralytic ileus
3. Establish an adequate airway with good oxygenation
4. Insert an intercath, preferably a No. 16
5. Administer dexamethasone (40 to 50 mg.) intravenously every 4 to 6 hours
6. Administer hyperosmotic solutions—urea or mannitol in the acute phase of injury may decrease spinal cord edema
7. Insert a Foley catheter—urinary retention develops at once after every severe cord injury.
8. Carefully record and send the neurologic evaluation to the facility receiving the patient. Include information concerning the accident and mechanism of spinal injury plus the x-rays documenting it.

Types of Spinal Injuries

The types of injuries are first discussed briefly and then the more severe or potentially disabling entities are covered in more detail according to anatomic regions.

Strains. Muscles and joint structures have inherent elasticity, which permits a definite range of passive motion exceeding the range of active motion. If motion is forced beyond this passive limit, the muscles and joint ligaments and capsules sustain strain injuries, which are painful for a few days to a few weeks, but the structures return to their pretraumatic state without permanent damage. Treatment is supportive and the patient should be reassured.

Sprains. Joint structures and associated muscles sustain sprain injuries when they are forced so far beyond their passive range of motion that they are stretched, torn, or avulsed from their attachments. These injuries result in hemorrhage and traumatic inflammation. Healing of the sprained soft tissue structures takes place by the formation of fibrous scar tissue, which is less elastic and less functional than normal tissue. Sprains, therefore, result in permanent damage. The injured part should be at rest while healing ensues. Treatment, therefore, could include use of a soft cervical collar, cervical traction, rest, heat or ice (whichever is most beneficial), and analgesics. Severe sprains may require hospitalization. The patient must be warned that the symptoms may persist for several weeks or even months. Gradual improvement is the rule.

Subluxations. Incomplete displacement of the articular surfaces of a joint is called a subluxation. It is a common neck injury resulting from a fall on the head, such as in diving, or from a sudden flexion motion of the neck. The cervical vertebral body is shifted forward on the vertebra below it. The articular facet is subluxed but there is no overriding of articular processes (dislocation). Spinal flexion x-rays are essential to document this injury. Adequate immobilization and treatment are necessary to avoid recurrent subluxation with consequent neuritis. Occasionally, chronic recurrent subluxation with pain may necessitate a spinal fusion.

Dislocations. Complete disruption of the integrity of a joint with deformity is called a dislocation. Severe residual damage results if the injury is not treated initially by the appropriate specialist.

Fractures. Forced hyperflexion or hyperextension of the spine causes a variety of fractures or disruption of the cartilage plates. Sudden forceful hyperflexion of the vertebral column causes compression fractures of the vertebral bodies and avulsion fractures of the joint facets. Forceful hyperextension may cause compression fractures of the interarticular isthmuses and of the upward lateral projections of the vertebral bodies. Fractures of the transverse processes usually occur in the lumbar spine as a result of sudden muscular contraction or a direct blow. Fractures of the spinous processes (clay shoveler's fractures) occur in the lower cervical and first thoracic vertebrae. These are avulsion fractures caused by violent hyperextension of the neck, usually while shoveling heavy materials. The mechanism of injury, therefore, is helpful in diagnosing as well as determining the position in which to immobilize spinal fractures.

Disc Injuries. The intervertebral disc structures are frequently injured and often undiagnosed. These injuries vary from a slight rent in the annulus fibrosus to complete avulsion with or without displacement. Any disc injury causes a disturbance in the motor unit of which the disc is a part. This leads to degeneration of the disc as well as the proximate joints.

Injuries of the Neural Structures. Compression or contusion of neural structures frequently occurs when the neck is forced into hyperflexion or hyperextension. Sudden deceleration, such as in vehicular accidents, is a common cause. The spinal cord, nerve roots, and sympathetic nerves may sustain varying degrees of injuries.

Vascular Injuries. The vertebral arteries are susceptible to traction or contusion injuries at the point at which they traverse the cervical foramina (except the seventh) of the transverse processes. The resultant spinal vascular insufficiencies vary in severity and duration.

Muscular Injuries. The paravertebral muscles are intricate and complex in structure and action and are subject to injury. Muscular strains and spasms have already been discussed and should be treated according to the degree of injury.

Stable vs. Unstable Injuries. Spinal injuries should be assessed to determine whether they are stable or unstable. This depends upon the integrity of the posterior ligaments, disc bonds, and vertebrae. If there has been a disruption of the posterior spinal ligaments, the injury is unstable. This is most common following a flexion or flexion-rotation injury. Certain fractures, including those of the neural arch and most laminar fractures of the fourth and fifth lumbar vertebrae, are likely to be unstable. One must also consider all fracture subluxations and dislocations to be unstable. The common anterior and lateral wedge fractures, if mild or moderate, are probably stable.

Cervical Spinal Injuries

The cervical spine is mobile but does not have great structural stability. The most significant anatomic structures providing stability are the thick neck musculature, the large, well developed ligamentum nuchae, the vertebral bodies and the intervertebral discs. The cervical spine is therefore susceptible to significant injury from sudden forces of acceleration or deceleration, such as those involved in motor vehicular accidents. Approximately 90% of cervical spinal disorders result from trauma, 85% of which involve motor vehicular accidents. As many as 10% of patients with cervical spinal disorders have neurologic evidence of spinal cord or root injury.

The type of fracture, dislocation, or soft tissue injury depends on the forces involved, *i.e.,* flexion, extension, or rotation. An understanding of the various cervical spinal injuries can therefore be obtained through knowledge of the pathodynamic forces and the local anatomy. For example, with a severe hyperflexion injury, the posterior ligamentous structures (ligamentum nuchae, interspinous ligaments, and ligamentum flavum) are disrupted. There may be facet dislocation or fracture associated with compression of the vertebral body. Often the intervertebral disc bond is disrupted with or without protrusion. Rotation injuries cause facet dislocation (unilateral or bilateral) with avulsion of the intervertebral disc. It appears that in hyperextension injuries, the sequence of pathological events is in reverse order to that in flexion injuries.

The atlantoaxial articulation is different from that of the other cervical vertebrae. Because of this variation in functional anatomy, the injuries are often unique. The atlas is composed of a simple bony ring. Embryologically, it contributes the odontoid process to the axis.[2] Great rotatory mobility is provided to the atlas and axis by means of shallow, broad, horizontal articular facets. These vertebrae are therefore susceptible to dislocation because of the lack of stabilizing structures. Such a dislocation may occur as a unilateral facet dislocation with the ring intact and no neurologic deficit. Dislocation may also be associated with a fracture through the isthmus or base of the odontoid process. There have been many reports of dislocations of the atlas and axis associated with infection, rheumatoid arthritis, and congenital absence of the odontoid process.[2] If the patient survives the initial trauma, these injuries usually do not require surgical fusion, nor do they result in serious neurologic difficulties.

The classic fracture of the atlas is a "bursting" fracture, which was first described by Jefferson in 1920. It results from a fall with the head held erect and a vertical load is transmitted along the spine. The energy resulting from the opposing forces is exerted laterally on the ring of the atlas. The passage for the cord through the atlas is large. When the fracture occurs, the fragments usually spread outward, increasing the circumference of the atlas. The fracture therefore "decompresses" the spinal cord, and neural injury is uncommon. Laminectomy is not necessary unless fragments of bone are driven inward. Patients without neural deficit do well with a period of skeletal traction followed by brace immobilization.

Fractures of the axis most commonly involve the odontoid process because the weakest and most vulnerable portion of the axis is the junction of the odontoid process and the atlas. The history usually reveals a fall followed by neck soreness and stiffness. Neurologic signs and symptoms are infrequent. Following external immobilization, these fractures heal by either fibrous or osseous union without serious sequelae. "Hangman's fracture" is a rare injury of the axis that occurs through either the pedicles or the laminae.[2] The cord may escape serious injury, but considerable spinal instability is the rule.

The most common fractures and dislocations are those between the third cervical and first thoracic vertebrae. Dislocations are unstable lesions in that they may be easily reduced by traction and gentle manipulation, but at the end of a reasonable period of immobilization they recur. Because there is a potential for serious neurologic damage, careful skeletal traction immobilization and reduction usually are followed by spinal fusion. Compression or vertical fractures involving one or more vertebrae between the second cervical and first thoracic vertebrae have a higher incidence of severe and permanent cord damage. Neural arch fractures are believed to be the result of rotation injuries, and many are associated with fractures of the transverse process. With displacement, the superior facet slides forward while the inferior facet retains its normal position. These fractures are frequently unstable.

The acute anterior spinal cord syndrome should be discussed with respect to cervical injuries. This condition, described by Schneider, occurs almost exclusively in the cervical region and represents anterior cord compression by dislodged intervertebral disc material, a bone fragment ("tear-drop fracture"), or actual destruction of the anterior portion of the spinal cord.[10] This syndrome is characterized by complete paralysis, hypoesthesia, and hypalgesia below the level of injury but with preservation of touch, position, and some vibratory sense. Prompt, extensive laminectomy and division of the dentate ligaments is recommended. Fusion at a later date is often required.

Dorsal and Lumbar Spinal Injuries

Nicoll reported that approximately 66% of dorsolumbar fractures involve three vertebrae, *i.e.,* the twelfth thoracic and first and second lumbar vertebrae.[8] These are of particular interest to the physician because most paraplegics sustain trauma to this segment. Unlike the cervical spinal fractures, these injuries are often the result of indirect trauma, such as a fall on the feet or buttocks. The impact is concentrated in the dorsolumbar region because this is the juncture between the mobile lumbar spine and the relatively immobile thoracic spine. This is also the level at which there is an enlargement of the spinal cord prior to termination in the conus medullaris at about the second lumbar vertebra with concentration of nerve roots. One skeletal segment represents a much greater difference in the functional level of neurologic deficit.[7] Without fracture displacement or dislocation of the posterior elements of the spinal column, neurologic damage seldom, if ever, occurs.

The compression fracture involves the vertebral body and usually is the result of sharp forward flexion. The anterosuperior corner of the vertebral body may be broken off; more commonly, the vertebra is subjected to compression forces and the cancellous bone is impacted into itself. If the compression is definite and is less that 25% of the height of the body, the patient should be observed for development of an adynamic ileus. Treatment should be symptomatic and the patient can be reassured that no significant disability is anticipated. If a greater degree of compression exists, an attempt at reduction is indicated except in the elderly. This involves local hyperextension in an attempt to elevate the fragment by the intact anterior ligaments. Once the vertebral height has been reestablished, immobilization is necessary until fracture healing occurs. Failure to correct a significant compression fracture may be disabling.

Fracture of the lumbar lateral processes is a common athletic injury. The lumbar vertebrae have spikelike lateral processes, some of which are thin or have narrow necks. These fractures are the result of a direct blow or violent muscular contraction or a combination of both. Fractures of multiple processes are almost always of the avulsion type. In any event, the significance of this fracture is related to the muscular injury and not the broken bone. There often is considerable separation at the fracture site and nonunion is common. Treatment depends upon the severity of the symptoms. Initially the patient should be placed at bed rest with local application of cold, followed by heat. After a few days, the acute symptoms should subside and support should be applied to the back. Ordinarily, the symptoms disappear within six weeks.

Vertebral arch fractures are potentially dangerous because of the possibility of neurologic involvement.[5] Once the fracture is recognized, the patient must be immobilized to permit it to heal because painful function may result if union is imperfect. This is a serious injury that should be treated as such.

Thoracolumbar dislocations and fracture-dislocations are unique injuries because almost all are unstable.[5] They have the potential to produce a neural deficit where initially none existed or to cause an increase in a previously incomplete neural deficit. It is not a rare injury and accounts for 4% of all spinal fractures.[6] Lumbar dislocation accounts for 10 to 20% of all thoracolumbar fractures. It should be pointed out that x-rays show only the displacement present at the time of the exposure and not the maximal displacement or the potential for redisplacement. The more unstable the injury, the more likely it is that placing the patient in the supine position to obtain the roentgenogram will accomplish partial or complete reduction. Flexion views should not be obtained to assess the degree of displacement. All apparent subluxations of the lumbar spine should be considered to have been dislocations at the instant of injury and should be treated as such. Back pain at the level of injury is a prominent feature of the history. The most reliable physical sign of lumbar dislocation is a palpable gap between the spinous processes, which is seen in approximately 8% patients. More than 50% have some degree of neural deficit. Conus function will return if the injury is a reversible anatomic lesion, such as edema, concussion, or mild hemorrhage.

Division of axons or crushing of neural cells results in an irreversible loss of function. The portion of the deficit due to damage of motor units may recover if the fibrous epineurium of the root fasciculi remains intact. This does not apply to the sensory components of the cauda equina because the sensory ganglion cells are located outside the spinal canal. Regeneration does not take place if the lesion is located between the ganglion cells and the cord.

Lap Seat Belt Injuries

The automobile lap seat belt has proven to be an effective means of reducing the severity of injury and the incidence of fatalities in vehicular accidents. A number of recent reports of specific visceral and musculoskeletal injuries in seat belt users warrant consideration. The injuries that constitute the seat belt syndrome are not unique to the seat belt wearer and in no way differ from injuries produced by other forms of severe blunt trauma.[12] A lap seat belt focuses collision forces on the abdomen, dorsolumbar spine, and pelvis. The spinal injury is characterized by marked spreading of the posterior elements without the usually expected decrease in vertebral height. This injury typically shows a seat belt contusion across the lower part of the abdomen at a level just cephalad to the anterior iliac spine. If an unstable fracture-dislocation exists, a palpable interspinous process defect and localized tenderness usually are present. This is potentially a severe injury, and a close examination for spinal fracture-dislocation, neural deficit, and associated abdominal injuries is imperative.

References

1. Bailey, R. W. 1964. "Missed" fractures of the cervical spine. *Wisconsin Med. J.,* 63:333–339.
2. Bailey, R. W. 1974. *The Cervical Spine.* Philadelphia, Lea & Febiger.

3. American College of Surgeons. 1972. *Early Care of the Injured Patient.* Philadelphia, W. B. Saunders.
4. Forrester, D. M., and Nesson, J. W. 1973. *The Radiology of Joint Disease.* Philadelphia, W. B. Saunders.
5. Holdsworth, F. W. 1963. Fractures, dislocations, and fracture-dislocations of the spine. *J. Bone Joint Surg.,* 45B:6–20.
6. Kaufer, H., and Hayes, J. T. 1966. Lumbar fracture-dislocation. *J. Bone Joint Surg.,* 48A:712–730.
7. Kelly, R. P., and Whitesides, T. E., Jr. 1968. Treatment of lumbodorsal fracture-dislocations *Ann. Surg.,* 167:705-717.
8. Nicoll, E. A. 1949. Fractures of the dorso-lumbar spine. *J. Bone Joint Surg.,* 31B:376–394.
9. Ruge, D. 1969. *Spinal Cord Injuries.* Springfield, Ill., Charles C Thomas.
10. Schneider, R. C. 1955. The syndrome of acute anterior spinal cord injury. *J. Neurosurg.,* 12:95.
11. Sharpe, J. C., and Marx, F. W. 1969. *Management of Medical Emergencies,* 2nd ed. New York, McGraw-Hill Book Co.
12. Smith, W. S., and Kaufer, H. 1969. Patterns and mechanisms of lumbar injuries associated with lap seatbelts. *J. Bone Joint Surg.,* 51A:239–254.

27

Initial Management of Injuries of the Hand

Robert M. Oneal

The importance of the hand to human function and well being is difficult to overemphasize. The hand together with the brain separates *Homo sapiens* from the rest of the animal kingdom. Even a casual analysis of the complex structure of the hand overwhelms the observer with its beauty of organization, its intricate interdependence of parts, and the wide range of its functional potential.

The hand is essential, and it is vulnerable to injury. The frequency and severity of serious hand injuries is impressive to anyone with experience in the field of trauma. The economic loss as well as the psychologic scars to the patient cannot be overestimated. Even seemingly minor wounds can lead to serious disability if the injuries are mismanaged.

The main purpose of this chapter is to present an approach to the evaluation of hand injuries by the primary care physicians and to provide a guideline for their management.

An understanding of the basic form of the hand and its anatomy is essential in evaluating injuries, but space does not permit a detailed description of the complex anatomy and its functional significance. The reader is referred to excellent texts and atlases on the subject.[1-5]

The digits are commonly referred to as the thumb and the index, middle, ring, and little fingers. Distal to the two rows of carpal bones of the wrist are five metacarpals, which articulate with the proximal phalanges at the metacarpophalangeal joint. The thumb has only two phalanges and their articulation is the interphalangeal joint.

The fingers each have three phalanges—proximal, middle, and distal. There are therefore two interphalangeal joints in each finger—the proximal and distal interphalangeal joints.

The metacarpal area of the hand can be considered as having a rigid central unit containing the second and third metacarpal bones with laterally placed movable units, the thumb metacarpal on the radial side and the ring and little finger metacarpal bones on the ulnar side.

The hand is both an intricate motor device and a complex sensory area. There are both extrinsic and intrinsic musculotendonous units. The extrinsic ones, which originate in the forearm and insert in the wrist and hand, include the muscles that flex and extend the wrist and digits. The intrinsic muscles, which originate and insert within the hand, are coordinating muscles of the hand and include the interosseous, lumbrical, adductor of the thumb, and thenar and hypothenar muscles.

The hand is supplied by three nerves (Fig. 27-1). The motor innervation follows a functional plan. The radial nerve innervates all the extrinsic muscles that extend the wrist and open the digits. These muscles prepare the hand for action. The median nerve innervates the extrinsic flexor, intrinsic thenar, and lumbrical muscles of the radial digital tripod.[6] This functional unit of the thumb and index and middle fingers is concerned with opposition, fine pinch, and manipulation. The sensation of the volar aspect of these same fingers is also supplied by the median nerve (Figs. 27-1 and 27-2). The ulnar nerve innervates the extrinsic flexor and intrinsic muscles of the ulnar hook, which includes the ring

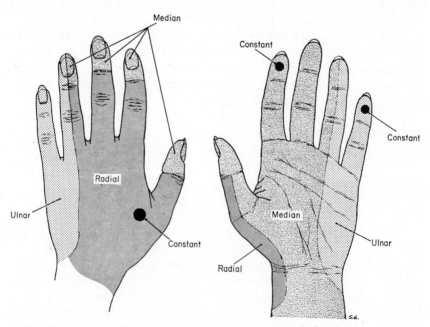

Fig. 27-1. Distributions of sensory innervation to the dorsal and volar aspects of the hand.

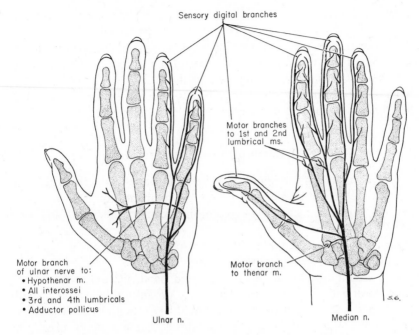

Fig. 27-2. Relationships of the volar mixed nerves of the hand.

and little fingers. This functional area is concerned with power grip. The corresponding volar skin on the fingers and palm are supplied by the sensory divisions of the ulnar nerve.

These motor and sensory units combine to provide the complex, co-ordinated functions of the hand that we are so dependent upon. As an example, a clenched fist employs the ulnar and median innervated flexor and intrinsic muscles plus radially innervated wrist extensors.

Finger flexion is mediated by the flexor profundus, which flexes the distal phalanx, and the flexor superficialis, which flexes the middle phalanx. They are intimately associated in the fibrous flexor sheath on the volar aspect of the fingers.

The extensor mechanism in the fingers is complex because it contains components of both the extrinsic extensor and the intrinsic muscles.[6,7] The extrinsic extensor inserts into the extensor hood, which encircles the base of the proximal phalanx and extends the metacarpophalangeal joint. Beyond this point, it divides into three bands—a central slip that inserts into and extends the middle phalanx at the proximal interphalangeal joint, and two lateral bands that are dorsal to the proximal inter-phalangeal joint and are joined by fibers from the interosseous and lumbrical muscles to converge and insert into and extend the distal phalanx. Because the interosseous and lumbrical muscles pass volar to the metacarpophalangeal joint before joining the lateral bands, they are flexors of the metacarpophalangeal joints as well as contributors to the extension of the proximal and distal interphalangeal joints. In the thumb, the intrinsic thenar muscles on the radial side and the adductor on the ulnar side contribute to the lateral bands, which with the extensor pollicis longus extend the distal phalanx at the interphalangeal joint.

Examination of the Hand

The examination for injuries of the hand begins with the whole patient. Careful questioning regarding concomitant injuries, significant medical problems, current or recent medications, allergies, and time when food or drink was last ingested is vital. The specific history of the injury should include the time, circumstances, and type of injury as well as details of prior first aid treatment.

For accurate examination of an injured hand, the patient should be lying down with the arm and hand resting on an arm board on a sterile towel. The first rule of examination should be to do no harm. The examiner should wear a mask and sterile gloves and use sterile examining equipment. He should handle the injured parts gently and proceed slowly with adequate explanations to gain the patient's confidence. The patient's cooperation is crucial for a reliable assessment of these injuries.

If the wound is massive or has significant arterial bleeding, hemostats should not be placed in the wound. Instead, pressure should be applied, the arm elevated, and a pneumatic tourniquet placed on the upper part of the arm and inflated to 300 mm. Hg in an adult and 150 to 250 mm. Hg in a child, depending upon the age. This will immediately stop the bleeding. A quick assessment of the injuries can be made, but in this type of injury, the patient will have to be taken to the operating room.

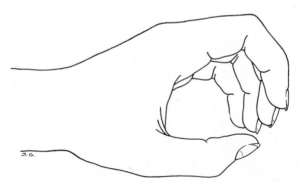

Fig. 27-3. Best functional position for immobilization of the hand.

The soft tissues should be gently reduced and the fingers placed in a position of function (Fig. 27-3). This position is maintained by a bulky dressing that incorporates the entire hand except for the fingertips. The tourniquet is then deflated and the return of capillary fill in the nail beds and fingertips assures the adequacy of circulation. The patient can then be sent for x-rays. Even without massive bleeding, an injured hand should always be dressed and splinted before the patient is sent to the x-ray department or the operating room to minimize the chance of further injury or contamination.

If the wounds are less massive, time can be taken for examination. In this case, one should have a plan to organize the examination. The entire hand should be examined because some injuries are subtle and can easily be missed.

Inspection. Always check for circulation. Check the capillary fill in each fingertip and check wrist pulses.

Observe the hand in the resting position, *i.e.,* in supination with the back of the hand on the table.[8] Normally, the fingers should assume a moderate flexed position increasing in degree from index to little finger. The finger position is similar to the position of function (Fig. 27-3), but the volar surface of the thumb is perpendicular to the volar surface of the fingers in the resting position. If the extrinsic flexors to one of the fingers are not intact, the finger will "rest" in an extended position, the degree of which depends on whether one or both flexors are cut. Ob-

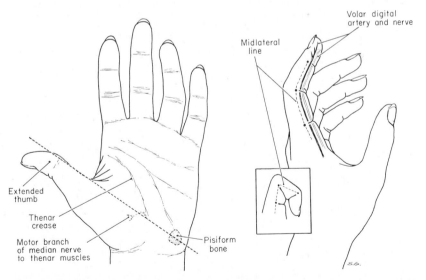

Fig. 27-4. Surface relationships of the motor branch of the median nerve (left); the relationship of the midlateral line of a digit and the neurovascular bundle (right).

serve this position in your own hand. Now, passively *flex* the wrist. Note that the fingers and thumb extend, demonstrating that the extensor mechanism is intact. These simple maneuvers are extremely helpful in children, malingerers, and uncooperative patients.

The location of wounds is a clue to the deeper structures involved. Lacerations on the dorsum are particularly likely to involve extensor tendons, and lacerations of the palm are likely to involve sensory branches of the median and ulnar nerves or the motor branch of the median nerve (Figs. 27-2 and 27-4).

Examination of Bones and Joints. Active flexion and extension indicate integrity of these structures. Note the presence or absence of bony prominences, localized swelling, and asymmetry. Radiologic evaluation is mandatory.

Examination for Nerve Continuity. *Never* inject a local anesthetic into a wound prior to a complete sensory evaluation, because anesthesia delays accurate assessment for several hours. In clean wounds, nerve repair should be carried out primarily in the operating room,[9] and accurate diagnosis is essential in making this decision. Sensation should be checked by pin prick. The areas depicted in Figure 27-1 are helpful. In more peripheral injuries, each finger should be individually treated. Note that the ring finger is innervated by both median and ulnar nerves.

There is no motor nerve function of the radial nerve distal to the wrist. The motor branch of the median nerve enters the thenar intrinsic muscles just beyond the distal end of the volar carpal ligament. Figure 27-2 shows its relationship to the sensory branches and Figure 27-4 illustrates the surface relationships. Injury to this branch can be demonstrated by an inability to abduct the thumb upward from the palm and then rotate it parallel to the palm. Contraction of the thenar muscles should be obvious during this action.

The motor branch of the ulnar nerve penetrates the base of the hypothenar muscles and innervates them; then it crosses the palm as shown in Figure 27-2. It innervates all the interosseous muscles and then the adductor of the thumb. The first dorsal interosseous muscle, filling the dorsum of the first web space, is easiest to palpate during abduction of the index finger radially. Adduction and abduction should be tested with the hand flat to negate the mild adduction and abduction caused by the extrinsic flexors and extensors.

These examinations are notoriously inaccurate in small children. Exploration of suspicious wounds in an operating room may be necessary for accurate diagnosis.

Evaluation of Tendon Function. The action of each tendon must be individually tested. There are no short cuts for learning the musculotendinous units, their locations, and their actions. With complete tendon disruption, there is an absence of motion, unless there are interconnections distal to the injury. This can be the case in the palm between the profundi to the middle, ring, and little fingers, and on the dorsum between the extensor communis tendons to the same fingers. Partial tendon disruption leads to weakness and can be difficult to diagnose. It is important to diagnose, however, because if missed, the partial disruption frequently becomes complete with unrestricted active motion.

When testing for integrity of the flexor profundus and flexor pollicis longus tendons, the proximal joints must be blocked. The test for integrity of the flexor superficialis tendons with an intact profundus is to block in extension the fingers not being tested, which inactivates the profundus to the finger in question. Proximal interphalangeal joint flexion is possible only with an intact superficialis tendon.

Be wary of injuries to the dorsum of the hand and fingers. Extension of the interphalangeal joints of the thumb and fingers is primarily a function of the extrinsic extensors, but there is also a significant contribution from the intrinsic muscles. Many times, direct inspection beneath dorsal wounds is necessary to establish the diagnosis. The results of interruption of this delicate mechanism are not always immediately apparent.

Principles of Treatment

The main objectives in the management of the injured hand are to salvage vital structures, prevent infection, repair injured parts, and restore function and form.

The following priorities of repair are helpful in planning a treatment program:

1. Adequate circulation
2. Satisfactory skin coverage
3. Well aligned skeletal framework
4. Good joint function
5. Restoration of nerve continuity
6. Proper tendon function

All definitive treatment should be carried out under the best possible circumstances. There should be good lighting, a well supported hand table with irrigation basin, and adequate assistance. The surgeon and his assistant should sit during the procedure. Proper instruments, an adequate assortment of fine suture material, a pneumatic tourniquet, a hand holder, and a Hyfrecator for electrocoagulation of small blood vessels are all essential. Milford's text discusses and illustrates these principles in detail.[3] All rings and other encircling jewelry should be removed. The entire hand and forearm should be prepared and draped. Thorough irrigation with large volumes of physiologic solutions is essential. Hexachlorophene and other strong detergents should never be used in open wounds. Povidone-iodine is an excellent solution for this purpose.

Once the correct diagnois is made, the next most important decisions are who will carry out the repair and where. In these modern times, with rapid communications and transportation, all patients with severe hand injuries should be initially referred to a physician trained and experienced in surgery of the hand. Severe wounds can be cleaned, dressed, and splinted in a functional position and referred promptly. Injuries of nerves and major blood vessels, open injuries of tendons, wounds resulting in significant skin loss, and major fractures and dislocations should be repaired in an operating room by an experienced surgeon. Anything less will probably lead to a very poor result.

The following hand injuries can, in general, be treated in adequately staffed emergency departments: (1) lacerations of the skin, (2) fingertip injuries and distal amputations, (3) infections of the subcutaneous tissues, (4) partial thickness burns, and (5) selected closed tendinous and ligamentous injuries.

Emergency department physicians must remember that their primary obligations in the management of patients with hand injuries are adequate first aid, careful assessment of the patient's general condition, and proper diagnosis of the specific injury. It may be more beneficial to the patient to postpone definite care for several hours rather than to proceed with ill-advised and ill-conceived treatment.

Anesthesia. *Local Infiltration.* One percent lidocaine can be infiltrated into lacerations for satisfactory anesthesia, and 1:100,000 epinephrine aids in hemostasis. Epinephrine should not be used around digital arteries and poorly vascularized tissue. When it is used, the maximal effect is not reached for seven minutes.

Digital Block. One percent lidocaine without epinephrine can be deposited around digital nerves at the base of the finger, in the web space, or in the distal part of the palm. In a badly injured and edematous finger, it is best not to inject the base of the finger but to use a block proximal to the web space. Anesthesia of the volar digital nerves is accompanied by anesthesia of the fingertips (Fig. 27-1). Additional proximal dorsal anesthesia can be provided by infiltration of the subcutaneous tissue dorsally at the base of the finger.

Wrist Block. Anesthesia of the median, ulnar, and radial nerves at the wrist is accomplished by perineural infiltration for the median and ulnar nerves and subcutaneous infiltration for the radial nerve. This technique requires knowledge of the specific anatomy and should be used only by those with experience. Wrist block combined with a tourniquet and mild sedation can provide a dry field and satisfactory anesthesia for 45 to 60 minutes in a cooperative patient.

Lacerations

With the exception of human bite wounds and massively contaminated wounds containing questionably devitalized tissue, primary closure of skin wounds should be carried out. (In clean wounds, closure can be carried out as long as eight hours after injury, particularly if antibiotics are used.)

The following procedure can be followed in the treatment of most wounds.

1. Decontaminate the wound
   A. Irrigate copiously with physiologic solutions
   B. Remove all foreign bodies
   C. Do not use pHisoHex in open wounds
2. Test for viability of skin flaps
   A. Check capillary fill
   B. Look for arterial bleeding from the end of the flap
   C. Use tourniquet test—release and look for reactive hyperemia
   D. Reexamine all questionable tissue in 24 to 48 hours
3. Debride obviously nonviable tissue
4. Using atraumatic technique, close wounds carefully and without undue tension
   A. Use properly placed simple sutures of 4-0 or 5-0 nonabsorbable suture to evert the wound edge
   B. Use an occasional vertical mattress suture if necessary to evert the edges
   C. Use a half buried horizontal mattress suture to close the corner of a flap
5. Splint the injured part in a functional position for five to ten days depending upon the severity of the injury
6. Elevate the injured part for 48 hours. Do not use a sling. Ask the patient to hold the hand up while walking and to prop it up while at rest
7. In most cases, do not remove sutures for 14 days

Skin Loss

Small areas of skin loss that are too large to close easily with minimal undermining can be covered with a split thickness skin graft. The graft should not be too thick and can be obtained with a small hand-held dermatome, such as the one made by Week and discussed by Goulian.[10] It is basically a straight razor modified to calibrate the thickness of the graft. The donor site should be prepared with povidone-iodine, lubricated with mineral oil, and held taut with wooden tongue blades. Selection of the donor site is important because the resulting scars can be quite noticeable. The lateral buttock area is the best site. The volar surface of the forearm is easily accessible but should not be used, particularly in women and children, because of the poor cosmetic results.

A split thickness skin graft will take on a well vascularized bed, such as subcutaneous tissue, fascia, or periosteum. Cortical bone, denuded cartilage, or tendon will not support a graft. Adequate hemostasis of the recipient site and immobilization of the graft are essential. A tie-over dressing is effective. The hand should be adequately splinted until the graft is healed, which takes seven to ten days. If there is any chance of bleeding under the graft, it should be inspected within 24 hours and the blood evacuated. Otherwise, the immobilizing dressing should be left undisturbed for seven days unless there are signs of infection.

Puncture Wounds

These wounds are potentially dangerous because they are converted to an anaerobic environment when the thick volar skin is sealed off after withdrawal of the puncturing object. A small cruciate incision should be made at the puncture site and the edges excised to convert it to an open wound. Careful observation, antibiotics, and antitetanus immunization as well as elevation and immobilization are important adjuncts. Many small wounds penetrate important deep structures and can lead to serious unrecognized infections, especially in children.

Foreign Bodies

The history of the nature of the foreign body is important. Organic foreign bodies must be removed and may require an operating room procedure with adequate anesthesia and a tourniquet. Inorganic foreign bodies, such as glass or metal, may be left *in situ* in healed wounds unless they are symptomatic or near vital structures.

Pressure Injection of Foreign Substances

Substances such as paint or grease when accidentally injected into the subcutaneous tissue of the hand produce tremendous inflammation leading to ischemic necrosis. The most important factor is recognition because wide incision and evacuation of the foreign material are necessary. The procedure must be carried out in an operating room.

Replantation of Amputated Parts

Skilled replantation surgeons can be found in many parts of the world. Whenever an emergency department surgeon is confronted with an amputation of an essential part of a hand, the possibility of replantation should be considered.

Specific types of amputations that might be considered for replantation include: (1) thumb of either hand, proximal to interphalangeal joint; (2) dominant index finger, or nondominant index finger, especially in a child; (3) multiple fingers, proximal to mid-middle phalanx; (4) whole hand.

The hand and amputated parts must be managed carefully. Place the hand in a dry sterile dressing. Send for amputated parts if they have not accompanied the patient. Place the part in moist gauze, if available, and then place it in a plastic bag. Put the plastic bag in ice water, but do not put the amputated part in direct contact with the ice because it may become frozen. Do not soak the amputated part in pHisoHex or similar solutions; do not perform any exploratory dissection.

The patient must be sent to a replant surgeon as quickly as possible. With cooling of the amputated part, successful replantation is possible as long as 24 hours after amputation.

Fingertip Injuries

Trauma to fingertips is one of the commonest injuries to the hand. The objectives of treatment are to restore adequate sensation, length, and stability to the fingertip. The fingertips, containing closely spaced specialized nerve endings, provide a sixth sense, as illustrated by the adaptability of the fingertips in blind people. Restoration of tactile sense and maintenance of length are particularly crucial on the ulnar side of the thumb and the opposing radial sides of the index and middle fingers. Although the tip of the ring or little finger can be lost without sacrifice of function in the laborer, in the skilled worker or musician the loss can be significant. In young people, efforts should be made to conserve all possible length in all fingers. In selecting the best method of treatment for a patient, the age, occupation, and right or left handedness must be considered.

16

Repair of Soft Tissues. All vascularized tissue should be preserved and sutured carefully in place. When the distal phalanx is fractured and the nail bed lacerated, one should leave the distal part of the nail attached and suture it to the proximal part of the nail for orientation and stabilization. Adequate splinting, protection, and elevation are essential in postoperative management.

Skin Graft. When skin is lost and an adequate amount of the tactile pad is left, a skin graft can be used. The technique for obtaining a split thickness skin graft has been described under lacerations. During the healing phase, the graft contracts and the defect becomes smaller. If the loss is in an area crucial for sensation, a full thickness skin graft can be taken from the hypothenar area.[11] A pattern is made of the defect and transferred to the donor site. The subcutaneous fat is removed from the dermis and the graft applied in a manner similar to that in a split thickness graft. Full thickness skin grafts provide more durable cover, have less tendency to contract, and tend to achieve better sensory regeneration, but their use should be reserved for ideal cases.

Spontaneous Epithelialization. When there is a small defect in a young child, it can be allowed to heal by secondary intention with a satisfactory result. Epithelialization is usually complete in 10 to 21 days if the wound is kept clean and well protected.

Replacement of Amputated Tissue. In young children, replacement of an amputated fingertip with sutures may occasionally be successful if the wound is sharply incised and if repair is undertaken within two or three hours. Use of magnification to align the fingerprints may be helpful in lining up the dermal circulation. The nail can be used as a splint because it is soft enough to allow passage of the suture needle. In older children and adults, replacement of amputated tips by suturing is so rarely successful that it is almost never recommended.

Local Flaps. When there is significant soft tissue loss and exposure of bone, a local flap is indicated and can be performed under local anesthesia, but a considerable amount of judgment and experience is required. A flap should be considered rather than resorting to shortening of an essential digit simply to obtain closure.

Depending upon the level and availability of adjacent skin, there are several choices of local flaps, including the volar V-Y advancement,[12] the lateral V-Y advancement (Kutler's procedure),[13] and the cross-finger flap.[14] The cross-finger flap can provide more tissue than the other two techniques and it is much more versatile, but an additional operation is required to divide the flap. The return of sensation is not as good with cross-finger flaps as with subcutaneous based local flaps.

The palmar flap is to be condemned. Its use requires an unphysiologic position for the recipient finger, which can lead to permanent stiffness in a susceptible elderly patient. The palmar scar is also frequently painful.

Revision of Amputation and Primary Closure. In a situation in which maintenance of digital length is not crucial, trimming back the bone and closing the soft tissue wound is an expeditious way to get a patient back to work.

When the amputation is through a joint, it is best to leave the proximal cartilage intact but to narrow the lateral prominences. All bone fragments should be removed. All rough edges of amputated bone ends should be smoothed with a rongeur. The digital nerve ends should be identified, dissected, cut off, and allowed to retract proximally to avoid neuroma formation. The flexor and extensor tendons should not be approximated over the bone ends. The skin flaps should be closed loosely.

Fingernail Injuries

These injuries are common and the sequelae of inadequate management are so deforming that a separate discussion is justified. Kleinert and co-workers' report is an important guide to evaluation and management of these injuries.[15]

The fingernail is an ectodermal appendage. The nail is attached to the nail bed, which is closely adherent to the dorsum of the distal phalanx. The proximal portion of the nail root is covered by a fold of skin, and the narrow band of epidermis extending onto the nail is the eponychium. Under the nail root, defined by the crescent shaped lunula, is the germinal matrix of the nail bed where growth occurs. About four to five months are required for complete growth of a new nail.

The nail provides protection and stability, facilitates handling of small objects, and is essential for a normal appearing fingertip. Deformities such as a split or thickened nail or partial or complete absence resulting from inadequate initial management are very difficult to reconstruct secondarily. The following guidelines may lead to better initial management and fewer deformities.

1. Always obtain x-rays to rule out concomitant injuries to the distal phalanx or distal interphalangeal joint.

2. Examine the hand carefully to determine the integrity of the extensor tendon insertion on the distal phalanx.

3. Look for subungual hematomas and drain them through the nail.

4. Accurately restore lacerated nail beds and surrounding skin folds. One can use absorbable sutures in the nail bed; fine sutures are necessary to approximate the tissues accurately. Frequently, the nail is

avulsed, in which case careful splinting and protective dressings are necessary.

5. If the nail root and matrix are avulsed, replace them beneath the proximal skin fold with nonabsorbable mattress sutures. This repositions the growth structures and maintains the pouch beneath the skin fold until nail regrowth occurs.

6. Replace avulsed nail beds with a dermal skin graft. Remove the epidermis from a full thickness skin graft before completely removing it from the donor site. This creates a dermal graft with a superficial raw area that will encourage nail adherence.

7. Support sutured skin folds with gauze placed between the repair and the raw nail bed to avoid adhesions and later deformities. Because of scar distortion, this is particularly important at the nail root.

Mallet Finger

Blunt trauma to the end of the outstretched finger, with forced flexion of the tip, can avulse the extensor tendon from its insertion into the base of the distal phalanx. An x-ray examination is always needed because this injury can be associated with avulsion of bone fragments at the level of attachment, which is part of the distal edge of the interphalangeal joint.

The injury is manifested by an inability to extend actively the distal interphalangeal joint. If there is no significant fracture, treatment can be nonsurgical. The joint should be splinted in slight hyperextension for six weeks and then at night for an additional four to six weeks. It is generally agreed that the proximal interphalangeal joint can be left unsplinted. This form of treatment for closed injuries can be effective even if not started until two or three months after injury.

Buttonhole Deformity of Extensor Mechanism of Proximal Interphalangeal Joint (Boutonniere Deformity)

Rupture of the insertion of the central slip of the extensor tendon into the base of the middle phalanx associated with buttonhole rupture of the dorsum of the extensor hood overlying the proximal interphalangeal joint unbalances the extensor forces acting at both interphalangeal joints.[6,7]

The injury to the dorsum of the extensor hood allows the lateral bands to slip volar to the axis of the joint and they become flexors of the interphalangeal joint. The proximal interphalangeal joint cannot be actively extended because of the loss of the central slip. In addition, the intrinsic muscles acting through the lateral bands now flex rather than extend the proximal interphalangeal joint. The lateral bands (the extensors of the distal interphalangeal joint) now become shortened and hyperextend the distal joint because of their volar dislocation. This flexion of the proximal interphalangeal joint and hyperextension of the distal interphalangeal joint is called the boutonniere deformity. It may not become apparent for several hours or days following the injury when the lateral bands slip volar to the proximal interphalangeal joint. It is important to suspect the injury, properly splint the finger in extension at the proximal interphalangeal joint, and check it in several days. Once the full clinical picture is developed, surgical repair is usually indicated. Because treatment of the late deformity is unsatisfactory, accurate recognition and prompt treatment of the injury are important.

Rupture of the Insertion of the Flexor Profundus Tendon

This injury occurs as a result of forces opposite to that producing a mallet finger. There is pain, swelling of the finger, and frequent hematoma on the distal part of the palm from bleeding into the tendon sheath. Lack of active flexion of the distal interphalangeal joint is incapacitating; prompt surgical advancement and reattachment of the tendon are therefore indicated. This procedure is always done in an operating room.

Dislocations and Ligamentous Injuries of Finger Joints

These injuries are common and frequently seem insignificant, but since joint stability is essential for proper hand function, the disability that results from the mismanagement of these injuries is significant. A carefully taken history and clinical examination should delineate most of these injuries. The dislocations can frequently be reduced under local anesthesia. Concomitant ligamentous injuries allow joint instability and can be diagnosed by lateral stress x-ray examination. Consultation should be obtained in most of these injuries to evaluate the need for surgical repair.

One of the commonest overlooked injuries is complete rupture of the ulnar collateral ligament of the metacarpophalangeal joint of the thumb. To demonstrate the joint instability in the acute, painful, swollen injury, local anesthetic is injected and an x-ray examination obtained with stress on the joint toward radial deviation as compared to the uninjured thumb. If this injury is unrecognized and unrepaired, marked instability in a thumb pinch will be the result. Early surgical repair is successful.

Burns

The treatment of burns is thoroughly discussed in another chapter. The point to be made here is that on the dorsum of the hand, the tendons and joints are superficial and are frequently involved in deep burns of the skin. The common deformity resulting from dorsal burns is hyperextension of the metacarpophalangeal joints and flexion of the interphalangeal joints. To counteract these forces, the hand should be splinted with the metacarpophalangeal joints in flexion and the interphalangeal joints in extension. Superficial burns of the hand should be treated carefully to avoid conversion into full thickness burns.

Infections

Infections of the hand are common because of its exposed position and the frequency of minor trauma in which pathogenic organisms are introduced beneath the skin. In addition to the specialized anatomy of the subcutaneous tissue of the volar aspect of the hand, there are many closed spaces (Fig. 27-5), which can easily be the site of infection, and, if unrecognized, have devastating results. Diagnosis at an early stage is particularly challenging because the original wound of entry may be in-

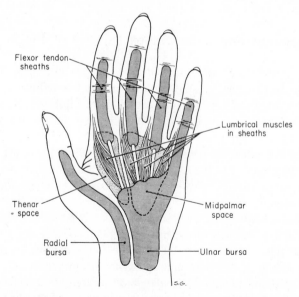

Fig. 27-5. Some of the closed spaces on the volar aspect of the hand that can be sites of infection and, if untreated, have devastating results.

significant or, with children, the history may be so inaccurate that the potential seriousness is not recognized. The early signs and symptoms are important to remember because early diagnosis is crucial.

Initial treatment of infections of the hand consists of putting the hand at complete rest, even for minor infections, by immobilizing it in the position of function. The extremity is then elevated and adequate analgesia supplied. Broad-spectrum antibiotic coverage and antitetanus protection are important. (Anaerobic organisms are common, in addition to hemolytic staphylococci and streptococci.)

If these early infections are recognized, taken seriously, and treated effectively, which frequently includes hospitalization, extension of the infection can be minimized. The greatest stimulus for spread is movement of the hand.

Felon. The tactile pad of the finger is a closed space and contains a network of fibrous septa extending between the skin and the volar aspect of the distal phalanx. Infections in this space are characterized by a tense, slightly swollen, exquisitely tender fingertip. A history of a sharp, penetrating wound (such as a pinprick by a diaper pin) usually differentiates infection from a hematoma resulting from a crushing injury. If this infection progresses unchecked, the pressure can lead to ischemic necrosis of the skin and osteomyelitis of the distal phalanx.

If it is seen early and aggressive initial treatment is instituted, the infection can be arrested. If not, prompt drainage is indicated. This requires a horizontal incision that divides all the fibrous septa, which means a lateral incision halfway between the volar surface of the phalanx and the volar skin. Care should be taken not to start too far proximally and as a result accidentally enter the distal sheath of the flexor tendon of the distal interphalangeal joint. If the incision is made deeply under the distal part of the phalanx, it is usually not necessary to extend it around the tip of the finger or to drain through to the opposite side. A small drain should be left in for 48 to 72 hours and a culture taken for anaerobic as well as the usual pyogenic organisms.

Paronychia. Infection around the periphery of a fingernail is common, and prompt treatment prevents extension of the infection around the base of the nail. If this does occur, drainage is necessary. If the infection has progressed and dissected under the nail root and detached it, the proximal portion of the nail must be excised to establish drainage. If there is an abscess under the more distal part of the nail, the portion of the nail overlying the infection must be removed to establish drainage and prevent further elevation of the nail.

Infections of the Volar Subcutaneous Tissue Overlying the Middle and Proximal Phalanx. Here, the more loosely arranged fibrofatty tissue allows for easier spread of the inflammatory exudate. It is important to differentiate this condition from acute tenosynovitis of the flexor tendon sheath. Early aggressive treatment is important to avoid spread, particularly to the web space from the more proximal infections. Drainage is usually done through a lateral incision, with the neurovascular bundle and tendon sheath being carefully avoided.

Web Space Infections (Collar Button Abscesses). The three web spaces between the four fingers contain loose fat, strands of palmar fascia, the tendons of the lumbrical muscles, and the deep transverse metacarpal ligaments. Infection can occur from direct puncture, extension from an infected blister or a callus volar to the metacarpal heads, or direct extrusion from subcutaneous tissue of the proximal phalanx. Although the infection usually begins on the volar aspect, the tissue is relatively unyielding, and the infectious process dissects dorsally where the physical findings are more prominent. Unchecked, this infection can spread into the deeper spaces of the hand, such as the midpalmar space (Fig. 27-5) and cause catastrophic damage.

These collar button abscesses, so called because of the narrow neck between the volar origin and the dorsal extrusion, require drainage in an operating room. The web space is never drained directly. Instead, two incisions are made, one on the volar aspect just distal to the distal palmar crease and a dorsal incision between the metacarpal heads. Through-and-through drainage is necessary for 48 hours.

Human Bite Injuries. These injuries commonly occur on the dorsum of the metacarpophalangeal joint when a clenched fist strikes a tooth. The tooth penetrates the skin and extensor mechanism and frequently enters the joint space, depositing virulent oral aerobic and anaerobic organisms. When the fist is relaxed and the metacarpophalangeal joint extended, the skin wound moves proximally, converting the aerobic wound to an anaerobic one. The infection then progresses to a septic arthritis, destroying the metacarpophalangeal joint.

Recognition of the seriousness of this injury and early aggressive treatment are essential if complications are to be avoided. The wound should never be closed. Instead it is irrigated thoroughly, and the patient is hospitalized for close observation and placed on appropriate antibiotics. The hand should be immobilized and elevated. The tendon is repaired secondarily after the wound heals.

Deep Space Infections. Early recognition of these infections is essential. The history is sometimes revealing. Any of the synovial sheaths may become infected but it is most common in the flexor tendon sheaths (Fig. 27-5). The diagnosis is based on the four cardinal signs and symptoms enumerated by Kanavel: (1) the involved finger is uniformly swollen; (2) all joints in the finger are slightly flexed; (3) any attempt to extend the finger passively causes exquisite pain; and (4) the area of maximal tenderness is over the anatomic outline of the tendon sheath.[3,4]

The diagnosis is not always clear but if a deep space infection is *suspected,* the patient should be hospitalized, initial therapy for infection begun, and prompt consultation with a hand specialist obtained.

If unchecked, this infection can spread rapidly into the adjacent spaces and bursae. From the little finger, the infection can extend proximally into the ulnar bursa and then into the radial bursa of the thumb. A high index of suspicion and prompt action will avert disaster in these serious deep infections.

References

1. Marble, M. C. 1960. *The Hand.* Philadelphia, W. B. Saunders.
2. Rank, B. K., Wakefield, A. R., and Mauston, J. 1968. *Surgery of Repair as Applied to Hand Injuries,* 3rd ed. Baltimore, Williams & Wilkins.
3. Milford, L. 1971. *The Hand.* St. Louis, C. V. Mosby Co.
4. Ciba Clinical Symposia. 1969. *Surgical Anatomy of the Hand,* Vol. XXI, No. 3. Summit, N.J., Ciba Corp.
5. Figge, F. H., and Sabotta, J. 1963. *Atlas of Human Anatomy,* Vols. I and III. New York, Hofner Publishing Co.
6. Harris, C., and Rutledge, G. L. 1972. The functional anatomy of the extensor mechanism of the finger. *J. Bone Joint Surg.,* 54A:713–726.
7. Littler, J. W. 1967. The finger extensor mechanism. *Surg. Clin. N. Amer.,* 47:415–432.
8. Grabb, W. C., and Dingman, R. O. 1963. The examination of the acutely injured hand. *J. Mich. Med. Soc.,* 62:271–275.
9. Grabb, W. C. 1968. Median and ulnar nerve suture. An experimental study comparing primary and secondary repair in monkeys. *J. Bone Joint Surg.,* 50A:964–972.
10. Goulian, D. 1968. New economical dermatome. *Plast. Reconst. Surg.,* 42:85.
11. Lie, K. K., Margargle, R. K., and Posch, J. L. 1970. Free full thickness skin grafts from palm to cover defects in fingers. *J. Bone Joint Surg.,* 52A:559.
12. Atajoy, E., et al. 1970. Reconstruction of amputated finger tip with triangular volar flap. *J. Bone Joint Surg.,* 52A:921.
13. Friedberg, A., and Manktelow, R. 1972. Kutler repair for finger tip amputations. *Plast. Reconst. Surg.,* 50:371–375.
14. Hoskins, M. D. 1960. Versatile cross-finger flap. *J. Bone Joint Surg.,* 42A:261.
15. Kleinert, H. E., et al. 1967. The deformed fingernail. A frequent result of failure to repair nail bed injuries. *J. Trauma,* 7:177–197.

28

Residency Training in Emergency Medicine

H. Thomas Blum

The use of emergency departments across the country is rapidly increasing. For the past 10 years the rate of increase has been 10% per year. The most important factor associated with this expansion is the increased utilization of emergency departments for general medical care.

There are many reasons for this changing pattern. The population increase has taxed many services in our society, including emergency department services. The lack of availability and accessibility of primary care are contributing factors. In metropolitan areas, particularly, there are large concentrations of low income people who have few options in seeking health care services. In our mobile society, many people of moderate income have not made use of private medical care. The emergency department is the main place where they seek medical attention.

The decline in number of physicians providing primary care in the rural and intercity areas has been a factor in increased utilization of emergency departments. Some physicians in practice are often unavailable in the evenings and on weekends. Many physicians are understandably reluctant to make house calls. Others feel more comfortable caring for the patient in the emergency department or referring the patient to the emergency department where facilities are more adequate than in their offices. Health insurance plans favor the utilization of emergency departments because coverage is not as easily obtained for similar services rendered in doctors' offices.

Because of specialization, many patients have become confused about the appropriate point of access to health care services. The hospital emergency service has become the focal point for in-patient care and some types of ambulatory care. There is an increasing tendency for patients to seek medical counsel when symptoms first appear. This pattern is nurtured by well intentioned publicity generated by health care professions. The hospital emergency department with its 24-hour service, therefore, has become the point of access to medical care for a significant number of patients. This manner of care has become attractive because the service is often rendered less formally than in a doctor's office and does not require an appointment. When discussing emergency services, therefore, the semantics create confusion because the designation "emergency room" or "emergency department" does not conceptualize the services rendered. These services could be more appropriately designated as functions of "departments of unscheduled or unpredictable medical care."

Ideally, in a more responsive, decentralized system, nonemergency cases would be better managed in a neighborhood health facility or a physician's office. Adequate reorganization of health care service to decrease the hospitals' burden of ambulatory and emergency care will probably not become a reality in the foreseeable future. Emergency care may be the most efficient way of rendering 24-hour service, even though decentralized services are aesthetically preferable. Health care manpower would be better utilized by developing more adequate transportation systems to major health care centers than by attempting to extend services into the neighborhood, especially in the evening and on weekends.

A compromise based on a lack of financial resources and health professionals may result in the continued use of hospitals for rendering unscheduled and unpredictable medical services. Emergency departments have become a fairly responsive component in meeting the public's needs within the present health care delivery system. In some respects, these units are an integral and major part of a newly developing system of health care delivery. The desirable features of this new arrangement seem to outweigh the deficiencies. Consumers appear to be more concerned about the availability of service than about the need for highly personalized service as long as the service is rendered with dignity and efficiency.

Responding to the need to render more health services in emergency departments are approximately 15,000 physicians who consider themselves to be either part-time or full-time emergency physicians. Some are older physicians seeking a less rigorous existence than that experienced in office practice. Younger physicians in interim situations are at the other end of the age spectrum. Between these extremes are a considerable number of part-time or full-time physicians with a wide range in qualifications, expertise, motivation, and interest. What are the implications of this range of skills and expertise? How does the patient know who is qualified and who is not? As in the rest of medicine, the patient does not know. He may know of a physician's reputation, which may or may not be well founded. Unfortunately, the emergency patient may learn of inadequately rendered care only after the fact. To compound the issue, physicians often are working with other health professionals who, like the doctor, have not been trained to handle the specific problems encountered in emergency departments.

There are a number of basic approaches to improving inadequately rendered emergency department care. Some of the important steps are: (1) to increase emphasis on emergency medicine in medical schools, nursing schools, and schools for allied health careers; (2) to establish residencies in emergency medicine; (3) to establish short-term postgraduate courses in emergency medicine; (4) to establish emergency department teams that include physicians, nurses, and allied health workers; (5) to improve and standardize emergency medical technician training; (6) to organize more efficiently emergency transportation and communication; and (7) to educate patients in the utilization of health facilities.

The University of Cincinnati Medical Center has focused initial efforts on upgrading emergency medicine in the student curriculum and establishing a residency in emergency medicine. There is now an elective course in emergency medicine for fourth year medical students in which they work with the medical and surgical teams in the emergency department, triage with the emergency medicine resident and nurse, and are exposed to rescue team work. The weekly emergency medicine lecture and film series is open to and enthusiastically received by the students. They find the course and the lecture series refreshingly relevant.

The medical center is also developing a sophisticated first aid course for first year medical students. The need for this instruction is apparent if one observes the graduates of many medical institutions who arrive for their first experience as physicians in the emergency unit. Many young physicians are not skilled in the rudiments of first aid and, therefore, lack credibility with allied health professionals, especially personnel who are involved in rescue and emergency services. Even more important is the effect this lack of skill has on the quality of care.

This lack of expertise is not limited to recent graduates of medical schools. In a recent survey, one of the questions asked of physicians was, "To what portion of your colleagues would you confidently trust your own life if you were a victim of an emergency?" More than half of the physicians replied that they would trust none of them. The consensus is that there is a great need for more expertise in the field of emergency care. Nevertheless, many medical schools still do not require training in emergency medicine. There is a clear need for improved curriculum content at the undergraduate and graduate levels of medical education. The need is equally great for short-term training courses for second career physicians who currently staff many emergency units.

In 1970, the University of Cincinnati Medical Center established the nation's first residency in emergency medicine with the following goals:

1. To train the physician to become an expert in managing the broad spectrum of medical problems encountered in an emergency setting
2. To develop the administrative skills necessary for the physician to provide leadership in this field
3. To stress the physician's role as a teacher in all aspects of emergency medical care
4. To encourage biomedical and health services research related to the improvement of emergency care.

The objective of the program is to train 12 (six first year and six second year) residents in a two-year program (in conjunction with the various specialty departments) to manage health care problems in the following areas:

Anesthesia
Tracheal intubation of adults and children
Airway management
Management of hypotension
Management of massive blood transfusions
Preoperative assessment
Use of regional anesthetic blocks
Diagnosis and treatment of toxic effects of local anesthesia
Use of respirators
Dynamics of pharmacology

Emergency Surgery
Diagnosis and initial treatment of patients with multiple injuries, gunshot and stab wounds, acute abdomens, and minor wounds

Intensive Care Unit
Appropriate management of acute respiratory and cardiac emergencies, including status asthmaticus, pulmonary edema, myocardial infarction, congestive heart failure, and acute respiratory failure

Medicine
Diagnosis and treatment of the common neurologic, hematologic, dermatologic, gastrointestinal, pulmonary, cardiac, and endocrinologic emergencies

Neurosurgery
Diagnosis of common head, neck, and spinal injuries

Obstetrics and Gynecology

Diagnosis and initial treatment of common obstetric and gynecologic emergencies, such as septic abortion, spontaneous abortion, labor and delivery, gonorrhea, pelvic inflammatory disease, tuboovarian abscess, and tuboovarian pregnancy

Orthopedics

Diagnosis and treatment of out-patient orthopedic injuries, such as uncomplicated fractures, low back pain, sprains, shoulder dislocations, bursitis, and "tennis elbow"

Pediatrics

Diagnosis and initial treatment of common pediatric emergencies with an emphasis on upper and lower respiratory problems, febrile seizures, and unexplained fevers

Emergency Unit

In the first month in the emergency unit, the trainee enhances his skill in minor wound care and serves on the surgery team. In the second month, the trainee takes a shift on the medical team in the capacity of a junior assistant resident in medicine. For two other months, the first year resident backs up medical and surgical teams. When the resident is ready, usually in the last two months of the six-month emergency unit experience, he assumes a supervisory role. In this capacity, in addition to caring for major emergencies, the resident helps the emergency unit run smoothly by being available to the nurses and other house staff physicians to handle problems. He deals with the overload of minor problems requiring increased triage to the medical "primary care section," suturing overload, specialty service not answering consultation requests, problems of patient placement, problems of interpersonal relation among physicians and other health professionals, scheduling problems, and consultations with other hospital emergency departments. While on this rotation, the second year resident in emergency medicine meets with the emergency unit director, manager, supervising nurse, social worker, and psychiatrist on a weekly basis to discuss particular emergency unit problems, to be involved in goal-setting, and to participate in the process of reaching predefined objectives. The emergency unit director and the second year resident scrutinize emergency department problems continually.

Psychiatry

Emphasis is placed on interviewing technique and evaluation of problems ranging from severe anxiety to psychoses. The resident is assigned to a psychiatry team (psychiatry resident, nurse, and psychiatric social worker) on duty in the emergency unit. Attending rounds are conducted by a staff psychiatrist.

Electives

The resident has two months of electives. The clinical electives include a month in the coronary care unit, a month in another emergency unit doing clinical work, or a month on any of the previous rotations. Nonclinical electives include a month in other emergency units doing health services research, a month working with the city hospital council and academy of medicine in emergency medical services development, or a month working with the city or volunteer life squads. Each resident is asked to take one or more nonclinical electives.

The trainee's performance is evaluated in the following way. Discussions are held with residents in emergency medicine who have been assigned to another department, two specialty staff physicians (usually including the departmental chairman), and the director of the emergency medicine residency. This group develops a syllabus. The residents who have been assigned to another department subsequently evaluate that rotation with the syllabus in mind. Likewise the specialist evaluates the resident against the syllabus. Discrepancies are discussed, and if the weakness appears to be on the part of the resident, consideration is given to having him spend an additional month on an elective in that specialty. If the weakness seems to be on the part of the department, efforts are made to improve that part of the rotation. In some cases the rotation has been changed. The resident is also evaluated for competency, responsibility, efficiency, cooperation, and courtesy to patients and their families and to co-workers.

The priorities of the program are: (1) to provide patient oriented care; (2) to strengthen the concept of the medical care team in the emergency unit; and (3) to improve community-wide emergency medical services.

Conclusion

Where will the trainees go when they finish the residency? What will their responsibilities be? The typical residents in emergency medicine at the University of Cincinnati have both clinical and organizational interests in emergency medical services. They anticipate running emergency departments somewhere. This kind of supervisory position entails clinical, administrative, and teaching responsibilities. The trainees are also interested in handling problems of emergency systems. They intend to develop and improve emergency medical services, e.g., acute coronary care systems, emergency department categorization and regionalization, and training of emergency medical technicians. The emergency physicians-in-training also learn how to approach the organizational problems related to the increasing demand on emergency departments for primary care.

In the future, will the emergency physicians perform procedures now done by specialists? The answer depends upon the availability of the specialist. If a patient with a fracture seeks care in an urban emergency department and an orthopedic surgeon is available, the emergency physician will triage the patient to that specialist. If the emergency physician is in an emergency department in a rural area many miles from the nearest orthopedic surgeon, the emergency physician will probably set the simple fracture. He will seek verbal consultation with the distant specialist if indicated.

What does the future hold? The recent surge of interest in emergency department problems and emergency medical systems will result in improved emergency and primary care in many areas of the country. The graduates of the University of Cincinnati Emergency Medicine Residency will provide some of the leadership in making these improvements. Other community-oriented medical centers will start emergency medicine residencies and short-term postgraduate training programs in emergency medicine.

Index